Second Edition

Orientation to Deafness

Nanci A. Scheetz
Valdosta State University

Allyn and Bacon
Boston • London • Toronto • Sydney • Tokyo • Singapore

Executive Editor: Stephen D. Dragin
Editorial Assistant: Barbara Strickland
Senior Editorial Production Administrator: Joe Sweeney
Editorial-Production Service: Walsh & Associates, Inc.
Composition Buyer: Linda Cox
Manufacturing Buyer: Chris Marson

Library of Congress Cataloging-in-Publication Data
Scheetz, Nanci A.
    Orientation to deafness / Nanci A. Scheetz. — 2nd ed.
        p.   cm.
    Includes bibliographical references and index.
    ISBN 0-205-32801-6
    1. Deaf. 2. Deaf—Psychology. 3. Deaf—Rehabilitation. 4. Deaf—Means of
communication. I. Title.

HV2380 .S33   2000
362.4'2—dc21

                                                                00-057627

Printed in the United States of America

10   9   8   7   6   5   4   3   2   1   04   03   02   01   00

To Richard
and my four daughters
Melissa, Marie,
Megghan & Monique

▶ Contents

▶ Preface

This text has been designed to provide the student with a broad overview of the field of deafness. In addition, it has been developed as a resource text for parents, educators, vocational rehabilitation counselors, interpreters, and other professionals who come in contact with the Deaf community. Issues that lie at the heart of the Deaf culture are discussed. Included in the chapters are a wide array of topics providing the reader with information pertaining to the unique characteristics of this population.

The text focuses on educational perspectives, psychosocial precepts, communication modes, vocational opportunities, support services, and recent technological advances. Further, it provides the reader with insights into one of the fastest growing populations today—the deafened adult. Throughout its chapters, myths surrounding deafness are dispelled and replaced with contemporary ideas. The broad scope of subject matter presented allows for flexibility and provides fresh material for new approaches to basic courses within the field of deaf education.

This book is designed as a teaching-learning vehicle. For this reason, basic concepts recur in varying situations, and illustrations and some concepts are repeated in diverging contexts to promote comprehension and enhance retention. It is a source book on the many dimensions of deafness. It is dedicated to a panoramic view of a complex field rather than an in-depth analysis of each major dimension. The chapters contain information giving the reader the opportunity to gain a more accurate portrayal of what the field of deaf education in the twenty-first century is all about.

This book is addressed to future and current educators, beginning with those who work with infants and continuing on to those who are faced with the challenges of the college student. Teachers who work with this diverse population are uniquely aware of the complexities of educating deaf children and deaf adults. This text is designed to furnish them with additional insights into the world of the deaf. Its intention is to provide a foundation for those students entering the field of interpreting and social work. In addition, its pages include information for parents and deafened adults who want to gain insights and understanding into the complexities of the world of the deaf.

The author wishes to extend special thanks to Ms. Heather Anderson and Ms. Mary L. Pitts for their assistance with research, and Ms. Diane Godin, Ms. Janet Shelfer, and Mr. Robert Fassett for their technical assistance with the manuscript. Their advice and suggestions have been very beneficial. The author also wishes to extend her thanks to her husband for his support, encouragement, and the many hours he devoted to reading the chapters, and for the suggestions he offered for enhancing the content. Special thanks are also due to the author's daughters, who so patiently helped with preparing the pages for this edition. Their skills, insights, and senses of humor have been invaluable throughout this project. And finally, thanks are extended to Steve Dragin and the staff at Allyn & Bacon for making this an enjoyable experience.

▶ 1

A Psychosocial
Perspective of Deafness

In our world a vast amount of information is conveyed through the medium of sound. The auditory channel affords those with normal hearing the opportunity to exchange ideas, gather information, and develop an ease in communicating with those around them. Sound also permeates our subliminal plane affecting our beliefs, attitudes, and opinions, thus influencing the way we respond to individuals and react to events occurring in our environment. These signals, which penetrate the subconscious level, are responsible for influencing how we respond to the messages we receive. Our perception, in part, is based on the voice quality of the sender, the choice of words, phraseology, and the tonal quality in which it is delivered.

Within this macrocosm, where sound is significant and communication plays a vital role, a smaller population of individuals exists, known to each other as members of the Deaf community. They are as diverse as those belonging to the much larger society; however, they share a common characteristic—they communicate visually and share a wide variety of interests based on the loss of their hearing ability (Schein, 1989).

Whereas the medical profession incorporates the terms hard-of-hearing, hearing impaired, and deaf to designate classifications of hearing loss, the term "Deaf," when capitalized, is used to refer to members of the Deaf community. Although members belonging to this group exhibit varying degrees of hearing loss, their disability reflects a similar characteristic in that generally their losses were incurred early in their development. The Deaf community is a concept, not a place, and those who cannot hear choose whether or not they want to belong. Those who join desire the companionship of individuals who have similar psychological and social needs and seek organizations that facilitate these interactions (Schein, 1989, p. 12).

Members of the Deaf community interact daily with those who can hear. As they mingle with hearing people, they begin to exchange ideas, gather information, and form perceptions regarding each other's worlds. It is through a lifetime of such interactions that all individuals mold their identities and find their places in society.

The establishment of self concept, that is, who one identifies one's self to be is critical in establishing the parameters for where one will ultimately reside, how one will cope with surroundings, and what contributions one will make during a lifetime. The manner in which identity is shaped is contingent upon two factors: first, those attributes that make each of us unique; and second, society's reaction to our uniqueness.

Individual differences are appreciated by the much larger group. These characteristics distinguish us from others and contribute to our uniqueness. However, when they become too extreme so that we are "set apart" or "stand out" from others, we are viewed as a curiosity. This is often the case with those who have a disability. If some part of an individual's body is not perfect, or certain characteristics of the anomaly become apparent, the person may be labeled, thus causing a stigma to be attached. This stigma generally carries a negative connotation and can remain throughout one's lifetime. It results in reactions that impact on the disabled person, forcing him or her to confront his or her identity. Through a series of these interactions, the self-concept begins to be formed and psychosocial development occurs.

When embarking on a discussion of the psychosocial aspects of deafness, it must be conducted by first exploring the much larger confines of the society containing this population. For although the discussion crosses the boundaries of the two communities, they are interdependent upon one other; each can only be fully understood as it relates to the other.

As members in the larger society interact with members of the Deaf community, responses are triggered that influence personal and social development. Thus, when examining personal growth, the interrelationship and interaction that transpire between the two communities is viewed, rather than focusing on a distinct "psychology of deafness."

The term "psychology of deafness" implies that deafness is a psychological variable that influences the behavior of deaf persons. Based on this, their life experience differs in some consistent ways from those who are not deaf (Vernon & Andrews, 1990). However, if members of the Deaf community are viewed as unique individuals who experience situations that are as diverse and varied as their responses to them, then insight into psychosocial development can be gained by examining those complex interactions that contribute to the shaping of the individual.

OUTSIDE THE DEAF WORLD: A HEARING PERSPECTIVE OF THE DISABILITY

The larger society in which the Deaf culture functions is comprised of a majority of hearing individuals who establish rules for social behavior, define the patterns for engaging in two-way communication, and ascertain which behaviors are acceptable. Hearing individuals operate from a certain body of assumptions and situations that become normative. Those individuals who deviate from these expectations cause them great concern or consternation. In today's society, people tend to move at a rapid pace, and anything that alters their established pattern is not viewed in a positive manner. Members are bombarded and influenced by stimuli produced by the media. They are led to believe that everything should be perceived as "perfect" and that one should live one's life "harmoniously." Thus, when situations or individuals are encountered that threaten to alter established patterns, they are viewed in a negative manner. Because deafness is a low-incidence handicap, hearing people may have very little, if any, contact with those who are deaf. However, when they encounter deaf individuals for the first time, they respond to them in a manner reflective of their preconceived ideas of what deafness entails. Members of the hearing society are conditioned to adhere to the mold prescribed by the norm. Attitudes are conveyed regarding how one should think, behave, believe, and, on a more concrete level, dress and act. Those who fail to exhibit compliance with these standards are viewed as being inferior or unusual. Once characterized in this manner by the larger society, a stigma is attached with the inference that one is odd, strange, or different; in our minds "the individual becomes reduced from a whole and usual person to a tainted, discounted one" (Goffman, 1963).

Once deaf persons are stigmatized, they may encounter a variety of responses. They may be avoided, ridiculed, punished, or reacted to in ways that indicate that they are thought to be less than fully human.

Stigma: Dealing with Those Who Are Different

Research within the area of special education indicates that those individuals possessing a physical disability are routinely stigmatized (Bender, 1970). In a society that cherishes health, beauty, youth, and physical abilities, those deviating from the norm are frowned upon. Although there are exceptions, historically speaking, disabled individuals have been treated as inferior beings by those who are nondisabled. One only has to review the literature to find reports of children with physical disabilities being left to die, included in "freak" shows, put to work in carnivals or, in later reports, institutionalized (Oberman, 1965).

Times have changed somewhat, and although what was once perceived as "brutal behavior" has diminished, the attitudes toward disabled individuals remain negative. Society continues to lack a basic understanding of handicapped individuals, and everyday interactions between physically disabled and nondisabled persons are typically strained, inhibited, and awkward (Higgins, 1980). Those who are nondisabled may be distressed with the emotions they find themselves experiencing. They may discover that they are responding to the deaf person with expressions of pity, curiosity, or indifference. They are faced with the dilemma of either acknowledging the disability or ignoring it entirely and pretending that it doesn't exist. These concerns and feelings may become so overwhelming that they influence the way individuals respond to the deaf individual. Instead of relating to the person as an equal with mutual respect and understanding, the interaction may be clouded with insecurities and inappropriate mannerisms. Upon leaving a situation of this nature, they may feel very uncomfortable and disillusioned. The disabled person, on the other hand, may leave the same situation with the impression that he is somewhat less than adequate.

The feelings that are conveyed by the nonhandicapped individual are reflective of the stigma that is attached to those who are disabled. When examining the stigmatization of the Deaf, there are five issues that merit special consideration. They include (1) the discrediting of the deaf through their signing, (2) viewing deafness as a master status, (3) the issue of spread, (4) scrutinization from the larger hearing world, and (5) acceptance in everyday encounters (Higgins, 1980, p. 126).

Discrediting of the Deaf

The term "discrediting" is used when referring to those nondisabled individuals who converge on particular characteristics of the disabled population for the purpose of mocking or ridiculing them. Within the area of deafness, this term is usually applied when focusing on manual communication.

Deafness can remain invisible, only becoming apparent with the onset of communication. When the conversation entails an exchange of information through the use of signs, accompanied occasionally by vocalic sounds, the persons involved in the interaction will draw attention to themselves. Because Americans are relatively reserved in their body movements, they may find the gestures and body movements of the Deaf community to be very alarming. The general public, when observing deaf individuals signing, may feel embarrassed or uncomfortable and thus resort to staring, mimicking, or mocking them. By focusing on this communication system, the Deaf are discredited; their failings in the realm of interaction with hearing people become obvious; and they are denied acceptance as "whole" or "normal" people.

Deafness as a Master Status

The term "master status," as defined by Higgins, has been utilized to illustrate the philosophy of the nondisabled as they direct their focal point to the failings of a particular group. The assumption here is that those on the outside looking in tend to focus on one characteristic, that is, communication differences between the Deaf and the hearing, and group all of the members who utilize the system as homogeneous. Individual characteristics go unnoticed and positive attributes are overlooked.

Spread

"Spread" is used to illustrate the following concept: When one has a disability that is perceived as negative, the part of the anatomy that is disabled is generalized to incorporate other parts of the body as well. Thus, hearing loss spreads to one's mental abilities and capacity to perform daily tasks. From a historical perspective, this is one of the reasons why the term "deaf and dumb" was originally coined. Although this term was used to refer to those who could neither hear nor speak, it further was given the connotation of being senseless (Higgins, 1980, p. 134). Today the phrase is not part of professional jargon. However, it still haunts the deaf individual as it continues to be utilized in the hearing community.

Scrutinization

The term "scrutinization" refers to the process of sizing a person up to be sure that he or she measures up to the task he or she is attempting. This form of stigmatization can be observed particularly when disabled individuals are hired by the work force or when one chooses to marry someone who has no disability.

Lack of Acceptance

Of all of the issues previously raised, the issue of acceptance is among the more critical ones, for at the heart of human existence is one's desire to be accepted. Through their daily interactions, deaf individuals frequently perceive that they are not accepted by or into the larger community. They feel that they are viewed as "tainted" people first and only later, if ever, as complete people. Many have faced ridicule, teasing, taunts, and neglect all of their lives, never feeling they are accepted for what they really are—people with hearing impairments. Thus, the need to be accepted may never come to fruition until they find their places within the Deaf community.

Lack of acceptance, feelings of failure, and irritation at being stereotyped are only some of the feelings stigma elicits. Deaf people find interacting with the hearing world to be full of misunderstandings, awkward silences, and unsatisfactory encounters.

As a result, deaf individuals usually find a haven within the culture of Deafness—an environment in which communication is taken for granted instead of becoming an issue, where the focus is placed on one's attributes instead of one's disability, and where a group with some shared characteristics can enhance each other's individuality. The last part of this chapter is devoted to examining the Deaf community in depth—the rationale for establishing a Deaf culture, the purpose it serves, and the impact on its members. However, before delving into this critical aspect of deafness, it is important to examine the effects society's attitudes have on the Deaf population, specifically with respect to their psychological development.

IMPACT OF DEAFNESS ON PSYCHOSOCIAL DEVELOPMENT: RELATING TO THOSE AROUND US

Members of a society have certain expectations for those residing in the group, and individuals deviating from the norm are viewed with apprehension. Such is the case when hearing individuals encounter the Deaf population. This apprehension projects itself in several ways. Those behaviors that society, as a whole, will tolerate at one point in time, may become totally unacceptable at another. The responses triggered by these various behaviors are diverse and they impact on the psychological development of the individual. Only by examining them can one appreciate their significance on social development as manifested in the psychological formation of the personality.

The Early Years

During the first few years of life, the influence society has on the deaf child is transmitted primarily through the parents. Because of the small number of deaf individuals, one may go through an entire lifetime without meeting anyone who cannot hear. Due to this lack of familiarity and knowledge, when confronted with a deaf child for the first time, those who can hear may base their perceptions of the child on obsolete stereotypes. Out of ignorance, society reacts in various ways. Its most immediate reactions are to minimize the differences and attempt to make the child appear similar to the "normal" person or to try and ignore the child completely. Society tries to make the square pegs fit round holes in order that the individual will blend in with society. If this cannot be accomplished, the end results are feelings of fear, dislike, pity, or avoidance. When encountering someone who is not "normal," we are faced with fears concerning our own normalcy and are not comfortable around those who are different.

Parents, when faced with questions from members in the community regarding their child's disability, must come to grips with their own feelings of guilt and the tensions that are created within the home environment. Thus, from the very beginning there are many adverse elements that impact on the parents, are transferred to the child, and are instrumental in shaping the child's development and socialization.

As the child continues to grow and develop socially, he or she may begin to exhibit traits that are not understood by the larger hearing community. The child's speech is frequently not comprehensible; therefore, the child may be labeled "retarded." Neighbors and friends may refrain from including the deaf child in their hearing child's activity due to his lack of "normalcy." The deaf child may fail to understand his parents' request and respond with a temper tantrum. This in itself may provide an impetus for labeling deaf children as having severe behavioral problems.

Society has a need for establishing a time frame designating when certain tasks such as toilet training, feeding, and dressing oneself should be mastered. When children deviate from the anticipated schedule and fall behind this time frame, community members view them as being developmentally delayed. This mindset, when conveyed to the parents, has a direct impact on the family. The mother may be faced with her own feelings of guilt and frustration, while simultaneously being influenced by the opinions of those with whom she has daily contact. These personal feelings, coupled with society's attitudes, will determine the manner in which she is able to relate to the child.

The Early School Years

School age marks an important time in children's lives, for it is here that they are publicly competing with their peers for the first time. Society views children and their accomplishments in school as an extension of the parents and as a reflection of the type of home from which they have come. Children are also observed as they compete with each other and are evaluated according to their scholastic achievement levels and their ability to master grade-level objectives.

Whether deaf children attend residential schools or day schools for the acoustically handicapped, they are nevertheless marked with the stigma of attending a "special school." Society continues to label them as "different," failing to acknowledge that they are typical children with special needs.

School is only one setting in which society observes and compares children. Behavior in public is where a different type of conflict may arise. Due to the nature of the disability, the method in which children are disciplined at home may be viewed as unacceptable while out in public. The parent's physical handling of the child in public may alone lend itself to criticisms, misunderstandings, and misconceptions.

Deaf children who attend residential schools are not afforded the same number of social contacts as their hearing peers. This is due in part to the school situation. Those attending residential facilities may return home only on the weekends during the school year. As a result they are not home during the week to participate in those daily activities that happen on a regular basis. Events such as baseball practice, dance lessons, trips to the video store, football games, running errands, family outings, and visiting neighborhood friends are all incorporated into the fabric of the child's home life. They, in turn, impact significantly on the socialization process. Children who are not encouraged by their parents to engage in social interactions will feel insecure and uncomfortable when asked to participate in family, neighborhood, and community functions. Those skills that are required to facilitate an exchange with society will be lacking, thus influencing the social climate in which they reside.

Another factor contributing to the impact society has on the child has been mentioned briefly before. For all children, role models play an integral part in their social and psychological development. During the early school years, these children may find few, if any, deaf role models to identify with and their opportunity to associate with hearing role models is equally reduced. This is due, in part, to the limited social contacts available to them. It is critical during early school age years to provide children with a variety of role models whom they can begin to mimic and imitate. Without an opportunity to do this, deaf children may deviate from those developmental patterns that are termed socially acceptable by those residing in the hearing community.

The Adolescent Years

During this time it is important to view the impact of deafness, both from the way society reacts and how the deaf individual responds. Given the same situation and environment, any two deaf individuals may respond differently to the way society treats them. The environment will impact heavily on the individual in the adolescent years. Psychologists agree that environment is of critical importance in the psychological development and adjustment of the individual. The theory is generally accepted that there is no psychology of man as he develops in a "vacuum," but only a psychology of man as he relates to his society.

To understand the development of the deaf adolescent it is important to note first the type of reaction he is most likely to encounter within his society. In the larger hearing society, people tend to respond negatively to anything that is different.

> *To the world at large, impaired hearing is an irritating block to quick, easy communication. If there is to be contact with the person behind the block, a barrier needs to be negotiated. But this takes patience and understanding— a patience that modern living is not geared to, understanding to which society has not yet attained . . . society commonly reacts with aversion to physical deviation, especially to such a mysterious one as impaired hearing that does not "show." And at the other extreme is society's naive faith in the magic of lipreading and the hearing aid to effect complete restoration, and the suspicion that ensues when the magic fails to produce the expected results in a given case. That there must be something worse wrong with the person is the public verdict. (Garrett & Levine, 1962, p. 304)*

In general, society may reject deaf adolescents because of a pervasive failure to understand "deafness" and its ramifications. Teenagers sensing this rejection may respond in three ways: First, they may choose to identify themselves solely with other deaf individuals; second, they may deny their deafness and seek their place among the hearing; or third, they may fluctuate between the Deaf and the hearing worlds (Schowe, 1979).

How individuals view themselves and what they are capable of accomplishing will determine which choice they will make. They may feel accepted into the hearing world and endeavor to become "hearing," or they may feel frustrated and rejected, prompting them to turn toward the Deaf community for support and opting only to maintain minimal contact with the hearing world. Regardless of which decision these individuals make, they will to some extent become part of the Deaf culture, a community where they feel they belong. Within this culture are churches, clubs, newspapers, sporting events, and other activities designed specifically for them. In addition, those belonging to this culture become involved in the vast array of social activities available to them. The majority of their social interactions occur within the confines of the culture. They socialize, interact, and typically marry an individual who is also a member. The extent to which individuals become involved with this culture is determined by their desire to obtain membership, their communication mode, and the educational setting in which they have been raised.

It is important to emphasize that during the adolescent years teenagers may feel alienated from their peer group, isolated from their family, and rejected by society. Frank Bowe expressed his feelings regarding high school and his social life in the article "Crisis of the Deaf Child and His Family."

*I was in high school yet not of it. I participated not at all in any school ac-
tivities. In four years of high school, I had just one date. I seldom left the
house, except occasionally for an athletic event. Even at home I rarely
sought out visitors, preferring (rudely!) to curl up with a book or magazine.
Although I did not recognize it as such, this was a crisis for me. Repeated
efforts by my family to draw me out merely angered me. I was starving for
deep, personal, committed interaction—and rejecting it. (Bowe, 1973,
p. 43)*

The difficulty adolescents experience as they are struggling to discover their
own identity and decide where they fit into society causes many deaf youth to withdraw. In their effort to become a part of the group, they realize that they can never
become "hearing" members of society. Shanny Mow, a deaf man, has stated this:

*. . . there remains an invisible, insurmountable wall between us. No man
can become completely a part of another man's world. He is never more
eloquently reminded of this impossibility than when there is no way he can
talk to the other man. (Mow, 1973, p. 22)*

Articulation problems, nasal or monotonal qualities, and mispronunciations
are all characteristics of the speech patterns common to this population. These
speech patterns tend to garble the message, creating misunderstandings. This results in a language barrier, hindering deaf adolescents as they strive to gain soci-
etal acceptance. They may be viewed as retarded or incapable of performing in the
hearing world. Deaf teenagers may feel estranged and withdraw into their own private world. However, they may encounter individuals in the larger society who
provide them with the link to the hearing world. These individuals are willing to
accept them for who they are and support them during this transitional period. This
affords them the opportunity to leave their childhood and embark on their adulthood with a positive outlook.

Those deaf individuals who feel a sense of acceptance from society have an
easier time identifying who they are and how they can become productive members
of their community. If they feel rejection, they will depend on others to make decisions for them and be unable to relate independently with the hearing society in
which they live.

Young Adulthood

By the time individuals reach young adulthood, they have begun to form their adult
identity and may seek to secure jobs in which they can find enjoyment and partners
with whom they can share their lives. Because many deaf students attend residential
schools, most of their social contacts are with other deaf individuals. They are
grouped together for a number of years and, therefore, tend to socialize within this

group. This, coupled with unsatisfactory attempts to become a part of the larger hearing society, encourages the formation of and participation in the Deaf culture.

Although deaf individuals choose to work with hearing people and live primarily in neighborhoods alongside hearing adults, they still elect to become integral members of the "Deaf community" or culture. This is the natural result of a people who seek their own kind with whom communication flows easily and mutual problems and interests can be shared. As deaf youth marry, they tend to form their own social group and function separately from the hearing society. They establish their own clubs, social, and athletic events. They remain in contact with hearing individuals but rely on the Deaf community for support and acceptance. Even though they may experience social difficulties on the job, they continue to have a tightly knit group where they can go for support. Through adulthood they may continue to feel that there is a certain stigma attached to them. Although their deafness may be perceived as negative by the larger community, within this culture a support group remains that fosters a sense of belonging and identity.

However, this tightly knit group can have a negative impact on those who do not conform to the norm of the culture. Individuals exhibiting deviant behavior within the group, or what others may interpret (perceive) as deviant behavior, may be faced with ostracism from the Deaf community. It is very difficult to alter or stop gossip within the network once it has begun. Members who lose "favor" with the group or become "blackballed" encounter isolation from the Deaf community and have a difficult time establishing their place in society. Although this seldom happens, it can be a shattering experience for the individual who is ostracized.

The Deaf culture is of critical importance to those who identify themselves with it. It has developed out of a need for camaraderie among a group of unique individuals who are seeking a place of their own in society. By exploring the impact the larger society has had on this population, greater insights can be gained into the impetus for establishing this culture.

A LOOK AT ERIKSON'S DEVELOPMENTAL MODEL AS IT APPLIES TO DEAFNESS

Society plays an integral role in the shaping of one's identity. Through our interactions with those around us, we are able to develop our personality. We have the ability to formulate a very healthy self-concept or to grow, developing the feeling that our personalities are lacking. Our environment and the experiences with which we interact provide us with the knowledge base and skills to cope with life's daily challenges. What happens to those individuals who are not given the opportunity to fully explore their surroundings, are not provided with the experiential base they require, and do not receive the positive reinforcement that is so critical to development? When this occurs, the effect on human development may be significant.

Various theories have been advanced that pertain to personality development. Each theory is unique, and yet all focus on those characteristics that impact and have bearing on psychological development. Although psychoanalytic and existential theories have been widely publicized and applied to deaf individuals, Eriksonian theory lends itself to examining the individual throughout the whole human life cycle. This theory developed by Erik Erikson is one of the classic models for studying human development.

Throughout his eight stages he traces human psychosocial development. Each stage has a crisis that must be resolved in order for the person ultimately to develop to his fullest potential. By examining these eight stages and the impact deafness has on each one, the psychological development of this population can be explored.

Before examining the stages and the impact of deafness on each one, it is critical to keep in mind the role communication plays in the developmental process. If deaf children are born to hearing parents and ease in interactive communication does not occur, the outcomes of each stage may be less than satisfactory.

However, when deaf children are born to culturally Deaf parents who actively engage in shared communication, the outcomes of each stage are reflective of those found in interactive environments between hearing children and their hearing parents. Table 1-1, included at the end of the section on Stage VIII, reflects the impact of deafness on development as evidenced by families with hearing and culturally Deaf parents.

Stage I (birth to 18 months): Trust vs. Mistrust

A foundation is established from birth that provides the basis upon which future development is built. This foundation is referred to as "Basic Trust." It is a time in one's life when "essential trustfulness of others as well as a fundamental sense of one's own trustworthiness" is developed (Erikson, 1968).

This general state of trust implies that the quality of the maternal relationship is critical to the early establishment of trust on the part of the infant. The words "maternal relationship" denote a key concept, and the importance of such a relationship cannot be overemphasized. Erikson further explains how mothers establish feelings of trust within their children by not only providing sensitive care for their individual needs, but by also projecting a sense of trustworthiness that they themselves have acquired through their community life-style. By presenting to the child a conviction that there is meaning related to their method of child care, a sense of mutual trustworthiness can be established.

In order for the mother to provide her child with those elements necessary for a mutual trust relationship to develop, she must first be free of conflicts within herself. Thus, the mother must be able to accept the child, thereby establishing a quality trust relationship. In the event that the mother's child has a disability, acceptance may come only secondary to her ability to sort through, comprehend, and accept her own feelings. The mother who is struggling with the emotional trauma of dealing with her child's disability may convert an otherwise warm, nurturing environment into a battleground involving emotional turmoil. As a result, the child may be subjected to tension and quickly sense those feelings of uncertainty that are projected by the mother. This stage may culminate with the mother feeling uncertain and alienated from the child, while leaving the child feeling "detached" and unable to form the bond that is critical for basic human development. The effects this relationship has on the psychological process within the confines of the family unit is discussed more fully in Chapter Three.

Stage II (18 months to 3 years): Autonomy vs. Shame and Doubt

The second stage in a child's life continues to be identified by rapid growth and enormous change. Babbling turns to audible language and desires are expressed more clearly. During this stage the child makes rapid gains in muscular maturation, in verbalization, and in the ability to discriminate and coordinate a number of highly conflicting action patterns. Characteristic of this stage is the child's ability to "hold on" and "let go," and although highly dependent on a primary caretaker, the child begins to project an autonomous will.

At this time the child can be viewed in different dimensions. He is beginning to perceive himself as a separate individual with desires of his own. At other times he is filled with doubt as to who he is and returns to his parents for support. This struggle between becoming independent while at the same time remaining dependent creates a crisis for the child.

One of the major areas of focus regarding "holding on" and "letting go" lies in the area of toilet training. The child becomes aware of his bodily functions and his control over them. He begins to establish feelings of "I" and "me" and may want to make his own decisions regarding bladder and bowel control. If the parent becomes too rigid, the child may rebel, thus withholding bodily functions until he is ready. Under too much stress to perform he may in turn take an alternate route, thus regressing into an earlier stage of childhood. The child wants to stand on his own two feet while at the same time he wants to receive parental support. "This whole stage then becomes a battle for autonomy" (Erikson, 1968, p. 108).

The child is striving to become the controller of his being, thus establishing feelings of self-worth and developing the aspect of self-esteem. If the child is not permitted this freedom of development and does not establish a feeling of self-worth, he will begin to be encompassed with feelings of doubt and shame. It is critical that the child sense that he has the freedom of expression and that his parents will not only permit him this avenue, but will also support him in his endeavor.

To enable the child to obtain a sense of "autonomy," he must first have acquired a sense of "basic trust." The child must be assured that regardless of what he says, he will continue to be loved and accepted. By conveying those feelings to the child he will feel comfortable when expressing himself, without the fear of being rejected. If the child does not establish this early feeling of trust, and the parenting techniques continue to incorporate a style enforcing rigid control, the child will remain dependent. Thus, his feelings of self-worth will be minimal and his preponderance of doubt overwhelming. These feelings of doubt are established early in life. They are precipitated by the indignities of punishment and restriction so often delivered by parents who are frustrated in their marriage, in work, or in their attempts to relate to society.

The parents themselves must have a sense of autonomy to grant the child the freedom to develop his. If the parent is involved in marital problems or experiencing feelings of self-doubt he will not be able to provide the supportive base the child needs.

This stage is critical to the child's development in that it is here for the first time that the infant is seeking emancipation from the mother. To accomplish this he must have developed a sense of trust and a feeling of worth. The deaf child who has not bonded closely to his mother may enter this stage lost in the parent's realm of uncertainty. He may be unable to acquire a feeling of "autonomy" due to the fact that he has not established feelings of self-worth and basic trust. As he progresses through the second stage of life, it is possible for his foundation to be weak and his development to be slower. If the parents are overprotective, they may refuse to give the child the freedom he needs to begin establishing feelings of self-worth. Due to the lack of language and communication at this very early age, emotional development as well as socialization may be hampered.

Stage III (3 to 6 years): Initiative vs. Guilt

Between the ages of three and six many events are occurring within the child's life. Physical growth, although still rapid, is slower in comparison to the first three years. Her verbal and locomotive skills are expanding and she is developing from the preschooler into the world of the elementary school pupil.

As the child enters into the third stage of her life she has achieved a certain degree of "autonomy" and is beginning to focus on other aspects of his environment. "The task of childhood—three to six years—is to develop a sense of initiative with a feeling of purposefulness of life and of one's own self" (Schlesinger & Meadow, 1972, p. 15). At this stage the child is convinced that she is a separate individual and is now striving to identify the type of individual she can become.

According to Erikson, there are three developments that support this stage while also serving to bring about its crisis. These developments can be summarized as follows: First, the child learns how to become more mobile and thus establishes a wider environment in which to explore; second, her sense of language expands and she is able to comprehend and ask an incessant number of questions, often acquiring just enough information to thoroughly misunderstand; and third, her language and locomotion permit her the ability to expand her imagination.

The child is beginning to be less concerned with her physical parts and is more concerned with what she can do as a total person. She is less preoccupied with the fact that her legs enable her to walk, but rather focuses on her body as a whole and uses her legs for running. No longer must basic functions demand concentration—she is free to explore what she can do creatively. She is not only expressive in her physical actions but also in her verbal abilities.

During this stage the child becomes aware of the various occupations in which people are employed. She begins to assimilate the role of an individual she is familiar with and mimics that role. In essence she imagines himself to be the doctor, the police officer, or the teacher. The child becomes somewhat aggressive at times, questions everything, and enters into the realm of infantile sexuality. She is constantly seeking answers to new experiences and events. The child is absorbing all that is around her while at the same time deciding where she fits in.

A key factor in developing this sense of initiative lies in the element of conscience.

> *The child . . . hears the "inner voice" of self-observation, self-guidance, and self-punishment, that divides [her] radically with himself: a new and powerful estrangement. This is the ontogenetic cornerstone of morality. (Erikson, 1968, p. 119)*

The child is becoming more adventuresome and in so doing she is continuing to look for parental permission and acceptance. While actively engaging in a new event she is also establishing feelings of right and wrong and developing her conscience. The child must be given the freedom to explore and identify with the role of an adult in order to conquer this crisis. The child is generally given the opportunity at this age to be out in public more, and through her increased experiences and her unending range of questions she begins to identify with various adult roles.

At this time not only is the family an important institution, but the school is beginning to have an impact on the child also. For the deaf child who has not established a positive rapport with her family and finds school to be unsatisfactory, the results can be devastating.

Between the ages of three and six the child's task is to develop a feeling of purposefulness for her life and to develop a sense of initiative. The child is characterized by her motor exuberance and her endless myriad of questions. She begins to use her imagination to project herself into adult roles and mimic their behaviors. The child is continually experimenting with new things while simultaneously seeking parental acceptance and approval for her actions.

Preschool and elementary school become a part of the child's world at this time. She begins to interact and socialize with other children her age, while building the basic foundation for education. The child's creativity and imagination are stimulated as she is introduced to a variety of new materials to manipulate.

The deaf child again may be more restricted at this stage due to her parents' control and overprotection. She may not receive the same sense of freedom that the hearing child has, and may feel constricted in her activities. The lack of verbal communication continues to erode her curiosity and her endless questions may go unasked and unanswered.

Early school experiences for deaf children may bring about additional feelings of confusion and emotional trauma. Those attending residential schools must cope with the loneliness of being removed from the home environment. Although academic programs offered by these facilities may be excellent and the children can participate in athletic and social events, those residing within the dormitories may feel confined as they are required to adhere to the rules of the institution.

Due to the very nature of the disability the child may not be given the freedoms or opportunities that are vital to this stage. Subsequently, she is denied the avenues necessary for developing "initiative." Encouragement for experimenting with her imagination may be delayed until later. She lacks the opportunity to make her own decisions and assume responsibility for, and take pride in, her actions. Overall, many of the developmental experiences characteristic of this stage may not be afforded deaf children.

Stage IV (6 to 11 years): Industry vs. Inferiority

Developmentally, when the child has reached this stage he has made various associations with a variety of adult role models and is now ready, in his own way, to experiment with the way things work. His sense of identity is transferred from his ability to utilize his imagination to his ability to learn to make things work. The child becomes enthralled with the mechanical aspects of how objects are made and put together and his sense of accomplishment comes from being able to construct things himself. The child begins to create and design a variety of playthings and thus his individuality becomes recognized. The importance of this building behavior lies not with what the child makes, but rather with the recognition he receives for making it. During this time period, children are encouraged in their efforts to make, construct, and build practical things. They are allowed to finish their products and are praised or rewarded for their accomplishments, thus establishing a sense of industry within the child.

Through this recognition children begin to feel good about themselves. These feelings are internalized, hence enhancing this concept of self-worth and self-esteem. However, if they do not have the opportunities to experience a sense of accomplishment for those tasks they undertake, they may begin to regard themselves as inferior.

When children are placed in situations where they are continually faced with tasks they cannot accomplish easily, they become frustrated and may fail consistently. As a result, feelings of inferiority may develop. However, those who are praised for their efforts and are the recipients of positive reinforcement will develop a solid foundation, increasing in importance as they grow older.

> ... this is socially a most decisive stage. Since industry involves doing things beside and with others, a first sense of division of labor and of differential opportunity—that is, a sense of the technological ethos of a culture—develops at this time. (Erikson, 1968, p. 126)

The child is embarking on new projects at home as well as at school, and both parents and teachers will have a significant impact on him at this time. How he resolves this crisis of industry versus inferiority will be determined to a great extent by the environment in which he finds himself and by the way people respond to his behavior. The deaf child may encounter several stumbling blocks at this stage. His parents may withdraw from him, his educational experience may prove deficient to that of his hearing peers, and society may label him with a stigma. Due to these handicapping conditions, the child may emerge from this stage with strong feelings of inferiority.

Stage V (11 to 18 years): Identity vs. Role Diffusion

As the individual enters this stage she develops a heightened awareness of the world around him. She has previously developed a basic sense of trust, a feeling for accomplishment and is now striving to become an independent person. During the first part of the seven years she will attempt to become emancipated from her parents, and toward the end of this time period she will direct her attention toward determining her role in society.

During the period of adolescence the individual can be seen as trying to establish her identity as different from childhood, but not quite into adulthood. During the early part of this stage the child is faced with problems surrounding independence, emancipation, and freedom from her family. However, during the latter part of this stage she focuses on her identity as a separate individual, apart from the family unit.

Throughout these years the adolescent attempts to compile all of the different roles she plays into one unified self. By doing this she is able to view herself as a separate individual, independent of her family and capable of finding a place for herself in society. In essence, she is integrating all of her previous experiences into a total person with which she can define her unique identity. During this time she struggles to bring together all of the things she has learned about herself while functioning in various roles such as a daughter, athlete, student, friend, and so forth.

It can be difficult for the teenager to establish this sense of "identity." Often times the adolescent will become confused as to which role types are acceptable and which behaviors are the most desirable. Previously, she has largely been influenced by parents and educators and the realm of society has had minimal influence on him. The teenager has primarily been taught to look to her parents for role models, and as her horizons broaden to include the vastness of society confusion may encompass her. She may be provided with one set of values from her parents and other sets from society. As a result, she is faced with the challenge of determining what she should believe and how she should behave. The teenager may continually feel she is on display and that she is being evaluated for her actions. She may expend a great deal of energy wondering what people are thinking of her. Quite frequently the adolescent becomes preoccupied with the way she is perceived in the eyes of others, and begins questioning how to connect others' perceptions of her relative to the way that she sees himself.

The adolescent begins to focus on her role in society. She becomes concerned with whom she can trust, what vocation she should pursue, and how she will be accepted by society and her peers. Previously, the child has attempted to achieve a feeling of trust in herself and those in her immediate environment. Now she is seeking individuals and ideas in which she can place additional feelings of trust. It is of paramount importance that she associate with those individuals who will grant her acceptance and avoid those experiences that will create embarrassment for her.

The teenager is unsure of herself during this period and may therefore go to great lengths to camouflage her uncertainty. She may find temporary sanction in the midst of a peer group while she sorts through her own values and identity. Parents and educators continue to provide the parameters for this development as the teenager seeks her role in society.

The very essence of adolescence constitutes a tremendous change in the child. Physiologically and psychologically she changes from the child into the young adult. With these changes come the need for the young person to identify who she is, where she fits in, and where she is going in the future.

The deaf adolescent who is searching for this identity may find her level of stress increasing. For now she must confront her deafness and determine where she will feel the most comfortable within society. She must deal with the realization that she is "different" and will never be a fully functioning, "hearing member" of her community. In addition, she must determine if she wants to associate primarily with the Deaf community or hearing world or fluctuate between the two.

If, prior to this time, a caring, trusting, and accepting relationship has been established, the individual will be able to resolve this crisis. However, if she enters this stage with previous crises unresolved she may find this to be a very difficult time.

Stage VI (18 to 25 years): Intimacy vs. Isolation

With the individual's identity established, he enters into this stage with a heightened awareness of those around him. He has determined who he is, what his preferences are, and with which type of people he likes to socialize. He is now ready to concentrate on what he can give to others both in a work and love relationship. Parental attachment continues to decrease and the individual strives to establish his own place in society as a productive human being. During this stage, the mark of a healthy individual lies in his ability to develop a mature relationship with his surroundings, such as his work and his intimate relationships.

The individual who has attained a sense of personal identity will be able to begin interacting with others both socially and vocationally. He will feel confident about himself and secure about establishing intimate relationships with others. The term "intimate" is used in a broad sense here and entails various implications. Erikson uses this term to include much more than lovemaking alone; it is meant to incorporate his ability to share and care about another individual without the fear of losing himself in the process (Elkind, 1970).

For those individuals who have resolved the identity crisis, the one of intimacy will be forthcoming. However, those individuals who do not feel comfortable with their identity will be reluctant to become involved with others for fear of losing their own identity.

> *The youth who is not sure of his identity shies away from interpersonal intimacy or throws himself into acts of intimacy that are "promiscuous" without a true fusion or real self-abandon.*
>
> *Where a youth does not accomplish such intimate relationships with others—and, I would add, with his own inner resources—in late adolescence or early adulthood, he may settle for highly stereotyped interpersonal relations and come to retain a deep* sense of isolation. *(Erikson, 1968, pp. 135–136)*

At this point in one's life, it is essential for the individual to begin to feel that he is a contributing member of society. He must feel good about himself and want to share his positive attributes both in a social and vocational sense. If he cannot find friends or coworkers to be intimate with, he may experience an inner void, thus resulting in feelings of aloneness.

Those who have not established a sense of identity will tend to withdraw from those individuals who strive to maintain a personal closeness with them. They will attempt various methods of keeping others at a distance. Erikson refers to this as "distantiation," the counterpart of intimacy. It is "the readiness to repudiate, isolate, and if necessary, destroy those forces and people whose essence seems dangerous to one's own" (Erikson, 1968, p. 136).

However, if the individual has progressed through the previous stages successfully, he will have determined who he is and what he is capable of doing. At this point he will be able to accept himself and share his being with others. It is through doing this that he will experience "intimacy."

During this stage, deaf adults who have attended residential schools and/or are associated with the Deaf community may find themselves seeking "intimacy" within this culture as they examine their role in society. Those who have been unable to establish their own identity and to determine where they "fit" in both cultures—Hearing and Deaf—may find themselves experiencing deep feelings of isolation.

Stage VII (25 to 50 years): Generativity vs. Stagnation

As one becomes established in a vocational setting and selects a marriage partner, she begins to turn her interests to the children who will be the upcoming generation of working adults. During these years the adult needs to feel needed and that she is a valuable member of society. Through guiding and influencing her children she can feel that she is contributing to the total of society. Erikson refers to this stage as "generativity" where the primary concern is for establishing and guiding the next generation. This concept of generativity is meant to include such tasks as creativity and productivity.

The individual becomes interested and involved not only with her immediate family but with other young individuals as well. She is concerned with society in general and what the world will be like in years to come. At this point she has placed her interests outside the immediate family structure and into the larger realm of society. She becomes concerned with others who reside outside of her immediate family and focuses her attention on the livelihood of future generations.

For the individual who has secured her identity and feels comfortable caring for others, she will now be able to contribute to the betterment of society. She will take a strong interest in those activities that will contribute to the ongoing development of the world in which she lives.

If the adult has not been successful in resolving the previous crises, she will have a difficult time becoming involved in the task of this stage. In order for one to become involved in society, she must feel confident about herself. Otherwise she will expend all of her energies inward trying to determine who she is and what she is all about. She will block herself off from the world around her, and all of the events in society to which she could contribute and benefit from will be nonexistent for her.

When the individual is unable to generate an interest in the world around her, she tends not only to withdraw but also to stagnate. Daily living becomes routine, and one's sphere of new experiences becomes increasingly limited. The adult in this situation generally becomes very self-centered and acutely aware of her own individual needs.

The maturational level of the individual and the way she has adjusted to her new role in society will determine whether she will be a very "outward" oriented individual or a very isolated, "inward" oriented person. Concern for one's own children and society's children, in general, characterize the important task of this stage.

Stage VIII (50+ years): Integrity vs. Despair

During the latter part of the adult years, one usually retires or semiretires from his field of work and has time to reflect on his previous life experiences and accomplishments. It is a time for taking an objective look at the world around him and observing human problems at a distance. It is also a time for evaluating where one has been and what he would like to accomplish prior to his death. For those who have successfully resolved the previous tasks it is a period of continued growth and a time for the individual to feel good about himself and his life. "The sense of integrity arises from the individual's ability to look back on his life with satisfaction" (Elkind, 1970, p. 28). For those individuals who are able to assess their abilities and their limitations, and are comfortable with themselves, it can be a time of enjoyment and relaxation. They can still remain an active part of society but function in a less stringent fashion.

> *Those individuals who are not pleased with their accomplishments and who have not led a productive life will have a different perspective of themselves and the world around them. They will view their lives as wasted and feel that not only have they not accomplished what they would have liked to, but also that it is too late to try something new. For these individuals there is a deep feeling of despair for themselves and for what their lives could have been. Those enmeshed in despair have the heavy sense "that time is short, too short for the attempt to start another life and to try out alternate roads of integrity. (Erikson, 1968, p. 140)*

How one will live the latter part of his life will be highly dependent on how he has developed since infancy. For those who have become autonomous human beings this part of one's life can be lived fully. Those who have been hampered developmentally will reflect back on their lives with feelings of sadness. At this time one accepts his life for what he has or has not accomplished and will view his actions either as positive or negative depending on the criteria he has established for himself. By accepting the responsibility for one's life, the adult may experience a feeling of satisfaction as he reflects back on his accomplishments.

THE DEAF CULTURE

The development of a healthy personality and the ability to integrate fully into society is contingent upon the way one is able to relate to one's environment. As one begins to express ideas and thoughts and shares them with members of the community, the person receives feedback that will be influential in determining how he or she perceives his or her identity. Because of the communication barrier and the attitudes of the nondisabled population as they respond to those who are disabled, this avenue for development is somewhat restricted, thus affecting the development of a healthy personality. In order for the individual to explore his or her identity he or she must have the opportunity to be accepted as a whole person first, enabling those around him or her to focus on his or her positive attributes and negative characteristics.

Membership in the Deaf community is based on several factors. First, one must want to identify with the Deaf culture; second, one must be able to relate to experiences that are shared by other members; and third, one must share a similar communication base in order to facilitate the exchange of ideas. Deafness by itself is not a sufficient condition for membership into the Deaf community. One must want to be identified as part of the group; value the history, folklore, and traditions of the community; and actively participate in the group's events and activities. Upon closer examination of these factors, one can begin to gain a greater understanding of the culture in which deaf people choose to relate.

TABLE 1-1　**Erickson's Eight Developmental Stages: The Impact of Deafness in Relation to Hearing and Deaf Parents**

Stage	Deaf Child/ Hearing Parents	Deaf Child/Deaf Parents
Stage I Birth–18 Months Trust vs. Mistrust	Parents must come to terms with deafness.	Deaf parents accept deaf child and may be excited that they have produced "one of their own."
	Stress may overpower feelings of warmth and nurture.	Parents may readily identify and understand the needs of a deaf child.
	Parental tension may be conveyed to the child and thus interfere with the establishment of trust.	Self-fulfilled parents provide child with warm nurturing environment where trust develops.
Stage II 18 months–3 years Autonomy vs. Shame and Doubt	Child becomes mobile and wants to explore.	Child becomes mobile and explores environment.
	Babbling may cease due to lack of reinforcement.	Babbling is replaced by signing.
	Parental caregiver may become controlling out of fear of something happening to the child.	Communication develops between caregivers and child.
	Child may be physically put and placed into position rather than receiving verbal direction.	Child begins to develop a sense of independence from parents.
	Autonomy may be stymied as feelings of dependence are fostered.	Child begins to establish a sense of autonomy.
Stage III 3–6 Years Initiative vs. Guilt	Language development may be delayed due to gestures and minimum sign communication.	Child's sign vocabulary continues to grow.
	Environmental experiences may be restricted, depending upon parental acceptance of deafness.	Child's mobility continues with broadened environmental experiences (child may begin interacting with members of the Deaf community).
	Child may be restricted in asking questions due to limited sign skills.	Child asks incessant number of questions.

TABLE 1-1 *Continued*

Stage	Deaf Child/ Hearing Parents	Deaf Child/Deaf Parents
Stage IV 6–11 Years Industry vs. Inferiority	Child's adult role models may be limited to hearing adults. Child might not have expressive language to convey imaginative thoughts. Child may sense inferiority to his/her hearing counterparts.	Child forms association with adult Deaf role models. Child uses his or her imagination. Child begins to explore how things work. Child is rewarded for accomplishments and begins to feel sense of industry.
Stage V 11–18 Years Identity vs. Role Diffusion	Deaf teenager may only be aware of Hearing culture (if he/she has been the only deaf student in a main-streamed program). Learned dependency may flourish due to weakened communication skills. Teenager may feel ill equipped to deal with the hearing environment. Teenager may feel isolated from peer group (depending on school environment).	Deaf teenager is aware of Deaf and Hearing cultures. May begin striving to be independent from parents. May sense a struggle of where he/she wants to "fit" within the Hearing and/or Deaf cultures. May rely on peer group for support (depending on school environment).
Stage VI 18–25 Years Intimacy vs. Isolation	Deaf adult may become actively involved with the Deaf community. May seek a spouse. Enters the workforce. May associate with Deaf community more than family. Begins to make a contribution to society. May share accomplishments with family.	Deaf adult may become actively involved with the Deaf community. May seek a spouse. Enters the workforce. Associates with Deaf community more than family. Begins to make a contribution to Deaf community.

TABLE 1-1 *Continued*

Stage	Deaf Child/ Hearing Parents	Deaf Child/Deaf Parents
Stage VII 25–50 Years Generativity vs. Stagnation	Focuses energies on his/her own children.	Focuses energies on his/her own children.
	May struggle with contributions in the workforce (feeling of limited advancement may exist).	May struggle with contributions in the workforce (feelings of limited advancement may exist).
	Deaf adult may or may not become actively involved in Deaf community; this depends on communication issues and self identity.	Remains an active member in Deaf community events.
Stage VIII 50+ Years Integrity vs. Despair	Deaf adults reach retirement.	Deaf adults reach retirement.
	Look back on theirs with either a sense of accomplishment or feelings of despair.	Look back on their lives with either a sense of accomplishments or feelings of despair.
	Develop a sense of satisfaction if they feel they have accomplished self-perpetuated goals.	Develop a sense of satisfaction if they feel they have accomplished self-perpetuated goals.

American Sign Language

Language can be viewed as a tool that is instrumental in building communication links. These links open the door to an infinite number of interactions, affording us the opportunity to share our thoughts, beliefs and values, while being privy to the thoughts of others. These interactions, in turn, contribute to our self-esteem and provide us with a sense of our social identity. For some, spoken language is sufficient; for others, it is ineffective or virtually nonexistent.

Members of the Deaf community value their language. Through it they are able to converse with ease, share intimate thoughts, exchange humorous antidotes, and enjoy everyday discourse. Even though some may not master their language until adulthood, once it becomes ingrained, it opens up a whole new arena for shared experiences.

Patrick Graybill (1996), an accomplished Deaf actor and storyteller, has shared his thoughts on coming to terms with American Sign Language (ASL) as a "bona fide language." He states:

> *The more I learned about ASL and Deaf Culture . . . the better I felt as a*
> *Deaf person and the freer I felt to be an actor on the stage . . . I am cur-*
> *rently a proud member of the Deaf community. And I enjoy being with the*
> *advocates of ASL . . . I have compassion for . . . deaf people coming from*
> *schools where they have not been given an ASL base and who do not yet*
> *have a clear sense of identity. (p. 230–231)*

He further provides us with a heightened awareness of the role ASL plays in the Deaf community by commenting on the different perspectives Deaf and hearing individuals have regarding silence.

> *We deaf people have our own center, whereas hearing people have theirs;*
> *therefore, conflicts have arisen. For instance, our idea of silence and theirs*
> *are not alike at all. They think that silence means lack of sounds. As for deaf*
> *people, silence is feeling lost in a room of hearing people who chat with*
> *their mouths and do not use ASL. (p. 231)*

Identification

Individuals who accept their deafness seek to become part of a community where they can establish feelings of "involvement" and "wholeness." They feel more comfortable with deaf people than the hearing and strive to be with their "own" people.

However, it is important to note that not all deaf individuals identify with the Deaf world. If the child has attended public schools and has resided in primarily an "oral" environment, he may not be fluent in manual communication and view himself as a hearing person who has difficulty understanding some words, rather than as a "deaf" individual. He does not want to identify with this population and will not seek membership in the Deaf culture. Some of these people may choose to participate in activities hosted by the Deaf community but are not members. While audiologically they are deaf, socially they are not (Higgins, 1980, p. 40). Some deaf individuals who do not sign or are opposed to this mode of communication may be a source of ill feelings within the community, as they might not respect the identity of the Deaf culture.

Shared Experiences

Shared experiences are frequently at the core of understanding another individual's behavior. Such is the case within the Deaf community. Members of this group traditionally have experienced frustration in communicating with the larger hearing society, have encountered embarrassing misunderstandings, and have experienced the loneliness of being left out of interactions with family members, neighborhood acquaintances, and others residing in the hearing community. Shared experiences also include the sharing of folklore, historical antidotes, and a rich legacy of storytelling.

Through these exchanges, lessons are taught, Deaf pride is instilled, and feelings of camaraderie flourish.

Participation in Activities

Membership in the Deaf community entails a commitment to its events and activities. At the heart of their socialization is involvement in activities that are established by and for them. One can travel across the country and become engaged in those activities which are hosted by various Deaf groups. Once the individual identifies himself with the culture, he seeks out its members as he travels or when he relocates to other regions of the country.

This involvement in activities may take the form of Deaf clubs, sporting events, or religious services designed specifically for them. Once entry into this culture is established, it provides a network for those inclined to interact freely in their "society."

Diversification Within the Culture

Just as the hearing population is comprised of a heterogeneous group of people, the same amount of diversity can be observed within the Deaf community. This population contains differences in social class, educational attainment, religious preference, and communication modes. In addition, one's genetic makeup, family background, and degree of hearing loss will determine the diverse mixture of this group.

Those who view deafness from this perspective recognize the characteristics of the Deaf community. When discussing deafness, they focus on attributes rather than deficiencies and identify the characteristics that are associated with this unique population.

A poignant portrait of what it means to be Deaf has been presented by Lynn Finton (1996). Lynn, a hearing wife and mother is married to a Deaf ASL user. Their two hearing children are being raised in a bilingual/bicultural environment. Wanting to determine how her daughter viewed deafness, she posed the following scenario to her: If a Martian arrived on earth and had never encountered a Deaf person before, how would you describe to the Martian what it means to be Deaf. Her elementary-school-aged daughter, Erin, replied:

> *They sign. They can't talk . . . well . . . they can talk but they don't unless they are at home or with people they know well. They go to church with other Deaf people with a priest who signs like them. They can drive [with sarcasm], they watch TV, all that stuff and they use captioning. That's it! (p. 270)*

As Lynn comments, her daughter truly has a concept of Deaf culture. At the beginning of her narrative, she comments on the most "important and unifying feature of the culture," ASL. She further mentions the concept of community, and she identifies Deaf people as individuals who do "normal" things. Never once does she mention that they can't hear. This is a true commentary that she has an appreciation for the positive cultural aspects of deafness and that she does not view Deaf people from a medical/pathological perspective (pp. 270–71).

SUMMARY

Through a lifetime of experiences we develop, mature, and emerge as unique individuals. We are influenced by the people we meet, the situations we encounter, and the choices we make. These interactions impact on us as we cast our place in society. Our values, goals, and group preferences are all influenced by our perceptions of ourselves, characterizing the way we respond to those around us.

Those who are deaf evolve through the same process. Their insights into themselves, coupled with their perception of how society views their deafness, significantly impacts their overall development. Daily exchanges afford them the opportunity to formulate opinions regarding their deafness, the Deaf community, and their relationship with this culture. Consciously, they select their preferred mode of communication and determine the extent to which they will affiliate with the Deaf community. Their linguistic preferences and cultural identity, rather than their degree of hearing loss and their geographic location, become the salient characteristics of those seeking membership into the Deaf community.

Establishing a sense of identity and belonging is a lifelong process. Through our experiences we begin to gain insights into who we are and explore what we want to become. We search for individuals with similar values, concerns, and beliefs, and strive to find our place in society. Deaf and hearing alike seek out those communities that extend an atmosphere of acceptance and foster a sense of belonging.

▶ 2

The Art of Hearing

Sound continuously permeates the environment, providing the listener with an awareness of the events occurring around him or her. It serves as a communication link and provides humans with the ability to acquire knowledge, develop language, and enhance their intellectual functioning capabilities. There are sounds that provide comfort when one feels distraught and sounds that provide warning in times of danger.

What is sound and how is it generated? Once sound is propagated, how does the hearing process function to incorporate it into useful information? What can impede the hearing mechanism, causing impairments within the auditory system?

THE PROPAGATION OF SOUND

In order for sound to be created, some force must initiate vibrations, causing a sound wave to travel through a medium. As the sound wave travels, it may ultimately be received by the hearing mechanism and then transmitted to the brain where it can be interpreted accurately. For sound to be processed, there must be four components: a vacillation of some type; a force to generate vibrations; a medium through which sound waves are transported; and a hearing mechanism that has the ability to receive and unerringly perceive the sensation.

Sound waves have two characteristic phases or density levels: compression and rarefaction. Compression occurs as the sound wave travels and the molecules of the medium are forced against each other. When the molecules attempt to separate from each other, returning to the natural density level, the rarefaction phase ensues. As the sound-producing source continues to vibrate, another compression is transmitted, and the oscillation continues as alternating compression and rarefaction. This reciprocal movement characterizes the sound wave, originating from the sound source and radiating outward at a constant velocity. This process is illustrated in Figure 2-1.

Compression
(Region of high pressure)

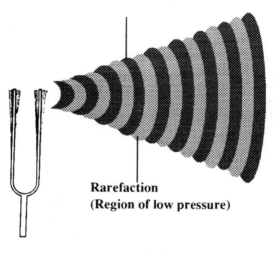

Rarefaction
(Region of low pressure)

FIGURE 2-1   **The Wave Nature of Sound**

When objects are made to vibrate they disturb the surrounding air in wave-like fashion, much like a water
wave is produced when you toss a stone into a pond.
Unlike the up-and-down motion of a water wave, however, a sound wave is a high pressure (compression) and
low pressure (rarefaction) alternation, as illustrated in
the sound wave produced by a vibrating tuning fork.
(Courtesy of Tom Fico and Wanda Hodnett)

The transmission of sound can be visually illustrated by imagining the following situation. Picture a group of elementary-age children lined up for lunch in the
school cafeteria. The boy at the end of the line loses his balance slightly and shoves
the child ahead of him. This causes the next child to push the next child and so forth,
creating a chain reaction. The child who initially lost his balance regains it and
straightens up as do all of the other children in the line. Suppose by the time the child
at the head of the line has regained his balance and has straightened up, the child at
the end of the line has lost her balance again and the process continually repeats itself. A wave of compression occurs each time a child is pushed, and a wave of rarefaction is instilled as each regains balance.

Sound moves through the air in typically the same way. The source of the sound
causes the air molecules to push against each other (compression), whereby they

bounce back to their original state (rarefaction), only to be pushed again (see Figure 2-2A). This process repeats itself consistently over a period of time. Sound waves can be measured in terms of intensity (loudness), by examining the height of the peaks, and frequency (pitch), by examining the distance between adjacent peaks. A complete succession of one compression and rarefaction constitutes a cycle. Therefore, the frequency of a sound wave can be determined by measuring the number of cycles that transpire in a second's time. Figure 2-2B reflects the frequency and amplitude of sound waves.

As the sound waves reach the ear, the mechanism for hearing responds to the stimulus, providing individuals with the ability to interact with their environment. This hearing process is an extremely complex one and can be better understood by examining the three parts of the ear: the external, middle, and inner ear, (see Figure 2-3) and their respective functions.

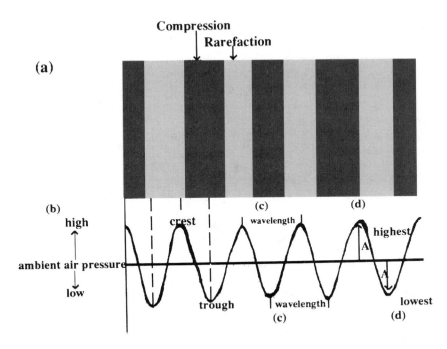

FIGURE 2-2A   **The Compressions and Rarefactions of a Sound Wave**

The compressions and rarefactions of a sound wave depicted in (a) correspond to the crest and trough, respectively, of a water wave in (b). The peak to peak (or trough to trough) distance shown in (c) is called the wavelength of the wave. The highest (or lowest) pressure variation from the ambient (undisturbed) air pressure shown in (d) is called the amplitude of the wave. (Courtesy of Tom Fico and Wanda Hodnett)

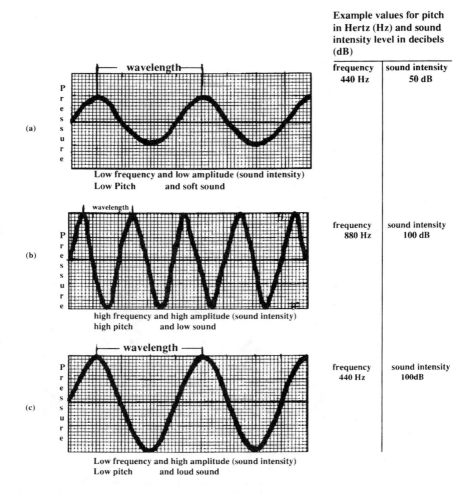

Example values for pitch in Hertz (Hz) and sound intensity level in decibels (dB)

frequency	sound intensity
440 Hz	50 dB
880 Hz	100 dB
440 Hz	100dB

FIGURE 2-2B   **Difference Between Frequency/Pitch and Amplitude/Sound Intensity (Loudness) in Sound Waves**

First note that longer wavelength of sound denotes a lower frequency and a shorter wavelength a higher frequency. (a) A sound wave of low frequency and pitch (440 Hz, for example) and low amplitude and sound intensity (50 dB, for example) compared to sound wave in (b) in which the frequency and amplitude are doubled (880 Hz and 100 dB, respectively). Compare the wavelengths and peak heights in (a) and (b). In (c) the frequency is the same as (a) (compare wavelengths) and the amplitude is the same as in (b) (compare peak heights). In this manner, one could imagine a sound wave of high frequency and low amplitude (high pitch, soft sound). For more information on sound measurements in Hertz (Hz) and decibels (dB) see section pertaining to audiological evaluation. (Courtesy of Tom Fico and Wanda Hodnett)

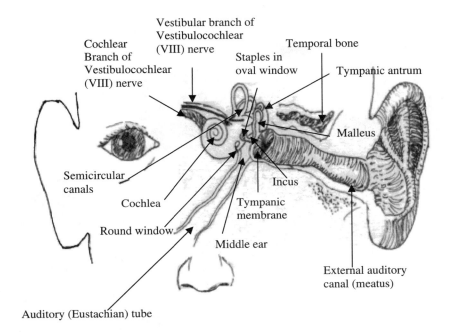

Vestibular branch of
Vestibulocochlear
(VIII) nerve

Cochlear
Branch of
Vestibulocochlear
(VIII) nerve

Staples in
oval window

Temporal bone

Tympanic antrum

Malleus

Semicircular
canals

Incus

Cochlea

Tympanic
membrane

Round window

Middle ear

External auditory
canal (meatus)

Auditory (Eustachian) tube

FIGURE 2-3 **Structure of the Auditory Apparatus**

Illustration depicting the left ear seen through the left side of the skull. The three divisions of the ear—external, middle, and internal—are portrayed.

(Courtesy of Marie A. Scheetz)

THE EXTERNAL EAR

The external portion of the ear consists of the auricle or pinna and the external auditory meatus, or ear canal. The auricle is the visible flap-like portion of the hearing mechanism and is connected to the side of the head. Its primary purpose is to receive sound waves and direct them into the external auditory meatus.

The ear canal is cylindrical in shape and ranges from 25mm to 35mm in length. It is approximately 7mm in diameter and enters the skull at a slight angle. It contains hair follicles and wax-producing glands. These elements serve to protect the tympanic membrane from foreign substances. The external auditory canal is larger at the auricular orifice and becomes somewhat smaller at the point at which it approaches the tympanic membrane (eardrum), the external boundary of the middle ear. Figure 2-4 illustrates the boundaries between the external middle and inner portions of the ear.

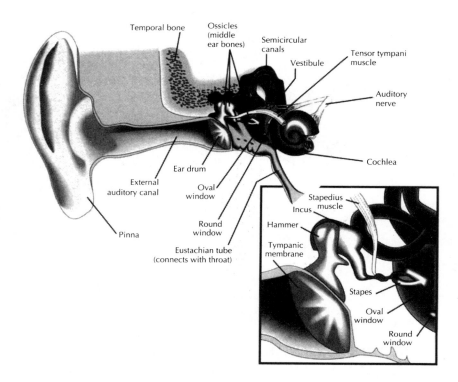

FIGURE 2-4 **The Auditory Apparatus**

(From *Physiology of Behavior,* Fourth Edition, by Neil R. Carlson, Copyright 1991 by Allyn & Bacon. Reprinted with permission.)

THE MIDDLE EAR

The middle ear consists of the tympanic cavity and is defined by the tympanic membrane on one boundary and the oval window on the other. The cavity, which is irregularly shaped, has a vertical dimension of approximately 15mm, varying in width from 2mm to 4mm. This cavity is housed within the petrous portion of the temporal bone and can be viewed in two sections. The topmost portion extends upward beyond the superior border of the tympanic membrane and is referred to as the attic, or the epitympanic recess. Because the tympanic antrum communicates with the mastoid air cells, there is indirect communication between these two cavities. The portion of the cavity that lies medially to the tympanic membrane is referred to as the tympanic cavity proper. This cavity is lined with a mucous membrane that also lines the tympanic antrum and mastoid air cells. A schematic diagram of the middle ear can be viewed in Figure 2-5.

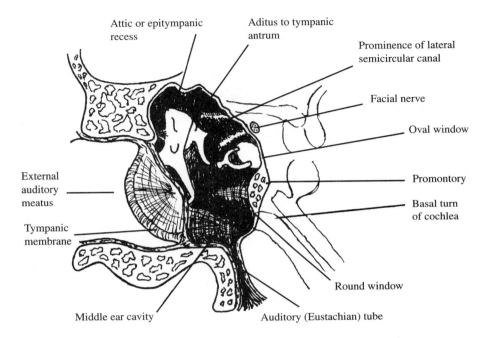

FIGURE 2-5 **A Schematic of the Middle Ear as Seen from the Front**

(Courtesy of Marie A. Scheetz)

Within the middle ear cavity and occupying a substantial amount of its space is the ossicular chain. The ossicles, consisting of the malleus (hammer), incus (anvil), and stapes (stirrup), are the tiniest bones in the body. The malleus, the largest of the bones, is attached on one side to the middle, connective tissue fibers of the tympanic membrane. Its other side connects to the incus. The incus links the stapes whose footplate is inserted against the oval window. This chain appears to serve two main purposes: first, to supply a vehicle for transporting sound vibrations to the inner ear fluids, and second, to provide a buffer to protect the inner ear from excessively strong vibrations.

In addition to the ossicular chain, two muscles occupy the cavity—the tensor tympani and the stapedius. They are the smallest striated muscles in the body. These muscles also serve a dual purpose. First, they enhance the movement of the tympanic membrane and the ossicular chain when the signal is weak; second, they inhibit the movement within the middle ear when intense stimulation is received.

There is a secondary safety device that operates within the confines of the middle ear. The Eustachian tube connects the air-filled middle ear with the mouth cavity. It serves as an air pressure equalizer and provides a means of ventilating this cavity.

When changes in air pressure occur, the Eustachian tube expands, thus permitting the middle ear to compensate for the changes in the outside air pressure. A detailed view of the inner ear is illustrated in Figure 2-6.

The round window and the oval window provide the boundary for the end of the middle ear and the beginning of the inner ear. They both serve an integral function in the transmission of sound from the environment on its path to the auditory center housed in the brain.

THE INNER EAR

The inner ear can be divided into two cavity systems. One segment houses the sensory organ required for establishing one's equilibrium, and the other provides the framework for the essential organ of hearing. These two organs share the same bony labyrinth and have the same fluid systems. The outer hard shell of the inner ear is referred to as the bony labyrinth, and the inner membranous portion is called the membranous labyrinth. The entire inner ear is filled with fluid. The membranous labyrinth is protected from the bony labyrinth by a fluid called perilymph, which is actually spinal fluid supplied from the ventricles of the brain. Endolymph, which is similar

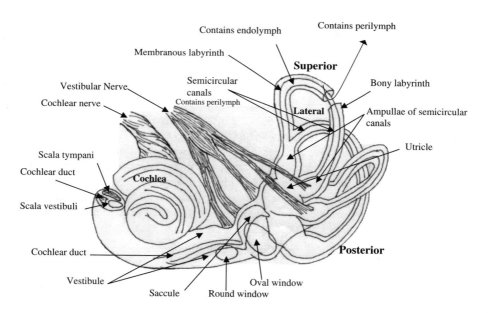

FIGURE 2-6 **Details of the Inner Ear**

(Courtesy of Marie A. Scheetz)

to perilymph but very viscous and differing somewhat in chemical composition, is the fluid that is found within the membranous labyrinth and is entirely separate from the perilymphatic system. Figure 2-7 demonstrates the fluid movement that occurs within this labyrinth.

That portion of the inner ear that is concerned with equilibrium is often referred to as the vestibular apparatus. Within the vestibule lies the utricle and the saccule, which both function as sensors for the pull of gravity and acceleration. The central portion of the vestibule communicates with the three semicircular canals; this bony structure also provides for the continuation of the cochlea, the snail-like shell within the inner ear.

The three semicircular canals, the anterior and posterior vertical canals, and the horizontal or lateral canal open into the vestibule through five orifices. They are located at right angles to each other and form the sense organ for turning in space. They, together with the utricle and the saccule, promote a sense of balance.

The cochlea, that is a continuation of the vestibule, consists of a base followed by two- and three-quarter turns. The canal is approximately 35mm long and ends blindly at the apex. Its basal end is nearest to the middle ear while the apical end is the farthest from it.

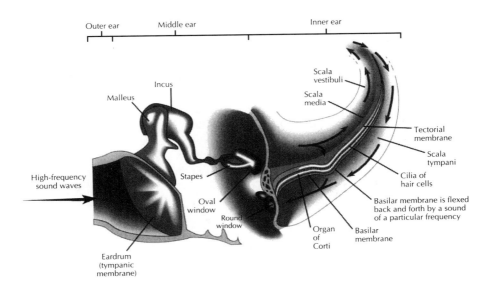

FIGURE 2-7   **Sound Waves Transmitted Through the Oval Window Deform a Portion of the Basilar Membrane**

(From *Physiology of Behavior,* Fourth Edition, by Neil R. Carlson, Copyright 1986 by Allyn & Bacon. Reprinted with permission.)

The canal is partly divided into two galleries or scalae—the upper portion is the scala vestibuli and the lower portion is identified as the scala tympani. The two chambers are separated by a spiral shelf of bone called the osseous spiral lamina. It consists of two layers of bone, each of which is continuous with structures that form the cochlear duct of the membranous labyrinth. The division of these two galleries is completed by a fibrous flexible membrane, the basilar membrane, that stretches across from the lower edge of the bony shelf to the spiral ligament that attaches it to the outer wall. The basilar membrane and the shelf both terminate approximately 2mm short of the end of the gallery. Thus, the basilar membrane completes the roof of the scali tympani and also forms the membranous portion of the floor of the cochlear duct. The roof of the cochlear duct is formed by an extremely fragile membrane, the vestibular membrane of Reissner, that extends obliquely to the outer wall of the cochlea.

The membranous tube that is located on the basilar membrane contains the sensory cells and their supporting structures known as the organ of Corti. The organ of Corti consists of four rows of hair cells that run parallel along the length of the basilar membrane. The inner row contains approximately 3,500 hair cells, and the three outer rows consist of approximately 20,000 slightly smaller hair cells. These hair cells are embedded in the tectorial membrane that extends over them. The tectorial membrane is composed of a rather viscous, slow-flowing jelly stiffened by a system of fibers that are attached at the outer edge to the solid limbus (border). It can move up and down in a somewhat stiff fashion. The tectorial membrane also attaches itself loosely to the organ of Corti before attaching more firmly again to the limbus. The organ of Corti and the tectorial membrane slide past each other slightly as they move up and down together. This movement bends the hair cells setting off nerve impulses in the nerve fibers. An enlargement and cross section of the cochlea depicting the tectorial membrane and the organ of Corti is contained in Figure 2-8.

The hair cells housed in the central core of the cochlea unite with the nerve fibers to form the auditory nerve, the acoustic branch of the VIII (eighth) cranial nerve. This auditory nerve passes through a channel in the temporal bone and sends impulses to the base of the brain. From there the auditory pathway extends through the brain to the auditory center of the cerebral cortex located in the temporal lobes of the brain. The auditory pathway is illustrated in Figure 2-9.

THE PHYSIOLOGY OF HEARING

Sound is transmitted to the human ear via air and bone conduction. However, the majority of the sounds we attend to are airborne since the mechanism of air conduction is more sensitive than the mechanism of bone conduction.

Sound waves traveling through the air are received by the pinna and are directed into the external auditory meatus where they impinge on the tympanic membrane (eardrum). The tympanic membrane is set into vibration by the moving air particles that are adjacent to it.

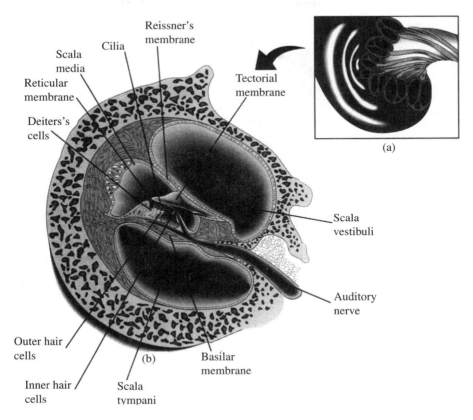

FIGURE 2-8 **A Cross Section Through the Cochlea, Showing the Organ of Corti**

(From *Physiology of Behavior,* Fourth Edition, by Neil R. Carlson, Copyright 1991 by Allyn & Bacon. Reprinted with permission.)

As the tympanic membrane begins to vibrate, the malleus, whose handle is embedded in the eardrum, sets the ossicular chain into vibration. As the ossicular chain continues to vibrate, the stapes generates movement within the oval window which produces a pressure wave in the perilymph of the vestibule. In addition to transmitting sound, the ossicles regulate the energy collected by the tympanic membrane into a movement of greater force with less excursion, or range of movement, thus matching the impedance of sound waves in air to that in fluid. In the event an extremely intense sound is produced, the stapedius and tensor muscles function as a damper for the vibrations, thus the chain provides protection for the inner ear.

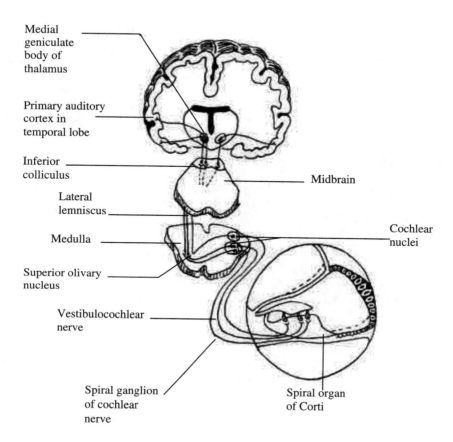

FIGURE 2-9   **Diagram of the Auditory Pathway from the Organ of Corti to the Brain: A Simplified Illustration A View from the Left Ear**

(Courtesy of Marie A. Scheetz)

As the footplate of the stapes produces pressure on the inner ear, the round and oval windows respond to provide relief from the increased pressure. The interaction of the two windows is complex but can be described simply. When the footplate is pushed into the vestibule, the round window is bulged outward toward the middle ear cavity. The reciprocal action of these two windows compensates for the compressibility of the perilymph and the movement of the ossicular chain.

The fluid motion from the oval window to the round window is transmitted through the cochlear duct. As the perilymph of the scala vestibuli is compressed, the vestibular membrane, or membrane of Reissner, bulges into the cochlear duct, causing movement of the endolymph and creating movement of the basilar membrane.

As the basilar membrane is displaced, there is a "shearing" action on the hair cells by the tectorial membrane that initiates nerve impulses. These impulses are carried by nerve fibers to the auditory portion of the VIII cranial nerve and then to the auditory center of the brain.

As stated earlier, sound can also be transmitted through bone conduction. Because the inner ear is encased in the temporal bone, vibrations of this bone will directly influence the movement of the fluid within the inner ear. As a result, those sounds transmitted by bone conduction are somewhat distorted. The nerve fibers compose a series of ascending and descending fibers that transmit the nerve impulses and "fine-tune" the signals. Once the auditory signal reaches the auditory cortex (brain), interpretation occurs and meaning is given to the transmitted signal. See Figure 2-10.

In bone conduction there are two modes of vibration: inertial, or translator motion, and compressional motion. Inertial motion can be defined as the process in that the bones resist acceleration caused by an external force. In turn, the compressional motion refers to that process when the surface is pressed upon and becomes smaller. When a low frequency sound is produced, the force and movement of the ossicular chain excites the hair cells, and the skull as a whole moves in response to the stimulation. However, when a high frequency stimulus is received, the skull does not move as a whole but rather vibrates so that opposite surfaces move in an out-of-phase relationship. The back and front of the skull move outward as the sides of the skull move inward. This movement produces a compression of the cochlea. As the fluid within the cochlea is compressed, the movement that takes place activates the nerve impulses.

One is not ordinarily conscious of sounds being transmitted through bone conduction as most of the sounds we are attuned to are airborne. However, when the head is in contact with a solid surface and the bones of the skull receive vibrations, one becomes more aware of the functioning of the bone-conduction mechanism. A summary of the structures of the ear and their functional roles is presented in Table 2-1.

CAUSES OF AUDITORY DYSFUNCTION

When discussing the various types and causes of hearing disorders one can begin by categorizing them into groups according to the age at onset of the hearing loss and the anatomical location of the dysfunction. Those dysfunctions that are present at birth are referred to as congenital losses, with those occurring after birth being labeled acquired losses.

The area of the ear in which the impairment occurs designates the type of loss possessed by the individual. Conductive losses are referred to as those in which the dysfunction occurs in the outer or middle ear with the inner ear functioning normally. If one's hearing loss occurs due to pathology in the inner ear or the auditory nerve, the term sensorineural loss is used.

FIGURE 2-10 **The Basilar Membrane Reflecting Resonance and the Activation of Hair Cells Found in the Cochlea**

(a) The cochlea is illustrated in a linear fashion enabling the viewer to observe how sound is transmitted. Low frequency sound waves (below the level of hearing) are routed around the helicotrema without exciting the hair cells. Higher frequency sounds create pressure waves that permeate through the cochlear duct and basilar membrane and arrive at the scala tympani. This creates vibrations in the basilar membrane in response to certain frequencies. (b) Reflects the varying lengths of basilar fibers found within different areas of the basilar membrane. (c) High frequency sounds create maximum excitation of the hair cells near the oval window and low frequency sounds excite hair cells near the cochlear apex.

(Courtesy of Marie A. Scheetz)

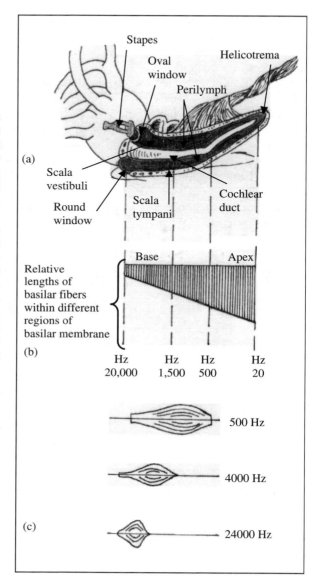

Conductive Hearing Loss

Conductive hearing loss refers to any dysfunction that occurs in the outer or middle ear in the presence of a normal inner ear (Newby, 1964). In a conductive loss the problem lies with the individual being unable to conduct sound to the remainder of the hearing mechanism.

TABLE 2-1   **Summary of the Structures of the Ear and Their Functional Roles**

Structure	Functional Role
External (outer) ear	Collects and absorbs sound waves.
Pinna (auricle)	Receives sound waves.
External auditory canal (meatus)	Transmits sound waves toward the tympanic membrane.
Tympanic membrane	When sound waves come in contact with the tympanic membrane, they cause it to vibrate, thus setting the ossicular chain into motion.
Middle ear	Converts sound waves into mechanical vibrations.
Auditory ossicles	Transmit sound waves from the tympanic membrane to the oval window.
Auditory tube (eustachian tube)	Provides a mechanism to equalize pressure on both sides of the tympanic membrane.
Inner Ear	Involved in the transduction of mechanical and hydrodynamic energy into neural impulses.
Vestibular aparatus Utricle Saccule Semicircular canals	Concerned with equilibrium Static equilibrium Static equilibrium Dynamic equilibrium
Cochlea	Consists of a series of fluids, channels, and membranes; responsible for transmitting sound waves to the organ of Corti (the organ of hearing) where nerve impulses are transmitted to the VIII (eighth) cranial nerve where neural impulses are transmitted to the auditory center of the brain.

Conductive hearing losses may be induced by the following:

1. Obstructions of the external ear canal
2. Impaired movement of the tympanic membrane
3. Restricted movement of the ossicles

When any of these situations occur, sounds are received by the inner ear at a reduced level of intensity due to the blockage or faulty mechanism operating in the outer or middle ear.

Very frequently, hearing losses that develop in children are conductive losses. Due to current medical advances, many causes of this type of loss can be cured readily. Individuals with this type of dysfunction tend to speak in a relatively quiet voice, function with generally unimpaired speech discrimination, can usually hear better in the presence of noise than can the person with normal hearing (medically referred to as paracusis Willisii), and can tolerate loud speech and other intense sounds that would normally cause discomfort in the normal ear (Newby, 1964).

Individuals with conductive losses function as if they were wearing earplugs and as a result tend to experience a similar loss at all of the varying frequencies. Occasionally individuals may hear higher or lower frequencies better; however, the majority of people receiving sounds perceive them with basically the same level of intensity.

Common causes of conductive losses include:

1. blockage of the outer ear (ear canal) by an excess accumulation of cerumen (wax)
2. atresia or an occluded auditory canal
3. anomaly in the middle ear evidenced by missing or malfunctioning ossicles or tympanic membrane
4. infection in the middle ear, characterized by otitis media
5. otosclerosis in which the typical movements of the three bones of the ossicular chain are prohibited. This affects women more than men and is frequently accompanied by tinnitus (a sensation of ringing or humming in the ears).

The prescribed treatment for conductive losses may be medical or surgical. Those experiencing a blockage in the ear canal can usually have the obstruction removed. For those who have a type of otitis media, antibiotic therapy can be prescribed. Those experiencing difficulty with the tympanic membrane can undergo a myringoplasty, a skin graft to repair the damaged area, or a tympanoplasty in which hearing is restored due to repair or reconstruction of the damaged parts contained in the middle ear. A stapedectomy (a surgical technique) may be employed when the dysfunction occurs with the ossicular chain. Use of this procedure allows the bones to become mobile again, thus increasing the individual's ability to hear.

Sensorineural Hearing Loss

Sensorineural losses, unlike conductive losses, occur when the dysfunction is located in the inner ear or along the nerve pathway from the inner ear to the brain stem. This type of hearing loss can be characterized by an individual's inability to perceive sounds at varying frequencies with the same level of intensity. Very frequently, the ability to hear high frequencies is lost. However, as in Ménière's disease, a type of sensorineural loss, the ability to hear low sounds is more greatly affected.

Individuals with sensorineural losses tend to speak with an excessively loud voice, even in situations where that degree of volume is not required; they do not possess the ability to hear their own voices in order to monitor them; they experience difficulty with speech discrimination and can generally receive sounds produced at the lower frequencies. Individuals may be aware that sounds are being produced during a typical conversation but have difficulty in differentiating which words are being spoken to them. In addition, those experiencing this type of loss do not receive protection from loud sounds as evidenced in a conductive loss. As a result, although faintly produced high frequency sounds may not be heard, other sounds that are very intense can be received and are powerful as well as painful. Therefore, the range of hearing for people with sensorineural losses is somewhat limited and narrow. The loudness of sounds tends to occur rapidly and "recruitment" follows. Recruitment is defined as the abnormally rapid growth in the sensation of loudness (Katz, 1985). Characteristic of this condition is the individual who complains one minute that he cannot hear and in the next breath is accusing others of shouting at him.

Persons experiencing sensorineural losses may also share the sensation of tinnitus (buzzing in the ears), commonly found among those with conductive hearing losses. Individuals usually complain of a buzzing or ringing sound that may be apparent in either ear or not localized at all. The ringing sound may be confused with external sounds, such as a doorbell or telephone.

Sensorineural losses may be attributed to causes other than Ménière's disease. It is well documented that certain drugs can damage the cochlea and the VIII nerve, thus causing a sensorineural loss. The most common drugs being used are aminoglycosides, such as streptomycin and gentamicin. Other causes include fractures, vascular occlusion, and inflammatory lesions that may be viral (e.g., mumps). Those diseases that involve the nerve cells that relay impulses to the temporal lobe cortex may also produce defects in hearing. In addition, intense noises from industrial sources as well as loud music are capable of creating permanent damage (Walter, 1982). Although the majority of babies born with a hearing impairment have incurred a sensorineural loss, this type of loss can occur at any time in a person's life. The causes for a sensorineural loss can be classified as congenital or acquired (adventitious).

Congenital Losses

Congenital losses are defined as those being present at birth. Although the dysfunction is present at birth, only one of every 2,000 live births or approximately 50 percent of the cases of profound childhood hearing loss are attributed to genetic causes (Konigsmark & Gorlin, 1976).

Genetic causes may be subdivided into three categories: single mutant gene disorders, chromosomal abnormalities, and multifactorial genetic disorders (Fischler, 1985).

Approximately 80 percent of these genetic abnormalities can be attributed to single mutant gene disorders. They are passed on to children either through an autosomal dominant, autosomal recessive, or an X-linked inheritance pattern (Jackson & Schimke, 1979). When a dominant condition occurs, only one gene in the pair is abnormal while the other is normal. As a result, the pair is heterozygous and the condition is passed on to 50 percent of the offspring. In turn those offspring that are affected will pass the disorder on to their children. Approximately 10 percent of the cases of childhood deafness can be attributed to dominant conditions (Jaffe, 1972; Konigsmark & Gorlin, 1976).

When a recessive condition is present, both genes in the pair are abnormal and a homozygous state occurs. Although both parents may have normal hearing, they are carriers of the mutant genes (heterozygous), and each contributes an abnormal gene to the affected child. When an autosomal recessive inheritance pattern occurs, the implication is that there is a 50-percent chance that the offspring will be carriers, a 25-percent chance that they will inherit a hearing loss, and a 25-percent chance that they will have normal hearing. Recessive conditions account for 40 percent of profound childhood hearing loss and are generally more severe than dominant ones (Jaffe, 1972).

Abnormalities within the chromosomes may occur either during meiosis (process of cell division resulting in forming the egg or sperm) or during mitosis (cell division that occurs in the fertilized egg). The chromosomes contain many genes, and small or large segments may be affected. In general chromosomal abnormalities produce multiple disabilities and the risk of inheriting these disorders increases in those children born to mothers thirty-five and older. An in-depth discussion of these disorders, as well as those caused by multifactorial genetic disorders, can be found in Chapter 11.

Nongenetic factors that may contribute to congenital hearing losses include prenatal infections, including viral, bacterial, and protozoal infections; or anything that causes damage to the embryo while it is in the uterus. Diseases such as rubella, incurred during the first trimester, or cytomegalovirus (CMV), can be transmitted to the fetus, contributing to significant sensorineural hearing losses.

Acquired Losses
Hearing losses that develop after a baby is born and occur anytime within an individual's life span are referred to as acquired (adventitious) losses. Causes may be attributed to trauma, disease, infection, VIII nerve and central nervous system tumors, high fever, and the aging process.

Trauma. There are two types of trauma that contribute to sensorineural losses. One type, although rare, occurs when there is a fracture of the temporal bone and damage is sustained by the inner ear (e.g., head injuries resulting from automobile accidents and wartime injuries). The second type occurs when the inner ear is subjected to intense noise; even a brief exposure can create a permanent and irreversible type of loss.

Meningitis. One of the leading postnatal causes of sensorineural losses in school-age children today is meningitis (Catlin, 1978). In the past, infants contracting this disease did not generally survive. Today the number who recover from the disease is on the increase, and the survivors are often left with severe hearing impairments and other neurological debilitating disorders (Mindel & Vernon, 1971; Gerber & Mencher, 1980).

Cytomegalovirus (CMV). Prenatal rubella was one of the leading causes of deafness; however, cytomegalovirus has taken its place (Vernon & Hicks, 1980). Annually, approximately 30,000 infants are born with the CMV infection (Pappas, 1985), and about 4,000 will possess a hearing loss ranging from mild to profound in nature (Moores, 1987).

Ménière's Disease. Another form of a sensorineural impairment, confined to the inner ear, is referred to as Ménière's disease. Characteristics include tinnitus, vertigo, and hearing loss. The primary cause is increased fluid pressure within the membranous labyrinth. Thus, this disease is also referred to as endolymphatic hydrops (Newby, 1964). An individual may experience violent attacks of dizziness, periods of loud tinnitus, and abnormalities in hearing. Although the deafness experienced is quite severe, there are periods of time in which the symptoms disappear; and the disease goes into remission. Ménière's disease generally affects only one ear, causing severe recruitment to occur.

Hearing Loss Due to the Aging Process. As individuals increase in age, their acuity for hearing higher frequencies is gradually diminished. This phenomenon, known as presbycusis, begins to develop during the thirties and becomes more apparent with each decade. Table 2-2 reflects the causes of hearing loss and the percentage of individuals affected by each one.

Central Deafness

Throughout the first part of this chapter, hearing impairments have been identified and defined as they relate to the outer, middle, and inner ear. However, not all types of hearing loss can be attributed to dysfunction within the ear itself. Problems may occur after the nerve impulse enters the brain stem or within the auditory center housed in the cerebral cortex. Anomalies related to the brain stem or the cerebral cortex are referred to as central auditory disorders. This type of hearing loss can be caused by a brain tumor, an abscess located in the brain, trauma-induced brain damage, or blood incompatibilities caused by the Rh factor.

Individuals with this type of hearing disorder have a normally functioning ear and are able to transmit sounds through the auditory channel with no amplification. However, once the sound travels beyond the acoustic nerve, the message becomes scrambled and cannot be accurately processed. One type of central hearing loss that occurs within the brain is a form of receptive aphasia, often referred to as auditory agnosia. As sound waves reach the hearing center in the brain, the brain must convert the signals that are received into meaningful information. When there is a lesion

TABLE 2-2 **Etiology of Hearing Loss**

Cause of Hearing Loss	Percent Due to Cause
Genetic/Hereditary	
Usher syndrome	0.6
Waardenburg syndrome	0.8
Treacher Collins syndrome	0.7
Other hereditary	34.8
Pregnancy Related	
Maternal rubella	2.8
Cytomegalovirus	3.8
Maternal drug/alcohol abuse	0.8
Medications taken by mother	0.3
RH incompatibility	0.7
Consequences of prematurity	10.4
Trauma	4.5
Other complications of pregnancy	7.7
Post-birth disease/injury	
Otitis media	10.8
Menningitis	13.8
Other infections	5.3
Medications taken by child	2.4
Trauma	1.9
Other post-birth	6.0

Gallaudet Reasearch Institute (1998, November). Regional and National Summary Report of Data from the 1997–98 Annual Survey of Deaf and Hard-of-Hearing Children and Youth. Washington, D.C.: GRI. Gallaudet University.

in the brain and this process does not occur, the receptive ability is hampered, resulting in auditory agnosia. Therefore, losses of this nature are not auditorily based but of a neurological origin.

Nonorganic Hearing Loss

When individuals experience a significant amount of stress or undergo deep psychological or emotional conflicts, the ramifications of the situations may manifest themselves in the form of a hearing loss. Disorders of this nature are referred to as psychogenic dysacusis, functional deafness, or nonorganic deafness. There is no malfunction in the auditory process itself. However, individuals may experience a partial or total inability to hear; they are not just pretending to assimilate the characteristics of a hearing impaired person. This is a psychological disorder and falls within the province of the psychiatric field.

AUDIOLOGICAL EVALUATION

Hearing loss can be divided into three primary categories: a conductive loss, a sensorineural loss, or a mixed loss. Although the categories are broad and inclusive, the effects on individuals may vary considerably. Thus, it is the audiologist's job to ascertain the existence of a hearing impairment and make judgments concerning the severity and influence of the loss on the individual, the location and configuration of the lesion responsible for the pathology, and to recommend possible solutions for remediation of the problem (Katz,1985). To accomplish these tasks, an extensive battery of tests must be administered.

Due to the medical advances made in the past several years, the knowledge base surrounding hearing impairments has broadened, and techniques involving test procedures have become both more exact and complex. Audiologists no longer depend on a tuning fork or the sole results of an audiogram to make their diagnosis. Today, most clinicians feel that the minimum audiological examination must consist of pure-tone testing, both by air and bone conduction, with appropriate masking, speech reception threshold tests, and auditory discrimination tests at superthreshold levels (Katz, 1985). By administering a complete test battery, audiologists are able to obtain information that helps them identify the problem area and describe how it impacts on the individual. Once this information is obtained, they can make appropriate recommendations for remediation.

Pure-Tone Testing

Pure-tone audiometric testing provides the examiner with a broad perspective on the type and pattern of hearing loss experienced by the individual. Information can be categorized into three general bodies of knowledge. First, one can determine how well the range of frequencies is transmitted through the entire auditory system. Second, the pattern of acoustic reflex abnormalities can be determined. Third, questions pertaining to the individual's auditory status can be addressed:

Is there a hearing impairment?
How severe is the loss?
Is the loss conductive, sensorineural, or mixed?

In order to obtain this information, a pure-tone audiometer must be used. This instrument is designed to test one's hearing level at 5 decibel (dB) increments and provides both qualitative and quantitative information. The machine is calibrated whereby a zero dB hearing level is established at each frequency representing the lowest intensity at which the normal ear can detect the presence of the test tone 50 percent of the time (Newby, 1964). Therefore, an individual's hearing loss can be determined by the number of decibels in excess of this zero point that the tone must be intensified in order for a person to recognize that sounds are being transmitted. In the audiometric test situation, tones are administered through earphones for air conduction tests, and through a bone-conduction vibrator to evaluate functioning abilities of the inner ear.

When audiologists evaluate these individuals' hearing, they assess their ability to hear sounds at varying frequencies. Frequencies that comprise the test battery generally begin in the range of 250 Hz through 8,000 or 12,000 Hz. The sound-pressure level required to make a sound audible for the average normal-hearing person is referred to as "zero hearing level." Therefore, one can identify a hearing loss by the number of decibels required to make the sound audible. The hearing level required to reach that threshold is the amount of the audiometer's calibration that equates to the amount of hearing loss. The maximum hearing level in most pure-tone audiometers is 100 dB HL (hearing level).

As with any other test instrument, the audiometer is only a tool and the results will only be as accurate as the skill level of the individual conducting this evaluation. The audiogram does not present a complete picture of an individual's hearing loss, rather an estimate based on the audiologist's observation of the person's behavior throughout the test situation.

In essence, the audiogram provides information in five areas. It:

1. illustrates patterns of hearing sensitivity for tones at various frequencies;
2. provides a comparison of air and bone conduction sensitivity;
3. reflects the individual's hearing in relation to the normative standard;
4. projects interaural symmetry or asymmetry; and
5. can be used to reflect the results of other pure-tone tests (Hannley, 1986).

Pure-tone testing is administered to the better ear first, beginning with the frequency of 1,000 hertz (Hz) or cycles per second (cps). After a threshold level has been established, testing continues at even octaves above and below 1,000 cps with 12,000 cps being the highest frequency tested. When a complete measurement is obtained on the first ear, the second ear is tested. If the thresholds of the second ear differ from the first ear by 40 dB, masking should be applied to insure that hearing in one ear is not being assisted by hearing in the better ear.

Bone-Conduction Testing

When a hearing loss is indicated through air-conduction tests, it is standard procedure to administer bone-conduction tests. The purpose is to determine whether the hearing loss is caused by conductive or sensorineural factors, or a combination of the two.

For example, to determine a conductive loss, the audiologist places a small vibrator on the mastoid process of the temporal bone behind the pinna of the ear to be tested. By conducting this procedure the examiner is able to ascertain if an external or middle ear lesion exists and further determine the extent of the conductive hearing impairment. It is assumed that the threshold for bone-conducted signals is a measure of the sensorineural system. When test results indicate that sounds are heard normally through bone conduction, it is inferred that the sense organ and the auditory nerve are normal and working properly. When air-conduction thresholds are obtained, they represent the functioning level of the entire auditory system. Therefore, when a discrepancy occurs in the threshold levels between air and bone conduction (air-bone gap), it is assumed that the difficulty must lie in that part of the mechanism that is responsible for the conduction of airborne sounds. However, when there is evidence that the loss is purely conductive, the bone-conduction thresholds will be normal (Dirks, 1964).

In essence, when both types of tests are completed, it can be determined if the loss is conductive or sensorineural. However, if bone-conductive measurements reflect losses that are equal to those obtained by air-conduction testing, the loss is sensorineural. If there is some loss by bone, but not as much as by air, the loss is termed a mixed one (Newby, 1964).

Hearing test results are plotted on a graph referred to as an audiogram. The two dimensions of an audiogram are frequency and intensity. The results of each ear are plotted separately by both air and bone conduction. The symbol *O* and the color red are used to plot the threshold points for each frequency tested for the right ear. An *X* and the color blue or black are used to identify frequencies and threshold levels for the left ear. A sample audiogram form is included in Figure 2-11.

Losses reflecting conductive, sensorineural, and mixed patterns are characterized by different configurations on the audiogram. Generally, conductive losses are evidenced by fairly equal losses at all frequencies, with perhaps slightly greater losses appearing at the lower frequencies. An audiogram depicting a conductive loss is reflected in Figure 2-12.

Sensorineural impairments are characterized usually, but not always, by close to normal hearing activity at the lower frequencies with rapid decreases at the higher frequencies. Bone- and air-conduction thresholds are approximately the same. See Figure 2-13 illustrating a sensorineural loss.

Individuals exhibiting characteristics of conductive and sensorineural losses are identified as having a mixed impairment. In the event a conductive loss is present and there is some secondary nerve involvement, the audiogram may depict a loss in both the high and low frequencies.

A typical mixed impairment will produce an audiogram that shows some loss by bone conduction but a more severe loss by air conduction. However, depending on the etiology of the mixed loss, it may manifest itself by demonstrating a conductive loss in the lower frequencies and a sensorineural loss in the higher frequencies. See Figure 2-14.

Classification of Hearing Loss

The degree of hearing impairment can be grouped according to five separate classifications, ranging from mild through profound. The classification can be made on the

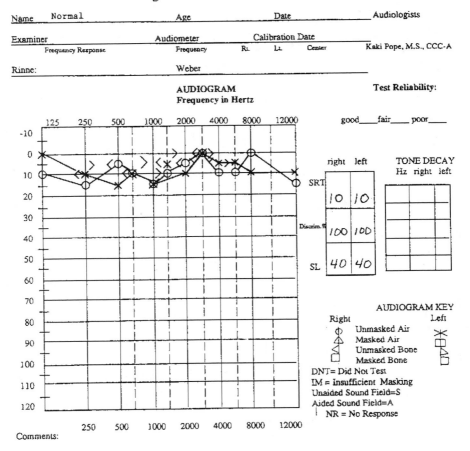

FIGURE 2-11   **Sample Audiogram Form Reflecting Hearing within Normal Range**

(Courtesy of J. Shelfer)

basis of sensitivity at a single frequency or on the basis of the average sensitivity of several frequencies—the "pure-tone average" or PTA.

Individuals experiencing mild, moderate, and moderately severe hearing losses are identified as hard-of-hearing. Through the use of amplification, auditory training, and speech and language therapy, they are able to engage in a verbal exchange of communication and receive information auditorily. The term "deaf," from an au-

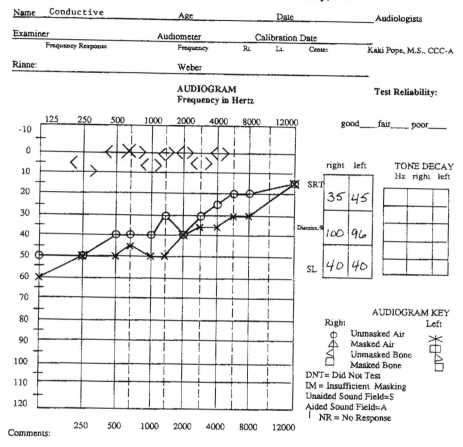

FIGURE 2-12   **Audiogram Reflecting a Conductive Loss**

(Courtesy of J. Shelfer)

diological perspective, refers to those individuals with a severe to profound hearing loss who cannot hear speech through their ears, with or without amplification. Although they may hear some loud sounds, they do not rely on their auditory mechanism as the primary channel of communication.

Table 2-3 includes the various classifications of hearing losses and the impact the loss has on the individual. Table 2-4 reflects the degree and prevalence of hearing loss found within the school-age population.

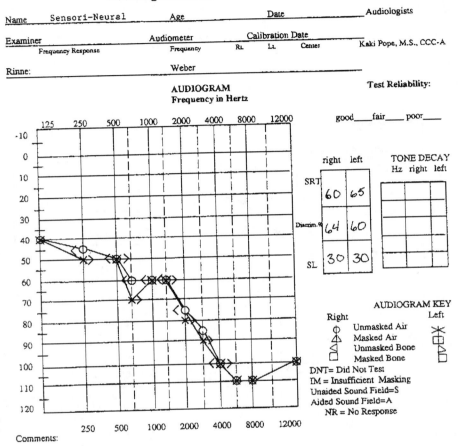

FIGURE 2-13   **Audiogram Reflecting a Sensorineural Loss**

(Courtesy of J. Shelfer)

Although these classifications have been established to aid the consumer and professional in understanding the severity of the varying degrees of loss, one must be careful not to "pigeonhole" or label someone based on this information. Labels and classification systems provide professionals with an avenue whereby they can discuss the various types of hearing losses and determine which services will contribute the greatest amount of benefit to the consumer. In this respect labels serve a very useful function. By providing professionals with terminology that can be used

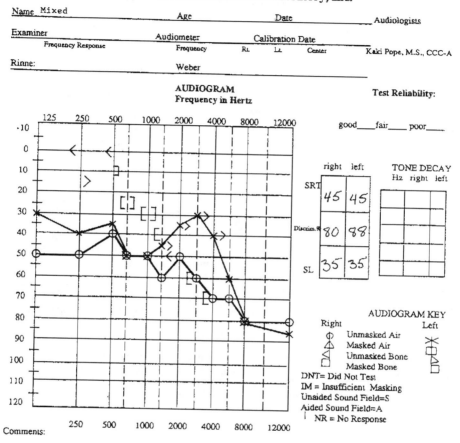

FIGURE 2-14 **Audiogram Reflecting a Mixed Loss**

(Courtesy of J. Shelfer)

for identification purposes, placements can be made and services secured. However, labeling of any group can have detrimental effects. Individuals may be misclassified, labels may be misunderstood, and stereotypes may occur. In addition, parents and consumers who are not well-versed in the vernacular of medical terminology may misconstrue what is said and misinterpret those services deemed necessary to enhance educational and personal development.

TABLE 2-3 **How Hearing Loss Impacts Spoken Communication**

Classification	Hearing threshold level*	Impact on Spoken Communication
Normal limits	−10–15	
Mild hearing loss	16–29	Experiences difficulty hearing faint sounds or speech from a distance; preferential seating is important; individual may benefit from speech reading instruction—possibility of benefiting from an aid
Moderate hearing loss	30–44	Has the ability to understand conversational speech at a distance of 3 to 5 feet. Can benefit from a hearing aid, auditory training, speech reading, and speech therapy—attention also must be given to preferential seating
Moderately severe hearing loss	45–59	Conversation will not be heard unless it is loud. Individual experiences difficulty participating in group discussions. This person will benefit from all of the above services; particular attention should be given to enhanced language instruction and possibly a class for the deaf and hard of hearing
Severe hearing loss	60–79	May identify environmental noises and loud sounds; can hear a loud voice about 1 foot from the ear; may distinguish vowels but not consonants; need the services of special education classes designed for the deaf
Profound hearing loss	80+	Does not rely on hearing for primary means of communication; may hear some loud sounds—needs the services of special education classes for the deaf

*1981 ASA reference, after Goodman, 1965. Based on charts compiled by Jack Katz, *Handbook of Clinical Audiology* (1986).

TABLE 2-4 **Degree and Prevalence of Hearing Loss within the School-Aged Population**

Mild	(from 27–40 dB, ANSI)	10.2%
Moderate	(from 41–55 dB, ANSI)	11.7%
Moderate severe	(from 56–70 dB, ANSI)	12.1%
Severe	(from 71–90 dB, ANSI)	17.0%
Profound	(from 91 dB and above, ANSI)	35.1%

Gallaudet Research Institute. (1998, November). Regional and National Summary Report of Data from the 1997–98 Annual Survey of Deaf and Hard-of-Hearing Children & Youth. Washington, DC: GRI. Gallaudet University.

In addition to the classification system, there are several other factors that determine how well individuals with any given degree of loss will function within their surroundings. The following list of factors is not exhaustive:

- the auditory environment in which listening occurs
- individuals' ability to utilize speech reading, speech, and residual hearing
- secondary handicapping conditions such as physical impairments and/or mental handicaps
- vocational occupation
- personal preference for life-style
- educational background
- etiological factors
- psychological adjustment to degree of hearing loss

Speech Reception Threshold Tests

Audiometric testing would not be complete without an assessment of the individual's ability to hear and understand speech sounds.

The focus of this testing revolves around the individuals' abilities to understand speech to the degree that they can repeat simple words or understand phrases or connected speech. Speech tests are ideally suited to provide evaluative data pertaining to central auditory disorders (those that occur in the brain or brain stem). The softest intensity level at which the individual can repeat words or understand phrases is referred to as the speech reception threshold (SRT). A common test administered to establish SRT consists of two-syllable words, which are referred to as spondees. One's SRT is defined as the hearing level at which the examinee can repeat 50 percent of the words accurately.

The ability to discriminate speech or words is also critical. Although some individuals have the ability to hear (i.e., detect) speech at increased amplitude levels, they may suffer an impairment in understanding what is heard. As similar sounds are produced, individuals may have a difficult time discriminating one sound from another and therefore cannot understand the spoken words.

To test word discrimination skills, phonetically balanced (PB) word lists are administered at least 40 dB greater than the individual's SRT. Each list contains fifty monosyllabic words, equally representing samples of speech sounds that are found in typical spoken English phrases and sentences. Scoring of this test is based on the percentage of words the individual hears correctly.

Social Adequacy Index

Speech discrimination tests provide information pertaining to the individual's ability to perceive speech sounds. However, the test scores by themselves are of minimal use to the clinician. It is essential to relate these findings to the individual's ability to function socially in everyday settings. At the present time there is no specific formula for equating speech discrimination scores with particular levels of social functioning. Rather, one must examine these scores as they relate to a multitude of variables. Those variables that have particular significance and contribute to communication performance include intelligence, motivation, experience, communication set, situational cues, expectation, redundance, and linguistic sophistication (Penrod, 1978).

Although valuable data is gained by administering speech discrimination tests, it is crucial that the findings be integrated with additional data previously obtained during the audiological test situation. It is of paramount importance that observations made by the clinician be coupled with the formal test results so that an accurate picture of the person's ability to communicate with his environment is established.

SUMMARY

The purpose of this chapter has been to acquaint the reader with how sound is transmitted, basic anatomy and physiology of the ear, causes of auditory dysfunction, types of hearing disorders, and the components of the audiological test evaluation.

Although this has been designed to provide only an overview of these topics, one can begin to see the complexities involved in the transmission of sound and one's ability to receive and perceive meaning from it.

The ear can be thought of as a "gateway" to one's environment. When the auditory system becomes impaired, the impact on the ability to relate to one's surroundings becomes greatly affected. The ear provides the communication link for us with our language and thus our culture, community, and society. Without the ear's ability to function accurately, the perception of one's surroundings is drastically altered.

▶ 3

Family Dynamics

A REFLECTION ON HAVING A DEAF SON: ONE FATHER'S PERSPECTIVE

Parents deal with the reality of deafness from the moment the diagnosis is made. They grapple with communication issues, educational choices, and what it means to have a deaf member in the family.

Below a father shares his feelings on raising his deaf son.

When our youngest son, Brian, was six months old, he contacted spinal meningitis. For some time, the doctors feared that he would not survive the illness, but he did, and over a period of several months seemed to fully recover. We had been warned that deafness, as well as other problems, could result from his illness. We were, therefore, observing Brian very carefully for any sign of a problem. Soon, my wife, Leslee, and I began to question Brian's ability to hear.

Our suspicions were strong enough that we began to take Brian to ear specialists in our home town and in the surrounding area, but none of them made a diagnosis of deafness. One doctor told us that Brian did not have a hearing loss, so he must have some other problem. Although the doctors were not diagnosing Brian's deafness, my wife Leslee was convinced that Brian could not hear and refused to give up until she knew for sure.

Several months later, on the day Jimmy Carter was elected president, Brian was diagnosed as being profoundly deaf (off the charts as the doctor put it). Our whole world turned upside down that day. It is difficult to describe the pain that Leslee and I felt when we got the news. As much as we had known the truth, we were not prepared for its reality.

Neither Leslee nor I had any knowledge of deafness and felt completely lost as to what to do for Brian. We knew that he needed to begin his education as soon as possible but we had no clue what that meant. The battle between the proponents of oral and manual communication was raging at that time, and we didn't know which way to turn. As hearing people, our inclination was to do whatever we could to help Brian become "normal," so the oral approach seemed to be the best route to follow. In addition, oralism was essentially our only option in rural south Georgia at that time.

Brian was soon enrolled in a multicounty oral program in a neighboring county. We started with high hopes that were quickly dashed as we saw no sign of Brian developing speech or acquiring language. Leslee was determined to do whatever it took to allow us to "talk" to our son. We took Brian out of the oral program and enrolled him in a special education kindergarten class. Brian received some brief sign instruction during the day, and our family went to classes at the speech and hearing center at night.

As Brian approached school age, Leslee and I knew that we faced some very difficult decisions. Little did we know just how difficult those decisions would be.

When Brian was five years old, our whole family, except our oldest son, attended a "Learning Vacation" conducted by Gallaudet University. This week long program was designed to orient families with young deaf children to the reality of deafness. We had our first opportunity to interact with deaf adults during that week and to get their perspective on life in general and deaf education in particular. At the end of the week, Leslee and I both knew that Brian needed to be in a residential school setting where he could be exposed to language on a consistent basis. We also recognized that Brian would never have the opportunity to be fully integrated into school life in Moultrie, Ga., our small home town.

We enrolled Brian in the Florida School for the Deaf (FSD) and Blind in St. Augustine, Fl., when he was six. It was without a doubt the most difficult decision we ever had to make concerning any of our children. As we watched Brian go from a frightened, homesick child to a confident, well-rounded young man, we knew that as difficult as the decision had been it was the best one for Brian.

Brian confirmed that for me one day when he was about fifteen. He was active in sports and was scheduled to travel to Ocala with the wrestling team. The day before the wrestling match, I drove the 200 miles to St. Augustine after work to spend a little extra time with Brian. I walked into his dorm room and saw him sitting on the bed hanging out and carrying on an intense conversation with several of his friends. That conversation could never have happened had he been mainstreamed because there was no deaf peer group for him in Moultrie. FSD had given him the opportunity to be involved in all aspects of student life, and he had indeed grown up to be a "normal" young man.

The stress of trying to cope with Brian's deafness as well as raise two other children put a tremendous strain on our marriage and our family. We loved him and wanted the very best for him, and deafness didn't fit that picture. Leslee and I dealt with our grief in very different ways and that created a great deal of tension and misunderstanding between us. We also got caught up in the trap of focusing entirely too much attention on Brian to the detriment of our relationship with Lara and Brad, out other two children. We seemed to have lost a sense of balance, and it took us quite some time to regain it.

As difficult as Brian's deafness has been for all of us, the positives far outweigh the negatives. For me, personally, the struggle to overcome the communication barrier forced me to be a better father to Brian than I was to Lara and Brad. In order to communicate with Brian, I had to be very intentional, something I suppose I took for granted with his sister and brother. Our individual struggle to deal with the ramifications of having a deaf son eventually caused Leslee and me to draw closer to one another and to God, to whom we finally released the struggle. Unfortunately, the marriages of many hearing parents of deaf children do not survive the tremendous stress put on the family.

For years, we made the 400-mile round trip to St. Augustine twice a weekend so that Brian could be at home with us on Friday night and Saturday. That, in itself, had a major effect on our lives for thirteen years. The hardship was made more than worthwhile when, during his valedictorial address at graduation, Brian thanked us for the sacrifice of sending him off to school.

After graduating from FSD, Brian went to Gallaudet University in Washington, DC, where he should graduate this spring. His goal is to teach and coach at a residential school for the deaf, where perhaps he can be a positive influence on the younger deaf population. He has fallen in love with a precious deaf girl, Dena, and they plan to marry soon.

Until I had a deaf child, I had absolutely no understanding of deafness or Deaf culture. I have come to love and respect the Deaf community. Their language is beautiful and intriguing, their openness and honesty is refreshingly different, and their humor is hilariously unique.

I am happy to say that I no longer see deafness as a horrible disability. Deafness is not horrible at all—it's just different.

From the onset of conception, parents are filled with wonder and anticipation of the arrival of their offspring. Through the months of waiting, their minds dwell upon images of a healthy newborn, equipped with all of the physical and mental attributes that comprise a perfectly healthy, functioning infant. Occasionally, the possibility of a child being born who is less than perfect enters the parents' minds. However, it is generally pushed aside by more pleasant thoughts surrounding the parents' image of the "ideal" child. Generally, expectant parents assume that their baby will be normal at birth.

When parents receive the diagnosis that a disability such as deafness exists, the report can be devastating, shattering their dream for a "normal" child. As they struggle with the diagnosis and attempt to comprehend what the disability entails, they may question the effect that their youngster's hearing loss will have on the parent-child relationship. These thoughts may spark memories of their own childhood and of the early gratifications they experienced within the family unit. Memories such as these, combined with the diagnosis, invoke feelings of remorse. Parental expectations about the perfect child are destroyed, and the parents begin questioning how they will relate to their infant. Furthermore, they may ultimately wonder what effect this relationship will have on their youngster's development (Martin, 1987).

The psychodynamics that ensue are critical, impacting significantly on the family unit. Numerous variables influence the parents, thus contributing to the manner in which they will respond to their child. These variables include parental personalities, the quality and stability of their marriage, their relationship with their own parents, the birth order of the deaf child, and their understanding of the disability. The interplay of these factors is critical, influencing the direction in which parents will proceed as they begin to cope with the reality of having a deaf child in the family (Mindel & Vernon, 1987).

DEALING WITH THE DIAGNOSIS OF DEAFNESS

Because of its invisible nature, deafness may go undetected for one to three years. From the physicians' standpoint, it is very difficult to clinically confirm a hearing loss in the early stages of life. Often they are reluctant to make a diagnosis or prognosis until the child is two or three years of age. The parents may initially suspect that there is something wrong with their child; but when the anticipation becomes a reality, shock and bewilderment frequently occur (Meadow, 1980). Even though the majority of parents realize that they can produce a disabled child, the possibility of it happening remains remote, and the concept of the "ideal child" remains foremost in their minds. When the suspicion becomes reality the parents may experience conflicting and irrational feelings of guilt.

Literature on the birth of disabled children, as reviewed by Ross (1964) and Wright (1960), indicates that mothers undergo various stages as they cope with the realization that their child has a disability. The stages involve feelings of grieving, denial, guilt, sorrow, anger, and, ultimately, resignation (Moses, 1985).

Grieving is an ongoing process, not an end result or a product. It continues throughout one's lifetime as a person "separates from a significant lost dream, a fantasy, or a projection into the future" (Moses, 1985, p. 87). Parents have dreams for their unborn children; when these dreams are shattered, a grief response may be triggered.

Denial can serve a constructive purpose, providing parents with some time to absorb the implications of the diagnosis. Parents may manifest signs of denial in different ways. They may initially deny the fact that a disability exists, or they may concede the disability but deny the implications of the diagnosis. Other parents may acknowledge the disability and its ramifications but deny that it has any effect on them, thereby severing themselves from their feelings.

Feelings of anger surface when parents feel they have been dealt an injustice. They may question what they have done to merit the birth of a less than perfect child. In an attempt to rationalize this consequence, they may examine their lives, feeling guilty about what they have done or failed to do while expecting their child.

Circumstances that surround the birth of a deaf child can differ significantly. Unlike those occasions when a child is born with an obvious physical handicap, deafness can remain hidden for extended periods (Rodda & Grove, 1987). Therefore, the parents assume that their child is "normal." When the diagnosis is finally confirmed, these parents also experience a broad range of emotions. The sentiments they share correspond to those experienced by others upon discovering that their child has a physical or a mental handicap.

As the parents, particularly the mother, struggle with their own feelings, they may fail to relate to the youngster, imbuing the child with feelings of uncertainty and isolation. According to Levine, "the waves of disturbance experienced by many hearing parents of a first deaf child commonly find release in various types of psychological defenses: overprotection, denial, rejection in different guises, open rejection, cure-seeking, doctor shopping and outright consternation" (Levine, 1981, p. 59). The parents' behavior may fluctuate daily as their moods change from denial to concern and from concern to anger. These fluctuations create stress within the family unit and may bewilder the child.

Often upon receiving the diagnosis, parents find themselves blaming each other or themselves for the child's deafness. Accusations may be converted into multidimensional feelings. These feelings are then expressed in the form of anger, guilt, or hurt feelings. Although the parents attempt to conceal them, they surface from time to time and explode into unfounded accusations. Parents respond to their emotions in several ways: They find themselves questioning why they are being punished by being given a handicapped child; they vacillate between overprotection and rejection of the child; and they may respond with a life-style reflective of self-sacrifice and martyrdom, all for the sake of the child (Schlesinger, 1971). Parental feelings concomitant with their perceptions of deafness will influence how they will respond to the child. Hearing parents who are faced with the uncertainties of raising a deaf child may initially set unrealistic goals, discovering later that they must modify their expectations (Quigley & Kretschmer, 1982).

Dealing with negative feelings and the child's disability tend to strain marital relationships. Not only the deaf child suffers, but parents and siblings suffer also (Moses, 1985, p. 94). When raising and nurturing a child, the parents or primary caretakers anticipate that they will be confronted with a series of challenges. However, when the family unit enters into this same process with a disabled child, these typical experiences become intensified. Parents must resolve their feelings about the handicap and devise techniques that will enhance communication. When this occurs, familial stress is reduced and the deaf child is woven into the fabric of the family unit. In the event these issues are not resolved, the stability of the family unit can be threatened.

Once the diagnosis is confirmed and the needs of the deaf child are identified, the parents may begin to inadvertently focus their attention exclusively on this individual. Other family members may feel their needs are being overlooked or that their concerns have become secondary to those of the deaf child. As they feel their placement in the family is threatened, they may begin competing for attention. This provokes a series of crises that occur within the family setting. The family dynamics that follow may create a strain on the marriage, producing periods of stress or contributing to its dissolution. Other potential threats include the inability or refusal to accept

the deaf child into the family, parental disagreements regarding disciplinary procedures and techniques, pressures from the extended family, and barriers to routine verbal exchanges resulting in breakdowns in communication (Bowe, 1973).

During this period when the establishment of a healthy maternal relationship is
critical, the bond between the mother and the deaf child may be strained. This, in turn,
may cause the family unit to be thrown into a stressful situation. The child may be
sensitive to the tension and quick to pick up on the unsettled climate. In lieu of a
warm, nurturing environment, the child may be cared for in a mechanical fashion.
The mother's childhood experiences, her parents' attitudes toward disabled individuals, and her close friends will all influence the way in which she copes with the reality
of the disability. If the mother's close friends and family members are accepting, the
outside influence on her will be positive. Their support and encouragement provide
her with an avenue whereby she can vent and explore her feelings. This frequently
eases the stress that occurs throughout this transition period. If, however, the mother's
close associates express an unfavorable attitude, it may have a negative influence on
her and the family, thus creating a more stressful situation for both parents.

The Early Years: Recognizing the Disability

Parents frequently suspect something is wrong with their child long before a professional diagnosis is made. Often their suspicions are not confirmed until the infant is
three years of age. Haas and Crowley conducted a survey in 1982 that indicated that
in 80 percent of the cases, deafness was first suspected by parents, relatives, and
friends; in only 7 percent of the cases was a doctor the first to detect the disability
(Haas & Crowley, 1982).

Although parents may suspect something is wrong, they may avoid admitting it
to themselves or to others. Later, when the diagnosis is confirmed, they may experience several emotions. Initially, they may feel terror, helplessness, guilt, severe loss,
and depression. Because these are often such intense feelings, parents may adopt a
form of denial and use it as a coping mechanism. Through the process of denial they
are able to continue with their daily routines, while temporarily obscuring those
acute feelings induced by the diagnosis (Martin, 1987, p. 92). Eventually, some are
able to confront their suspicions and admit that their child is deaf. When this occurs
and the parents' initial emotions are allowed to emerge, they may be able to begin
resolving their feelings.

Although hearing parents may find this diagnosis to be overwhelming, deaf parents generally respond in a more accepting manner. This can be attributed to their
ability to cope with their own disability and their ability to comprehend the implications of deafness. Deaf parents are frequently familiar with and choose to be part of
the Deaf subculture. They prefer communicating through a form of manual communication and have experienced society's reaction to their deafness (Sisco & Anderson, 1980).

In most cases, by the age of three, the final diagnosis has been made; the parents
are confronted with the ramifications of deafness. Frequently, the professional who

makes the determining diagnosis tends to mislead the parents in an attempt to "soften the blow." This in itself can create additional heartache for the parents in the months and years to come. The parents may be informed by the professional, whether it be a doctor, audiologist, or teacher, that the child is unable to hear, but no explanation is provided regarding the effect this will have on the child's speech, English language development, reading ability, or socialization skills. Often the parents are led to believe that the child will eventually be okay or that he will grow out of his deafness (Mindel & Vernon, 1987).

Parents are also led to believe that with the assistance of a hearing aid and speech therapy, their child will develop a command of the English language that will enable him or her to communicate clearly and fluently. When the child falls short of these expectations, parents may become discouraged and return to the professional for advice. When faced with the parents' concerns, the professionals may respond in a negative manner. Frustrated by their inability to "fix the child," they may become insensitive to the parents' needs. Instead of providing them with encouragement and reassurance, they may tell the parents that they are not doing their job and that they are not working correctly with their child. This increases the parents' feelings of trepidation and frustration (Gallagher et al., 1983). As they continue to struggle with these feelings, they are faced with the realization that their child will never be "normal," that is, able to function as a hearing individual.

As parents become cognizant of the fact that their child has a disability, they begin to recognize some of the differences between their child and those who can hear. Their attitudes pertaining to deafness begin to crystallize and are later projected through interactions with their child. According to Myklebust there are four general ways parents express their attitudes to and about the child: 1) wholesome acceptance, 2) overprotection, 3) the wishful attitude, and 4) the attitude of indifference.

Wholesome Acceptance

Parents who embody an attitude of wholesome acceptance accept their children and are realistic about their handicapping conditions. They are aware of what the disability entails and realize that they can cope with problems that may develop. This is the ultimate goal all parents strive to obtain.

These parents develop successful strategies for communication. They include their children in the daily routines and solicit their input when planning meals, activities, and family vacations. They expect them to be active participants in the family unit, while remaining cognizant of their unique differences.

Many of these parents seek out Deaf culture activities for themselves and their children. They recognize the value of the Deaf community and look to members for support and for role models for their children.

Overprotection

When parents have a propensity toward overprotection, they are inclined to shield their child from those everyday situations and experiences deemed crucial to the developmental process. Without these experiences, their child is not afforded the opportunity to mature or become self-sufficient. Parents may unwittingly incorporate an attitude of overprotection. It may occur as they attempt to disguise their own feelings of shame, embarrassment, and/or resentment.

Other parents are afraid to "let go." They may become overly anxious that their child will get hurt or suffer some form of injury if allowed the option of exploring the surroundings. These overpowering feelings of concern are frequently transferred into expressions of overprotection. As this occurs, parents become reluctant to allow their child to participate in the usual variety of early childhood activities. These feelings, compounded with those of guilt, set the stage for a parent/child relationship in which the parents are engaged in an internal struggle. When this occurs, they discover that it is very difficult for them to relate effectively to their youngster.

When children are subjected to parental overprotection and are not allowed to do things for themselves, they gradually learn to expect people to wait on them. This can develop into a pattern that can last throughout their lifetime.

The Wishful Attitude

Parents exhibiting this attitude refuse to admit that their children are deaf and act as if deafness is not a handicap. In this instance, no allowances are made for their children's handicap and they are expected to act as if they were normal.

When parents reflect the "wishful attitude," children begin to feel insecure and unhappy because they cannot live up to parental expectations. There is keen evidence of this within the area of spoken communication. Parents of deaf children are not afforded the luxury of communicating through the verbal channel. Therefore, spoken messages may become misconstrued and cannot be easily clarified for the deaf youngster (Stokoe & Battison, 1981). Effective verbal communication requires that either of two events must transpire. The participants must hear and understand the words being spoken or they must be able to speech read the message being delivered. Both conditions have inherent problems. Within the English language, between 40 and 50 percent of the speech sounds are not visible on the lips. Some of the sounds are homophonous (sounds that appear similar on the lips). Also, one must have a fairly extensive English language vocabulary to engage in effective communication (Bevan, 1988). All of these factors determine how well children will understand the message. If they cannot see the words, the words look alike; if they do not have a meaning to attach to the words they see, misunderstandings will occur.

When parents relate to their children under the pretense that they can hear, those parents are operating under artificial conditions. The special needs of their children are ignored, and the expectations placed on them are unrealistic. This produces disillusionment in the parents and creates a stressful situation for the child.

The Attitude of Indifference

This attitude is especially damaging to the child. Indifference implies that the parents are unable to show the child real affection. The parents are lacking in sympathy and genuine understanding. Children raised in this type of family setting often experience feelings of isolation and despair (Myklebust, 1960).

Developing a Sense of Independence

Throughout the early years parents are faced with the trauma and the realities of dealing with a disabled child. While they sort through their feelings, their children progress through their own developmental tasks. They begin to develop self-care skills and become adept at dressing and feeding themselves. In addition, they begin to develop their own identities and see themselves as separate from their mothers.

Hearing children begin to make strides in toilet training, feeding, dressing themselves, and responding to demands of a verbal disciplinary nature. Speech and language are developing rapidly with an increase in intercommunication between the child and adult. The hearing child is beginning to establish a true sense of "individuality."

In contrast, deaf youngsters may be delayed in developing their sense of autonomy. This is evidenced within the speech and language area and in those areas pertaining to self-help skills, such as toilet training, feeding, and exploration of the environment.

Two or two-and-a-half year olds are often encouraged to cooperate with toilet-training routines when they know a reward is forthcoming. This provides them with a stimulus to accomplish the task. The responsibility of communicating the relationship between expectations and rewards may be an arduous task. It can become even more difficult for parents who are trying to convey this message when the auditory channel is dysfunctional. Although deaf children have the ability to comprehend the request, the manner in which it is presented may cause confusion and thus create delays in the child accomplishing the task. These delays may become apparent in developing skills, such as toilet training and dressing, and may overflow into the area of socialization as well.

Hearing parents may encounter difficulties clearly explaining safety concerns and rules to their deaf child. Consequently, they may sense a need to impose stringent protective measures. The child may be denied various activities, and those that involve roughhousing may be prohibited. As the children mature, their parents may refuse to let them play with neighborhood friends, ride bicycles, or engage in street play (Levine, 1981, p. 62). Due to the degree of parental overprotectiveness, it may become difficult at times to determine the child's true capabilities.

There are several factors that impact on deaf children as they strive to become independent. These include parental attitudes, familial relationships, and environmental influences. These factors are interdependent and are all intertwined with communication.

During the first few years of life, the child's primary source of communication emanates from the parents. They become their children's first teachers, providing them with a wealth of information, thus enabling them to expand their horizons.

Communication Between Hearing Parents and Their Deaf Children

Parents occasionally feel that because their child has a disability, he should not be expected to attend to his needs. At other times parents base their perception of their child on the premise that because they cannot hear they cannot understand.

They may equate the quality of their child's speech with his ability to comprehend, thus failing to realize that speech and language are two separate functions. Some assume that if their child is inept at speechreading and cannot produce sounds accurately, he will be incapable of benefiting from the spoken communication process. To compensate for this, parents may initially rely on gestures and structured phrases when addressing their child. Later, however, as the scope of their messages becomes more complex, parents may become frustrated. They realize that the concepts they are trying to convey mandate that a more elaborate form of communication be incorporated.

From the onset, hearing babies receive a stream of spoken language, and the verbal sounds begin to be associated with their conceptual equivalents. As they develop, the sounds they hear become recognized as words. Babies begin to attach meaning to these sounds as they relate them to familiar concepts or experiences. As Levine so eloquently states it, "eventually language and concept fuse, and the child is well on his way to the developmental benefits bestowed by hearing" (Levine, 1981, p. 55).

Unlike hearing babies, deaf infants rely on their visual channel to grasp information that surrounds them. They try to extract meaning from facial expressions, verbal clues, gestures, and those activities that occur within their environment. Initially, they may transmit their messages through pantomime and gesture. However, as they progress through early childhood they discover that this form of communication is not adequate.

Parents who elect to communicate with their deaf children through an oral mode focus their energies on speaking clearly and selecting appropriate word/sentence construction choices. Likewise, they encourage their children to respond to them in a similar manner.

The Effect of Oral Communication

Eye contact is imperative when conversing with deaf children. In an attempt to convey information, parents may become oblivious to their child's activity, seize them and proceed to communicate. Unfortunately, if these interruptions occur repeatedly, they may interfere with those activities that are designed to augment a sense of independence. That space, that is so critical for developing a feeling of separateness, may be lost in the quest to establish communication.

While most hearing children experience the freedom of physical movement under the direction of verbal instruction, when engaging in dialogues deaf children are faced with physical restrictions. Physical handling may be substituted for verbal instruction, and they are confined to the boundaries of their visual field. Directives and discipline that take the form of "verbal handling" provide children with the impetus to seek initial emancipation from their mothers.

Because of the difficulties imposed by the communication barrier, deaf children are periodically "trained" rather than educated by their families. They may continue to receive their instruction in the form of physical directives. Oftentimes these directives replace spoken exchanges, subjecting them to excessive amounts of autocratic control. This form of control can have a negative impact on them, thus thwarting their attempts at developing feelings of self-esteem.

The deaf child does not receive verbal warnings to stop actions that are unacceptable. Therefore, when physical punishment is administered, it may appear to be unwarranted. When this occurs, children sense they have done something wrong but may be oblivious to the nature of their mistakes. This situation may be compounded when there are hearing siblings in the family. Limited to their visual channel, deaf children may observe comparative differences in discipline and freedom. Unable to hear what is said, they may misinterpret the form of discipline that is administered between them and their hearing siblings. Discipline is only one area in which effective communication is critical; building one's self-esteem is another. In the event children do not make the association that rewards are given for a task well done, their motivation may be stifled. They lose their desire to cooperate and see no need to become independent.

Conveying messages of rewards and punishments of a concrete nature is difficult at best; but when one is confronted with the challenge of expressing feelings of love and affection either verbally or nonverbally, the task becomes more difficult if not altogether impossible. The mother's ability to impart emotions to her child is integral to the bonding process. Hearing provides a primary channel through which expressions of love, closeness, and individualization are transmitted. Communication becomes the vehicle for socialization and training. It plays a critical role in the process of separation/individualization that occurs between parents and their child (Altshuler, 1974). It is crucial that children feel they are loved and accepted by their parents. They need to sense parental love and affection, thereby establishing their own sense of independence and autonomy. Children must be permitted a certain degree of physical freedom affording them the opportunity to explore and define their boundaries. If parents retain too rigid a control, their children will remain dependent, unable to develop feelings of self-worth.

Communication lies at the crux of this problem: Speech and language become its integral parts. Without some form of language, communication becomes impossible; in one's effort to understand and be understood, frustration and anger may emerge. Speech and language are very important to hearing parents, and when there is a deficiency in this area the results can be devastating. Parents become annoyed when their child doesn't understand what they are saying, even with the realization that it is not the child's fault. The stress incurred leaves the parents with feelings of anger, which in turn can permeate the entire family structure.

The parents want their wishes to be comprehended, and at the same time they want to understand their child. Speech becomes of paramount importance and the parents may spend considerable time trying help their child to develop clear and precise speech. "It may be that many children perceive such insistence as punitive and react by rebellious muteness" (Schlesinger & Meadow, 1972, p. 15). These children may fail to recognize the importance of the emphasis on speech training. At this age they have their own agenda to follow, complete with activities and exploration. They may be baffled by the hours devoted to a skill perceived by them as meaningless. Commonly at this stage of attempting to establish a separate identity, they may wage a battle over communication. This battle can create a delay in communication as well as interfere with emotional development.

The Use of Simultaneous Communication

Spoken exchanges are only one way in which hearing parents communicate with their deaf children. Some elect to incorporate additional methods of expressing themselves and select a form of manual communication. Subsequently, parents discover that there are a variety of sign systems. They are designed to be implemented while one is speaking, hence providing the listener with a form of simultaneous communication.

The concept of using simultaneous communication with young deaf children became popular during the 1970s and continues to be used widely today (Jordan, Gustason, & Rosen, 1979). Simultaneous communication is embedded in the philosophy that messages can be delivered and understood more clearly when a bimodal form of communication is utilized. Professionals encouraging this form of communication have theorized that simultaneous communication strengthens parent-child relationships, thus providing an avenue for more elaborate conversational exchanges. In the past decade, the topic of sign language has received considerable attention. However, only a limited amount of research has been conducted pertaining to the use of simultaneous communication with deaf preschoolers. The most notable research in this area has been conducted by Greenberg (1980) and Meadow, Greenberg, Erting, and Carmichael (1981).

Greenberg's study examined the attitudes and stress encountered by hearing families who have a profoundly deaf preschool child. He compared the differences between two kinds of dyads: mothers who used an oral approach with their deaf children and mothers who conversed through simultaneous communication. Results from his study indicated that 1) there were no significant differences between simultaneous and oral mothers regarding attitudes of parental acceptance, 2) there were no significant differences between communication methods in regard to profound communicative and interactional problems, 3) mothers who signed engaged in extended and more complex interactions with their children than their oral counterparts, and 4) they were more responsive to their children's behavior. In addition, mothers in the oral group indicated that they felt somewhat more stress and felt that they had less control over their child's behavior than those mothers in the simultaneous group (Greenberg, 1980).

An additional study conducted by Meadow et al. (1981) produced similar results. In this study a comparison was made of four groups: 1) deaf children of deaf parents, 2) hearing children of hearing parents, 3) oral deaf children of hearing parents, and 4) signing deaf children of signing hearing parents. Videotaped interactions between the mother-child dyads were investigated to determine which groups had the most frequent and functional interactions when communicating.

The results indicated that deaf children and hearing mothers relying on an oral only form of communication spent significantly less time engaged in interactions than did mothers in the other three groups. Furthermore, these interactions produced the least amount of child-initiated conversations and the highest proportion of nonelaborated conversations. This study further illustrated that deaf mothers and deaf children engaged in similar interactions as those dyads consisting of hearing mothers and their hearing children. Those dyads involving hearing mothers utilizing simultaneous communication participated in more spontaneous forms of interactions than did mothers who utilized an oral only approach. However, those interactions utilizing simultaneous communication were not viewed as complex or as extended as those that occurred between the deaf children and their deaf mothers (Meadow et al., 1981). In order for children to grow and develop emotionally, they must have a communication bond with those around them. Hearing parents rely primarily on spoken communication, with its systematic means of expressing ideas and feelings, to convey this bond. When speech and hearing are affected, the process is altered. Subsequently, this may affect children in their endeavors to identify their feelings and develop a sense of closeness with their parents. During this time children are struggling with forming their own identity. If they do not perceive a warm and caring attitude and are not permitted the latitude to explore who they are, they may begin to personify those traits characteristic of unreasoning, rebellion, or blind obedience.

It is critical that parents transmit attitudes of warmth and caring when they interact with their child. When children perceive a caring attitude, they become eager to please and are motivated to cooperate. This results in a reduction of parent-child confrontations. If this caring relationship is absent, the development of conscience and self-control may be hampered, and the child will not emerge with feelings of self-worth or self-esteem.

Throughout this time the child enters into several arenas where power struggles occur. However, because of the additional restrictions parents place on them, many deaf children go through this period with feelings of intense negativism that may interfere with the normal maturation process. Both the child and parent find themselves struggling for what each feels is best. The child is simultaneously "holding on" and "letting go" while trying to establish a feeling of "I" and "me." The parent is coping with his own feelings of guilt and frustration while at the same time acknowledging the ramifications of deafness.

The Use of American Sign Language

While some parents adhere to a strict oral philosophy, others seek out, or by chance, discover the language that is embraced by the Deaf community. These parents, through classes in ASL and frequent visits to Deaf community events, become exposed to

American Sign Language. Although some develop only a rudimentary understanding of the language, others become proficient in it and can engage in extended conversations with their children.

The Formative Years: Coping with a Difference in the Family

As children continue to grow and develop, they begin to explore their environment with a thirst for understanding and knowledge. Their homes become an arena for instruction, and communication provides the tool for gathering insights. The roles of the parents become one of permitting their children the freedom to pursue locomotor and manipulative intentions while providing answers to their endless questions.

The element of communication cannot be overemphasized. Through this channel knowledge is transmitted, and the beginnings of socialization take place. When there is a barrier in the communication channel, the system itself is blocked and weakened (Rodda & Grove, 1987, p. 315). On those occasions when the parents cannot understand their children and their children cannot make their wishes known, the result is frustration coupled with feelings of inadequacy and disappointment.

When examining the socialization process, it is critical to consider the needs of the parents. Parents produce children for a variety of reasons and have several preconceived ideas of the experiences and rewards parenthood will bring. They may feel that they are not receiving the type of gratification they thought would be forthcoming. They may discover that their child does not comprehend what they say and are therefore reluctant to engage in verbal exchanges. They may sense that their attempts at communicating are misunderstood and therefore refrain from expressing themselves orally. As these misunderstandings continue to occur, parents and children alike may find that their attempts to communicate with each other are stymied. As a result deaf children may avoid asking questions, not realizing that important information is not being transmitted to them.

When faced with the communication dilemma, parents may become so frustrated that they either withdraw or resort to other methods when attempting to convey their message. In a survey conducted with parents, 63 percent of the mothers of deaf children indicated that they encountered some degree of frustration that could be specifically related to their child's deafness. Over half of those polled commented that the difficulties they faced could be attributed to the complexities of the communication process (Schlesinger & Meadow, 1972). The dilemma this process imposes takes its toll in influencing mothers as they interact with their children.

Unlike mothers of hearing children who can engage freely in verbal interactions with their children, mothers of deaf children may become more controlling and less flexible (Cheskin, 1982). The children's freedom for adventure may be restricted, and their curiosity about their environment may be dampened. When this occurs, deaf children may view their mothers differently than do their hearing siblings. They may interpret her lack of flexibility as a sign of parental nonacceptance and thus falsely perceive her as being extremely didactic, inflexible, and controlling.

Parents who have hearing children can communicate effortlessly with them. However, because deafness hampers verbal communication, those children who cannot hear may find they become tense while struggling to converse with other family members. Through interactions such as these, the mother, in particular, may appear to be less compliant and creative. The children may feel they are either being constantly told or shown what to do and are not provided with the opportunity to have any input. Deaf youngsters may feel restricted as they attempt to initiate actions and assume responsibility. Furthermore, they may find that they are not afforded the opportunity to express their opinions or contribute to the decision-making process. Later, when they are faced with the dilemma of viewing themselves as separate individuals, they may feel perplexed. As they become older it is important to focus on the attitudes they develop. The manner in which family, society, and school react to deafness, and therefore respond to them as individuals, will contribute significantly to the way in which they will view themselves. During this time they begin to realize that their hearing loss distinguishes them from hearing children, and they may begin to question their deafness. This realization typically occurs around the age of eight. At this time deaf children begin to indicate that they realize they are "different" from their family and friends. Deaf youngsters are faced with a paucity of deaf adult role models. As a result, they may experience difficulties as they try to identify with who they are and imagine what they might become in the future. During the school years they continue to search for their identity and seek out future role models.

Many parents report that during this period they are again confronted with those feelings they experienced when the initial diagnosis was made. As their children continue to sculpt their identities, the parents may again attempt to resolve those feelings that they have harbored inside. The feeling of "differentness" affects the child as well as the parents. The relationships that children establish with their family, friends, and environment will determine how they will view this concept of "differentness." Those who have not found acceptance and do not feel part of the family unit may view the difference as very negative. This may instill in them feelings of inferiority. The parents, while sensing this difference, may in their own way withdraw from their child. This withdrawal may be inadvertently displayed in many and varied situations. Deaf children may feel left out of conversations at mealtimes and not included in the planning of family activities. Their overall development may be hampered because of their lack of social involvement; thus, they may feel deficient as they try to interact with others.

Due to the ramifications of deafness, children, while attempting to speak, may not articulate clearly, thus making spoken communication extremely difficult. In an attempt to clarify their requests, they may behave in a manner deemed unacceptable by society. When this occurs, especially in public settings, hearing family members may become uncomfortable or embarrassed. Parents may become so overwhelmed by this that they either withdraw from their child or fail to explain to them what they are doing wrong. This leaves their children feeling even more isolated and confused. They begin to experience a form of environmental deprivation as they struggle to become involved in meaningful familial relationships—the very relationships that are so critical to the development of one's primary self-concept.

At this time children must experience a sense of accomplishment. In order for them to feel that what they have done is good, they must receive positive feedback from those around them. If parents are alienated by the child's poor speech and vocalizations, they will usually respond to the child in a negative manner. When this happens, children will realize that their accomplishments fall short of their parents' expectations. They may feel inferior and begin to develop a poor self-concept.

Social Interactions and Family Dynamics

One must be mindful that speech is only one area in which the child may sense a feeling of inferiority. The fact that many deaf children perceive that they are isolated from family activities can singularly precipitate feelings of loneliness and inferiority. Shanny Mow, a deaf man, expresses the feelings he experienced with his family when he was a young child.

> *You never forget that frightening experience when you were Brian's age. You were left out of dinner table conversation. It is called mental isolation. While everyone is talking or laughing, you are as far away as a lone Arab on a desert that stretches along every horizon. Everyone and everything is a mirage; you see them but you cannot touch or become a part of them. You suffocate inside, but you cannot tell anyone of this horrible feeling. You do not know how to. You get the impression nobody understands or cares. You have no one to share your childish enthusiasm and curiosity, no sympathetic listener who can give meaning to your world and the desert around you. (Mow, 1973, p. 24)*

Instead of being provided with the opportunity to develop through family interactions, they may remain confused and lonely in their "own little world." It is not at all uncommon to ask deaf children what goes on at home and hear them respond "nothing important," as that is the explanation they have been given to their numerous questions.

The family unit provides an avenue for children to express what they have done during the day and receive either praise or criticism for their actions. Through this exchange their insight into what they can accomplish is strengthened. If children are not included in the barrage of words and the exchange is blocked, their development will also be delayed.

How the family relates to the child at the dinner table is as important as the social situations to which the child is exposed. It is not enough for any child to visually assimilate a situation. They must become an active part of it in order to grow and mature. The extent to which deaf children are accepted and allowed to participate in social situations will have a direct bearing on their abilities to develop positive self-images. Frequently, they are not encouraged to participate in social activities with their peers and remain on the outside, observing daily activities. Oftentimes, they are provided with little, if any, explanation of the situation and are left to provide their own interpretation of the events that have transpired (Rodda & Grove, 1987, p. 325).

Due to their experiential deprivation, their assessment of the situation may be inadequate or inappropriate. In order for them to develop a positive self-concept of themselves as they relate to the family and other social situations, they must have repeated successful experiences. However, this does not occur if they remain on the sidelines. In order for deaf individuals to feel that they can succeed, they must be given the freedom, direction, and encouragement to try. If they are not given the opportunity to accomplish tasks at which they initially expect to succeed, they will feel not only frustrated but also inferior. When the avenue to success is blocked, children begin to develop the "I can't syndrome" as opposed to the "I can" attitude, and the feeling of accomplishment so critical to this age is replaced by feelings of inferiority.

The way in which the parents and other family members view the child's deafness will determine how the child will view himself. This parental view will also play a major role in influencing the parents' selection of the school they feel is best for their child. The parents must make a choice as to whether their child will attend a day or residential school and whether he will be permitted to use Total Communication (using speech and signing simultaneously) or be restricted to oral communication. The choice parents make, in addition to the parental attitude toward the child, continues to impact heavily on the deaf individual. These two influences remain extremely important throughout the school years.

It becomes quite apparent at an early age that parents and educators play a vital role in the development of young deaf children. If the parents can resolve their own feelings and respond to their children in a loving and nurturing manner, deaf children will be able to emerge from their silent world as psychologically healthy youth. However, if parental feelings are not resolved and parents remain hostile, overprotective, domineering, or rejecting, the results can be devastating. The child, upon being subjected to these attitudes, will internalize them and project them outward in the form of emotional immaturity, learned dependency, passive indifference, hostile attitudes toward hearing individuals, and environmental ignorance. The parents' ability to resolve their inner conflicts and respond to their deaf child will determine how adept their child is at accepting and coping with the disability.

Based on the premise that the psychological development of deaf individuals is commensurate with that experienced by all individuals, it becomes apparent that environmental influences, rather than the condition of deafness itself, will determine how well individuals are able to develop healthy personalities (Levine, 1981, p. 52). The influence parents and family members have on their child cannot be overemphasized. However, at this stage children's hours in school begin to increase, and not only their teachers but their peers have an important effect on them.

Adolescence can be a restive time for any parent-child relationship, and the exacerbation of deafness can make this an even stormier period. Teenagers experience varying degrees of stress while trying to formulate an identity, and their uncertainties are projected to their parents.

The teenage years are considered the hallmark of the third time in which we might expect to find the deaf child confronted with an identity crisis. During adolescence children may undergo a great deal of stress as they attempt to discover their own identities (Cohen, 1978). As previously described, parents are primarily affected during the first two periods of crises. However, this period of reflection and interaction becomes extremely difficult for them as well. Teenagers struggle to establish their identity, and parents attempt to mold the adolescent into what they feel is an "ideal" young adult. The "ideal youth" visualized by the parents will be determined by their hearing status. Whether the parents are hearing or deaf will determine what expectations they have for their child. This factor will also influence the type of experiences to which they subject their children.

Deaf Adolescents of Hearing Parents
During the adolescent period, one of the most significant problems confronting deaf individuals is that their hearing parents are afraid or ashamed to admit to the consequences of their deafness. Even as their child enters adolescence, the parents may continue to deny their child's disability, creating an atmosphere of nonacceptance in the home. At this time parental influence becomes less direct, but the importance of a loving and trusting relationship remains intact. The parents, who in the past have found communication difficult, will sense an increasing amount of frustration when dealing with the issues, trials, and tribulations of this age. As the parents become increasingly frustrated with the situation, they may avoid communicating with their child, leaving the teenager with feelings of anger, resentment, and isolation.

> *Perhaps it would shock you to realize that many deaf children have never had a satisfactory, truly meaningful relationship with a hearing adult. . . . Far too many parents of deaf children seem pathetically unable to deal constructively with their children's behavior, and far too many deaf children harbor a feeling of burning resentment toward the family that has unwittingly, perhaps, but blatantly shut them out. Deaf children are tired of being non-participating, non-voting members of the family. Deaf teenagers are tired of being handed a five dollar bill and the car keys by parents who do not even know the manual alphabet. (Denton, 1971)*

One of the main components of development during this stage is providing adolescents with the opportunity to make choices and decisions regarding their lives. By engaging in the decision-making process, they continue to explore and establish the boundaries of their own identity. Frequently, parents refuse adolescents this freedom.

This may occur for two reasons: First, parents may feel that because of the disability the teenager is unable to make contributions or decisions regarding family activities; second, because deaf adolescents are unable to express themselves in the form of precise verbalizations, parents may feel that engaging in conversation with them is too difficult, if not a total impossibility.

The teenager may continue to experience feelings of resentment toward the family and with this growing resentment to develop a further sense of estrangement within the home. Through this estrangement the teenager may become more isolated while the parents may continue to live in a "storybook world," seeking the "ideal" nonhandicapped child.

Many parents continue to cling to the "hearing ideals," hoping that their child will one day appear "normal," will speak using grammatically correct English instead of manual communication, will perform academically on a par with his hearing counterparts, and will marry a hearing spouse. Parents, by continuing to believe that there is nothing wrong with their children, will have unrealistic expectations for them. This can place additional stress on teenagers as they struggle with their own concept of what they are expected to do and how they are expected to act. If parents continue to struggle with their own fears and nonacceptance, they will be unable to help their deaf teenagers through their own crises. These teenagers may again find themselves confused about their identity and the role they are expected to play within the family structure.

One of the widely accepted components of this stage is that teenagers become increasingly aware of how other people perceive them. They are generally in tune to parental expectations and may feel that they are letting parents down when they fail to meet those standards. This feeling of inadequacy compounds the stress previously experienced by teenagers as they attempt to establish their identities. As they continue to deal with their perceptions, the parents reexamine their expectations. In doing so, they respond to their child in a variety of ways.

Sometimes the parents will try to bind the adolescent more closely to the family, although generally this is a futile effort. Other responses include clinging to hopes that their child will "catch up" and be able to function like a hearing child. An additional and even more detrimental response includes projections of rejection as the parents wrestle with the reality that their child will never be able to live up to their expectations.

If teenagers perceive that they are not meeting the expectations of their parents and if they are not included in family activities, they may have a difficult time integrating the various roles they are required to play. Thus, role confusion may occur. In this type of family situation it is possible that the teenager continues through these adolescent years with unaccepting parents and a minimal level of communication, resulting in reduced family involvement. As a result, individuals may emerge from this situation with an ambiguous picture of their identity and a delay in their ability to engage in decision-making skills.

Deaf Adolescents of Deaf Parents

The deaf individual whose parents are deaf has progressed through the various stages of development in a manner similar to that of the deaf child whose parents are hearing. However, because of the parents' deafness, two major factors are altered. First of all, deaf parents are generally accepting of their child's disability, and that child is able to establish a place within the family structure. Second, there is a common channel of communication used so that both parties can converse. Teenagers with deaf parents have a definite advantage, as they can communicate their concerns and anxieties with individuals who can comprehend. This understanding and acceptance is an important asset for the teenager who is attempting to establish a solid foundation for adulthood (Benderly, 1980).

However, the Deaf family structure can have negative implications. Because of the overwhelming contacts with other deaf individuals, the adolescent's perspective on the hearing world may be distorted. They may react with a sense of shock when they realize that the majority of the people in their surroundings are hearing and that the educational and occupational world is dominated by those who can hear. If deaf adolescents have grown up in residential schools and return home to deaf parents who maintain a social environment dominated by deaf individuals, adolescents may grow up thinking that most, if not all, people are deaf. This, in turn, may produce an element of uncertainty as they encounter the reality of the hearing world, and they begin questioning their identity.

Another drawback deaf adolescents of deaf parents may encounter is their parents' limited awareness of resources available to them. They may not be familiar with those agencies and benefits that are designed to assist them and their children growing into adulthood (Benderly, 1980, p. 87). One such disadvantage may occur in the field of employment possibilities. Due to their handicap, the attitude of employers, and their skills and previous training, the parents' vocational choices may be limited. Once employed they may find they remain in entry-level positions and do not accelerate up the career ladder. This, in turn, influences both their economic situation and their social contacts (Welsh & Walter, 1989).

By comparing deaf and hearing parents, one generally finds that hearing parents have more social, educational, and economic resources at their command. This can be attributed to the unfortunate underemployment and low educational attainment within the Deaf community. It is further exacerbated by the social isolation they suffer; this stems from the linguistic handicap that is associated with their auditory loss (Schlesinger & Meadow, 1972, p. 114).

Being raised in a deaf environment may produce a warm, accepting atmosphere, but the realities of the hearing world may be distorted. Then, as teenagers become aware of the implications of the hearing world, they may have to reevaluate who they are and what they can realistically accomplish. How well they can assess the situation will depend not only on their family situation, but their school environment as well.

SUMMARY

The art of parenting can be one of the most challenging careers that the individual ever undertakes. Those wanting to be successful in this endeavor are forced to rely upon their ingenuity, creativity, and sense of humor to survive the childhood years.

Infants depend on their parents for their livelihood, and later, after the bonding process is complete, for stability and guidance. Through the years children will grow to develop their own identities, drawing from their parents' experiences, beliefs, and values. The home environment will impact significantly as they develop their self-concepts. Those who are fortunate enough to be raised in a warm, nurturing setting will have the opportunity to develop to their fullest potential. However, those entering the world with a disability are frequently greeted by parents who are struggling to cope with their disappointment at producing a baby who is disabled. From the on-set parental attitudes will impact heavily on the child's development and leave an imprint that will remain with their offspring for a lifetime.

The way in which hearing parents will relate to their deaf baby will differ significantly from the interactions that occur if both the parents and the child are deaf. Modes of communication will vary, incorporation into the family unit will be different, and the selection of an educational environment will be viewed from a distinct perspective.

▶ 4

The Educational Environment

Education functions as a mechanism through which values are transmitted and accumulated knowledge is imparted to members of a society. Beginning with infancy and continuing through adulthood, it furnishes us with insights into our culture, while molding our actions into appropriate behaviors. Through this process information is absorbed, skills are mastered, and individuals are prepared for their eventual role in society.

Education assumes the guise of informal as well as formal instruction. In many instances wisdom acquired outside the classroom is commensurate with learning that occurs within the formal setting. Parents, family members, teachers, and peers all function in an educational capacity. They provide the source through which a lifetime of learning emerges.

Many parents have educational aspirations for their children long before they are born. They have preconceived ideas of what the educational system can, and should, do; they also are prepared to take an active interest in their child's scholastic development. From the onset they become involved in early childhood programs and maintain an avid interest as their children progress into adulthood.

Although parents, in general, may be concerned with their child's educational formation, those who have a child who is deaf are confronted with a unique set of challenges. Oftentimes the diagnosis is not confirmed until the child is approaching preschool age. Once parents accept the fact that their child has a disability and cannot be "fixed," they begin coping with the reality of the situation. They begin searching for appropriate educational opportunities based on their expectations and perceptions of their child's capabilities.

This becomes a critical time for parents and their deaf children. As they enter the crossroads of formal instruction, they are confronted with a multitude of choices.

Unlike parents of hearing children, those selecting the most beneficial learning environment for their deaf child must make decisions pertaining to these aspects:

- mode of communication
- residential vs. day programs
- self-contained vs. mainstreamed settings
- facilities and activities providing an emphasis on Deaf culture vs. integration into activities revolving around hearing students

MODES OF COMMUNICATION

Upon enrolling in school, deaf children have the option of receiving their instruction through a variety of communication modes. While some are registered in programs that foster a form of oral communication, others attend classes that utilize a method incorporating Total Communication. Furthermore, a few students have the opportunity to receive classroom instruction through a bilingual-bicultural approach. The school's philosophy of deaf education is reflected in the mode employed in the classroom. A brief synopsis of these communication modes is provided below. (See Chapter 5 for additional information.)

Aural-Oral Communication

When this method of communication is adopted, the major emphasis is on developing the child's auditory and visual senses (Ling, 1984). This approach may incorporate the early use of amplification and auditory training. In addition, emphasis may be equally placed on the development of speech-reading skills (Sanders, 1982). However, one of the primary goals is the development of intelligible speech.

Cued Speech

Cued Speech is used in conjunction with speech. Eight handshapes are utilized in four positions on or near the face to supplement the spoken signal (Martins, 1987, p. 56). By incorporating the handshapes, one is able to distinguish between speech sounds that look similar when produced orally.

Total Communication

Total Communication is a philosophy that embraces all aspects—visual, gestural, auditory, and written—to convey messages. Educational programs purporting the use of Total Communication incorporate one of the manual systems in conjunction with speech when conversing with deaf children (Vernon & Andrews, 1990, p. 112).

Schools may select a form of manually coded English referred to as Seeing Essential English (SEE I) or Signing Exact English (SEE II). In addition, they may elect to use Signed English (SE) or Contact Signing. Others prefer to relate to children through American Sign Language (ASL).

Seeing Essential English (SEE I)
This system has been designed to provide a morphological representation of standard English (Quigley & Paul, 1984). The selection of signs or sign markers are determined by English word sounds, spellings, and meanings.

Signing Exact English (SEE II)
SEE II is derived from SEE I and there is some overlap in the use of the sign markers. They both follow the same rules for word sounds and spellings. However, they differ in their definitions of a root word or, in linguistic terms, a free morpheme. Therefore, several of the words are signed differently (Martins, 1987, p. 57).

Signed English (SE)
Signed English has been designed to provide a language environment similar to the one available for hearing children. Developed by Bornstein and his associates, it contains signs that represent the most commonly used inflections and words of preschool and lower elementary schoolchildren. Signs are selected based on their relationship to the meanings of English words traditionally found in the dictionary. If a word has two meanings, each is represented by a different sign (Bornstein et al., 1983).

Contact Signing
Contact Signing (sometimes referred to in the literature as Pidgin Sign English, [PSE]) is a method used for communicating when individuals from two different sign backgrounds want to converse. Frequently, this involves a fluent ASL signer and an individual who relies on a sign system for his or her means of expression. Referred to as a pidgin in some languages, the term implies that vocabulary is extracted from both languages.

American Sign Language (ASL)
American Sign Language is a language with its own syntax and vocabulary separating it from other foreign languages. Its linguistic structure is different from English. Signs represent words, while nonmanual cues such as facial expressions, head tilts, body movements, and eye gazes, can be incorporated to express specific grammatical functions in the language. ASL is not designed to use in conjunction with spoken English. Nonmanual cues inherent in this language are used instead to convey important linguistic information.

Bilingual-Bicultural Approach (Bi-Bi)

The philosophy of incorporating a bilingual-bicultural approach into classrooms that serve deaf children dates back to a case study conducted by Judy Williams in 1968 (Stokoe, 1980) as cited in Vernon and Andrews (1990). However, it has only been in the mid-nineties that it has received much recognition.

Within the confines of a Bi-Bi approach, "ASL and written English are used in parallel." (Kuntze, 1998, p. 2). Students are provided with instruction in the content areas via ASL, and English is reserved from use in the language arts area where the focus is placed on developing reading and writing skills.

By using ASL as a natural language base, English is taught as a second language. Students are exposed to communication strategies that differ from the oral and the total communication approaches. Programs stress the cultural affiliation of the deaf child and incorporate the use of deaf instructors in the classroom (Stewart, 1992).

According to Vernon and Andrews (1990), Bi-Bi programs stress six goals. They are the following: 1) consider ASL/Pidgin as a first language; 2) consider English as a second language; 3) give deaf teachers an important role; 4) include the history, culture, and literature of deafness in the school curriculum; 5) ground classroom practice in learning theory; and 6) promote interactive learning strategies (p. 241).

The Effects of Bilingual-Bicultural Education

Strong (1995) examined nine sites where Bi-Bi programs were either actively in existence or in the process of being established. Although he notes that his survey is not comprehensive, his findings merit discussion. Of the nine programs cited, four were housed in residential schools, two were day programs, one was not a school but a plan for a school, and for two schools no designation was made. Although each program is unique, they all share similar beliefs regarding deaf children and communication philosophies.

Even though it is too soon to collect evaluative data on all of these programs, assessment results produced by one of the programs, the Sign Talk Children's Center in Winnipeg, are promising. Staff members, involved with that program report that when initial assessments were made on preschoolers entering the Center in 1988, 70 percent of them reflected delays in language in both ASL and English. However, in 1992, after being enrolled in the program for four years, only 20 percent of the children showed language delays. Staff members were optimistic, stating that "all children . . . have the potential to develop effective bilingual/bicultural skills when exposed to the appropriate language models" (p. 90).

EDUCATIONAL ENVIRONMENTS FOR DEAF CHILDREN

Communication mode is only one consideration when parents search for an appropriate school placement. The parents' perceptions of deafness, coupled with their philosophy of education, will also directly influence the educational setting they select for their child. Parents who receive the diagnosis before their child reaches primary school age may be faced with the decision of choosing an appropriate preschool program. Others, who receive confirmation after their child has entered elementary school, may be faced with the dilemma of whether to leave them in their existing environment or move them into a specialized classroom, thus providing them with an alternative learning experience. Parents may be required to make these decisions throughout the preschool or elementary school years, and the choices they make will play a vital role in shaping the child and the family unit.

The educational milieu provided for deaf children varies considerably from instructional settings developed for hearing children. Program modifications are frequently required, support services may need to be added, and teaching strategies designed to circumvent the auditory channel are often incorporated. Depending on the educational environment, any or all of these modifications may be implemented.

Educational programs for deaf and hard-of-hearing children are generally classified within two general categories: Special Schools and Regular-Educational Programs. Special Schools may be designed as a residential facility or established as a day school. Regular-Educational Programs include day classes, resource rooms, and itinerant services. In addition, day classes may foster a mainstreaming approach or be structured in the form of self-contained classes.

SPECIAL SCHOOLS

Residential School Programs

Residential schools may be publicly or privately funded. They are designed following a boarding school concept and offer students dormitory facilities.

Residential schools grew mainly out of the need to provide special education services to the small and scattered population of deaf youngsters residing outside of the metropolitan areas (Levine, 1981).

These schools are designed with the Deaf population in mind and employ staff and teachers who have been specifically trained in the area of deafness. Several of them are located in metropolitan areas. Bus service is provided for children living outside of the residential school areas. This gives them an opportunity to visit their families on weekends and during the holidays.

Day Schools

Day schools are public schools that have been established to accommodate deaf students who live at home. Faculty and staff are specifically trained to work with this population. The majority of these schools are located in metropolitan areas and their curricula are generally structured to meet the needs of the deaf and hard-of-hearing.

REGULAR EDUCATION PROGRAMS

Prior to the formal primary school years, regular education programs occasionally offer additional educational opportunities for deaf preschool-aged children. These programs may take the form of Early Intervention Programs or Home-based Programs.

Early Intervention Programs

Early intervention programs operate on the same premise as preschools for hearing children. Youngsters attend school for a designated number of hours and then return home to be with their parents.

They are designed for deaf infants from birth through age three. These programs are provided by school systems and/or speech and hearing centers. They provide instructional services for parents as well as infants. Emphasis in the classroom is placed on the use of residual hearing, language development, and communication. Several of these programs also stress aspects of socialization that are so critical to child development. In addition, the teacher may work with the parents, providing them with methods, activities, and strategies for enhancing their child's speech, listening, and language development (Northcott, 1972).

Home-Based Programs

Preschool education is also provided through home-based instruction. When available, these programs may be found within metropolitan as well as rural areas. Itinerant teachers go into the homes and render one-on-one instruction to parents and their deaf infants. Instructional emphasis corresponds to that received by children attending day classes or enrolled in speech and hearing centers. The differences lie primarily in the location in which the instruction occurs and with the number of deaf children in attendance during instructional periods.

Day Classes

Day classes are provided for students who have mild to severe hearing losses. They are located in public schools where the majority of the student population has normal hearing. Classroom instruction may occur in self-contained classrooms, resource rooms, or in mainstreamed programs.

Self-Contained Classes

Some school systems designate specific classrooms for hearing impaired students and place them all together in one room for all of their classes. Although they attend public schools, they receive their instruction separately.

Resource Rooms

Resource rooms provide students with the opportunity to receive individualized instruction in various content areas. School systems utilizing these rooms generally hire an itinerant teacher to work with the students. Throughout the day they attend regular classes, returning to the resource room for instruction in English and in specific content areas.

Mainstreamed Programs

Mainstreamed programs came to the forefront in the mid-seventies when President Gerald Ford signed into law the Education for All Handicapped Children Act of 1975 (Public Law 94-142). This act emphasized placing students in the least restrictive environment. Students with varying degrees of hearing loss attend classes together with their hearing peers. They are provided with support services such as interpreters, tutors, and notetakers; the students compete in a regular classroom.

Parents are often faced with an arduous task as they attempt to select the most appropriate learning environment for their children. They want them to benefit from a sound curriculum while simultaneously developing friendships and engaging in extracurricular activities.

Most parents can postpone making a decision regarding school placement until the child reaches elementary school age. However, when they are confronted with the ultimate decision and must choose between a residential placement or a mainstreamed setting, they may have mixed reactions. Upon interviewing several parents, Ferris found they were filled with consternation upon rendering a decision about their child's school placement.

> For a long time we thought we should move to the same town where the state school for the deaf is located. We wouldn't have to be away from our boys all week. . . . We were told we were selfish not to move. We felt guilty. But this is our home. . . . My husband worked hard to get where he is at work. We talked with other families who did move and were disappointed. We decided not to move. It was a long and difficult decision to make. . . . (Ferris, 1980, p. 61)

> When we moved back to our home state, we first asked our town about an educational program for Terry. They had nothing. . . . Our town finally had to take Terry. Terry was six years old and legally had to be placed in a classroom. . . . At first [he] was the only child in the class. Now there are two 14 year olds who are deaf. . . . Should we keep Terry home in this program or send him back to the state school for the Deaf? It's scary not knowing if you are doing the right thing or not. (Ferris, 1980, p. 57)

Inclusion

In June 1997 Public Law 94-142 was reauthorized and became identified as the Individuals with Disabilities Act (IDEA; P.L. 101-476). This new mandate stated that "all children with disabilities are entitled to a (1) free and appropriate education which must occur (2) to the maximum extent appropriate . . . with children who are nondisabled (P.L. 101-476, subsection 1412(1), 1412(5)(B)" (Wright, 1999, p. 11).

Prior to 1997 students with disabilities were educated in self-contained classrooms and/or mainstreamed in select classes, sometimes only sitting next to nondisabled students for art or physical education. However, when students placed in self-contained classrooms were studied, the research indicated that there were negative effects associated with this type of classroom design.

Results indicted that disabled students were not reaching their full learning potential or being exposed to what life was like in the "real world." Furthermore, the nondisabled student population was not given the opportunity to associate with this group on a daily basis, thus restricting nondisabled involvement and hampering attempts to relate to the disabled (Jacobsen, Eggen, & Kauchak, 1999, p. 238).

As a result, schools were asked to establish the least restricted learning environment, where all children would be given the opportunity to grow academically and socially to the maximum extent possible. This mandate further requested that students be removed from the regular classroom "only when the nature and the severity of the handicap is such that education in regular classes with the use of supplemental aids cannot be achieved satisfactorily" (Section 612[5B]) (Jacobsen et al., 1999, p. 239).

Whereas mainstreamed programs were designed to provide academic instruction to disabled students in self-contained classes, inclusion advocates for a comprehensive approach to instruction. Each child is viewed as a unique individual with special strengths and needs. As a result, students with special needs are placed in regular classes, with appropriate support services to guarantee an adaptive fit (Jacobsen et al., 1999, p. 239). When carried to its fullest extent, deaf children who are included remain in the regular classroom with support services for all of their instruction.

The concept of inclusion is new, and its impact will be apparent throughout the next decade. Several studies have been conducted (Fox & Yesseldyke, 1997; Lewis, 1994; Wright, 1999), and more will follow as schools continue to grapple with providing the best education possible for all students.

RESIDENTIAL SCHOOL PLACEMENT

Parents consider residential school settings for a variety of reasons. If the child is residing in a broken home or has been unsatisfactorily mainstreamed into the public school setting, the residential school may appear to be the ideal solution. Deaf parents will customarily send their children to residential schools, as will those who live extended distances from any other quality school setting. If the family lives in a rural area or in a small community, a residential school may be the only answer to the child's educational needs.

Parents who are faced with residential placements find it difficult to send their children away at the age of six and only see them on occasional weekends and holidays. This separation may create feelings of guilt and depression. They realize that their children's educational development, as well as their social development, will be handled by someone outside of the family unit. They may be cognizant of the fact that their children may adopt the value base fostered by their peers in the residential environment, rather than the one that is advocated at home.

Once it has been determined that a residential placement is best, the parents must convey the concept of a boarding school setting to their child. In order to accomplish this, they must be highly skilled in communication strategies; even then deaf children may not comprehend what is happening.

During the early school years, communication between parents and their children may be difficult or weak at best. As a result, misunderstandings may and do occur. Children may not comprehend why they are being left at a residential school. Consequently, when the discussions become a reality and the children are left, many become confused and may experience feelings of fear and abandonment. This experience may have a tremendous emotional impact on them. Young children who are dependent on their mothers may perceive the situation to be a cruel act of abandonment.

Victor H. Galloway, in his essay entitled "Les Miserables," expresses the anguish he went through when being taken and left for the first time at a residential school. He paints a vivid picture of the emotional turmoil he experienced resulting from the misunderstanding involved in being "left" at school.

> *Although several attempts had been made by my grandmother to prepare me for life away from what had come to be home for me, my baptism into dormitory life was totally and wholly unexpected and completely confusing. She had repeatedly tried to prepare me for a long trip to get a pair of shoes. A trip for a pair of shoes? Being small and not possessing the background of language and life experiences that would facilitate lip reading, I found it difficult to understand why there was so much ado in preparation for this trip to get a pair of shoes. New clothes had been purchased; a trunk was then packed with new and old items; a package of home baked cookies had been prepared; and finally the car was loaded for the trip. The trip took all day in a steady downpour, lending an atmosphere of pervading gloom. The several small towns and villages along the route broke the monotony of the countryside drive. My bewilderment grew as we passed through each town, and in my own way I would attempt to verify verbally the plans to get a new pair of shoes. My grandmother, bless her departed soul, would nod back in seeming acknowledgment or agreement.*

Finally, in the distance loomed a few large and strange buildings. The car turned off the road and onto the green and rolling grounds surrounding these buildings. The travelers were met in the back of one of the buildings by a white-haired woman, seemingly bent and wracked by hard labor. I was led to one side by the stranger who incessantly talked to me and I simply could not understand a thing. One thing I did see and understand was that the trunk that I had seen packed with my new and old clothes and the package of home-baked goodies had been unloaded!!

Presently the car started to leave with all the people I knew in my life— my grandmother, my uncle and my aunt. They had abandoned me with this stranger! I made a mad dash for the car only to be restrained by this white-haired apparition. The long arduous trip to get a pair of shoes had suddenly turned into a nightmare . . . my people had merely planned long and hard to get rid of me! Thus was my baptism into dormitory life at the residential school for the deaf and the blind where I was to spend the next twelve years, a large chunk out of my childhood. Only, many, many years later and by reintegration of my experiences was I able to realize that my dear grandmother had tried to do right by preparing me for a long trip so I could go to school, *not get a pair of shoes. (Galloway, 1973, pp. 14–15)*

Oftentimes such misunderstandings occur. These children may be plagued by the fact that their families do not want them, while at the same time experiencing pangs of homesickness and feelings of isolation. At their young age, they have no way of comprehending why they are at school or why their families have deserted them.

Dormitory Environments

While attending residential schools, children attend class for approximately seven hours a day. The remainder of the time is spent outside the classroom in structured activities or in the dormitory setting.

They are usually grouped together with other children their own age and are supervised by houseparents. Houseparents are frequently responsible for monitoring behavior and supervising the children during the evening hours.

Interactions and experiences that the children have with their houseparents have a great impact on them, affecting overall development. Because the hours spent outside the classroom are as critical as those dedicated to formal learning situations, it is essential that the children establish a good rapport with their houseparents. These supervisors frequently become the sounding boards for the students' ideas as they engage in social activities. It is critical that students have the opportunity to participate in a variety of social situations. By experiencing feelings of success, they can develop a sense of accomplishment and self-worth.

Unfortunately, the individuals who are responsible for student development outside of the classroom are not always the best qualified people. Far too often houseparents are ill-equipped to communicate with the children. When this occurs the children may have no "parent figure" in which to confide feelings of homesickness and frustration, or express positive feelings of success and happiness. This is evidenced in the following passage as a deaf individual recalls his early experiences in a residential school.

> *The first houseparent I ever had was an elder woman with perpetually un-kempt hair. . . . As the clock is turned back, it is realized that she was ill-suited for the job of caring for thirty-plus boys between the ages of six and twelve. Many afternoons the boys were left alone to play while the "care-taker" leaned back on her chair and snoozed away for an hour or two. There were rarely any organized activities. It probably would have been dif-ficult for her to organize anything anyway because the small boys were not able to understand her very well. Communication for all practical pur-poses, was nonexistent. (Galloway, 1973, p. 16)*

Due to the very nature of the residential setting, problems other than those directly associated with the houseparent may be evident. Because of the large number of children in the dormitory, oftentimes rigid controls must be used in order to keep track of the children and to maintain a manner of discipline.

In addition, it is very difficult to provide them with the privacy they need, or to permit them the opportunity to become involved in independent activities or other situations in which they are encouraged to take responsibility for themselves and their belongings (Schlesinger & Meadow, 1972). Children, therefore, may not have the opportunity to develop feelings of independence and accomplishment. Rather, they may become somewhat coercively dependent on those around them and transfer the responsibility for their actions onto others.

Not only do they experience feelings of loneliness and frustration, but also due to the regimentation of dorm life, their freedom of exploration and testing boundaries may be somewhat stifled. They are rewarded for "doing" or "being" the same as the others. Little reinforcement is given for creativity or testing one's own initiative.

Residential school settings have some negative aspects that merit examination. They may provide a more structured program, they have a tendency to foster dependency, and students may have limited contact with their home communities.

Structured Environments and Learned Dependency

Due to the number of students attending these institutions, highly structured programs may be designed that enable administrators to maintain control over the students. Activities are planned both in and out of class. The students are told when and what they will eat, when they will go to bed, and when they must be up in the morning. Little, if any, opportunity is afforded the students to plan or implement their own decisions. When this type of structure is employed, individuals are permitted the opportunity to engage in few, if any, positive decisions. Therefore, independence is not encouraged. For individuals to mature socially they must become involved in decision making and unfortunately this is not necessarily the case (Tollefson, 1982).

Deaf individuals may grow up depending on others for their opinions and, consequently, they may remain rigid in their thinking. This rigidity is instilled to a large degree by the classroom teacher. Within the classroom setting many deaf individuals are led to believe that there is one and only one way to do things and, therefore, only one right answer to any given question (Furth, 1974). When teenagers express concerns regarding academic or social problems, they are often given an answer that does not readily lend itself to discussion. Therefore, decisions are made for the students and they are led to believe that the answer they receive is ultimate or final.

Limited Community Contacts

Students attending residential schools have one further disadvantage. Residential facilities traditionally limit the amount of contact students have with their community. As a result, they are not afforded the opportunity to compare their attitudes and behaviors with those residing in the hearing environment. What may seem to be "acceptable" behavior in a residential school may actually be viewed as "immature" behavior by society. Without some type of checks and balances with the hearing world, the child may deviate from the norm without even being aware of it and be labeled with society's stigma.

As they begin to mingle with different facets of society, questions may arise. They seek answers to their many questions but find there are very few resources available from which information can be drawn. Unlike their hearing peers who can solicit information from neighborhood friends, acquaintances, or strangers, deaf teenagers are limited in their social contact because of their spoken communication deficit. Strangers, or those who are unfamiliar with deafness, do not provide good learning resources for them. Only rarely are strangers easily able to handle the difficulties in these types of social interactions in which spontaneous communication is involved (Mindel & Vernon, 1987, p. 5). This is particularly true during the adolescent period.

If adolescents are searching for information regarding nonacademic issues, they will generally turn to their peers for advice. Oftentimes their peers will have limited contact with the hearing world, and the information they receive may prove to be faulty. One area in which this is prevalent is the information regarding sexual issues.

Because deaf adolescents rely on their deaf peers and the stereotypes presented through the media for information relating to human sexuality, they may be very ill-informed. When compared with hearing individuals at the same age, deaf adolescents appear to be more gullible and naive (Neyhus & Austin, 1978, p. 269).

Professionals frequently are known to share stories reflecting this lack of information on the part of deaf teenagers. Kisses may be interpreted to cause pregnancy, hugging can be misconstrued as rape, and so forth. Not only is their information limited due to the small realm of contacts they have, but the environment in which sexual development can occur may be restricted.

The monitoring of social behaviors becomes a difficult task for residential school personnel. They are given the charge to monitor those activities ensuing after school hours, and may feel pressure from the public and the parents to insure which the students are well cared for. Sometimes the schools are understaffed, forcing the administration to take a stand that may be counter to the needs of the developing adolescents.

When the students in residential schools are denied the same amount of freedom afforded those students attending public schools, their opportunities for developing social relationships are restricted. Typically, strictures against dating would fall in this category. This, in turn, hampers their social development, and their ability to deal with their identity is limited.

Sexuality is only one area in which the student does not receive adequate information or have the freedom for various experiences. Other nonacademic areas are also affected. Students who attend public school receive large amounts of information regarding the world as a whole from sources outside the classroom. The information filters in from society and from various sources within the environment. Information regarding living skills, employment, and social aspects are filtered down through the hearing media. The deaf student enrolled in the residential school setting, in essence, may be functioning in a "closed" environment, where utilization of many of the important life skills is not required.

Those students attending residential schools have limited exposure to events and situations occurring outside the school setting. As a result they form their opinions and mold their behavior conforming to those standards established by the Deaf subculture. They may be lacking a certain amount of social information that becomes apparent when they engage in interactions with the much larger hearing community. Those opportunities for dating and incorporating their decision-making skills so often taken for granted by their hearing peers may be restricted, if not nonexistent, for the student enrolled in the residential school.

However, residential living is not all negative for deaf children, for here they are in contact with other children their own age with whom they can identify. Although they may not have a parent figure at the school with whom they can relate, this void may be filled by having classmates and friends with whom they can interact. By attending this type of school setting, the child may experience a feeling of belonging and an even more important feeling may emerge that "It's OK to be deaf."

Classroom Instruction

Residential schools can provide students with a very positive learning environment. Instruction is usually presented through Total Communication, deaf students compete solely with their deaf peers, and deaf individuals may serve in a teaching capacity. All three of these factors can have a positive influence on the students.

The Effect of Total Communication

Students attending programs that embrace the philosophy of Total Communication have one more avenue of communication available to them. They are provided with the opportunity to concentrate on the content presented by the teacher instead of focusing on attempting to comprehend what the mouth movements are trying to convey. Because students can focus on the content, they usually absorb more. From the early school years, students exposed to a form of manual communication tend to score better on achievement tests when compared with students subjected to alternative communication modes. Research reported by Schlesinger and Meadow (1972) indicates that on Standardized Achievement Tests, those students exposed to early education utilizing a manual method scored significantly higher (approximately 1.44 years) when compared with their deaf counterparts who received their instruction through the oral method. Their research also indicated that children in the manual group received superior scores in the areas of reading, vocabulary, and written language. However, no significant differences were noted in the areas of speechreading or psychosocial adjustments.

Positive Aspects of Deaf Peer Groups

Within the residential school setting, students are placed in situations in which they are in constant contact with their deaf peers, and competition within the classroom is limited to those with a common disability. They do not sense a feeling of "differentness," and they generally have a better self-concept when compared with those deaf students attending public schools (Wang, Reynolds, & Walberg, 1989, p. 51). Students with deaf parents are most likely to have a higher opinion of themselves than those with hearing parents. However, students with deaf peer contact will have a much higher regard for themselves than those attending public school. This opportunity for identity development is one of the positive elements afforded students attending residential schools.

Research pertaining to self-image indicates that deaf students of deaf parents attending residential schools score significantly higher on tests assessing self-image than do deaf children of hearing parents attending that same type of school. They also score significantly higher than deaf students attending day schools. In addition, it has been determined that younger students attending day schools have a higher self-image score than their older counterparts. This suggests that during adolescence, when approval from peers is so critical, they may begin developing a negative self-image (Meadow, 1971). Being with deaf peers has a definite positive influence during the teenager's adolescent years.

Those who have previously attended public schools where they were the only student with a hearing impairment may respond positively to residential settings upon entering them for the first time. In the public school setting, they may have been ostracized or viewed as an anomaly. They may have had no one to communicate with and have been isolated from extracurricular activities. Within the residential setting they are surrounded by those with similar handicaps, can communicate with ease, and are able to build positive perceptions of themselves and their abilities. Not only are they fortunate to have deaf peers but deaf adult role models are often employed in these settings. They begin to learn in school, make friends, and are provided with those interactions that can foster the development of a positive self-concept.

Deaf Instructors in the Classroom

Students attending the residential school environment have the opportunity to learn in an atmosphere that employs deaf staff members. Approximately 12 percent of the teachers instructing hearing impaired children are deaf and most of them teach in the residential setting (Erting, 1978). This is relatively foreign to individuals attending mainstreamed or day programs. As a result, students who receive their education in the domain of regular education programs have little, if any, contact with deaf professionals serving in an educational role. As young deaf children grow, it is very important for them to have deaf role models, for in them they can begin to identify with the various adult roles. Also, they begin to realize that deaf people too grow up to become successful adults.

Overall, the residential school setting has both positive and negative aspects. It provides students with the opportunity to learn in an environment where their deafness is taken for granted and attention is placed on tailoring programs that will specifically meet the needs of the deaf. They are afforded the chance to compete in athletic events, become participants in student government, and socialize with a substantial deaf peer group. However, not all students with hearing impairments are comfortable in this environment and may seek alternative educational placements.

DEAF STUDENTS MAINSTREAMED INTO PUBLIC SCHOOLS

Prior to 1975, educational opportunities were somewhat limited for handicapped children. While the majority of them were sent to residential facilities, some attempted to attend public schools, while others remained at home. Although public schools admitted the students, they were not required to provide special services for them. As a result, many experienced failure and withdrew from the educational system.

However, this changed with the passage of Public Law 94-142 (The Education for All Handicapped Children Act of 1975). With the passage of this law, public schools were mandated to provide free and appropriate services for all handicapped children. The law specifically stated that educational programming had to be developed to meet the individual educational needs for each handicapped child. As a result, Individualized Educational Programs (IEPs) were designed and classes were developed (Mindel & Vernon, 1987). Furthermore, school systems began to receive increased pressure to provide mainstreaming programs for handicapped children (Meadow, 1980). The emphasis was placed on providing educational settings with the least restrictive environment, and school systems began initiating these types of programs.

There has been a significant change in the demographic pattern of the deaf school-age population since the passage of PL 94-142. From 1973 to 1984, private residential schools experienced a 65 percent drop in enrollment. Of the remaining 32 percent who attended residential schools in 1985, 1.9 percent of them were reported as being fully mainstreamed, and 6.2 percent of these students were partially mainstreamed. In addition, comparable data pertaining to students enrolled in public day classes indicated that over 67 percent of them experienced some form of mainstreaming (28.2 percent were fully mainstreamed and 39.28 percent were partially mainstreamed) (Wang et al., 1989, p. 50).

One can surmise that mainstreaming has become a popular trend in today's educational system. Students may be mainstreamed in classes with their hearing peers for all or part of the day. Generally, support services in the form of interpreters, tutors, and notetakers are provided as the students compete with their hearing peers.

There are positive and negative aspects of attending mainstreamed programs within the public school setting. Three of the most positive characteristics of day classes and mainstreamed programs center around the fact that the children can live at home, compete with hearing students, and may receive their instruction through a form of Total Communication.

The Opportunity to Reside at Home

Generally speaking, one of the most positive aspects of children attending public schools is that they can live at home and continue to grow, thus benefiting from their family setting. This in itself provides them with the routine of home life, individual attention, and a perception of what family structure entails. Interactions that occur within the family environment provide children with role models and a value base impacting on them as they develop their personalities. In this environment, it is easier for children to develop according to the dominant temperament established in the home. Subliminally, other benefits can be derived from this positive environment. If they are fortunate, they will have open, caring parents and will benefit from them as well as their siblings. This type of family situation can only be found in school settings where children return home at the end of the school day.

However, in order for deaf children to derive the maximum benefit from this setting, interactive communication must exist. Deaf children, like hearing children, need to feel that they are included in daily routines and that they are active participants in the family unit.

In the event that they reside in homes where parents or siblings do not make a concerted effort to foster interactive communication, they may grow up feeling insecure and inadequate and will thus isolate themselves from the family unit. If this occurs, the benefits of remaining at home can be stymied, and in some cases, virtually eliminated.

Competing with Hearing Students

Day classes provided by public school systems may also meet the special needs of this population. These special needs cover a wide spectrum. It may be something as minor as placing the child where he can see the teacher or as complex as utilizing a full team of special services, including itinerant teachers, tutors, speech therapists, and assistive listening devices. In order for deaf children to achieve academically in a day class setting, a valid assessment of their needs is essential. Children who have the potential to be the most successfully mainstreamed have less severe hearing losses (66 percent of the student population attending residential schools are classified as deaf [91+dB]), while only 18 percent of those in mainstreamed programs have equally severe impairments (Trybus & Karchmer, 1977). In addition, 2 to 5 times as many postlingually deaf students are enrolled in mainstreamed programs. Traditionally, they have highly developed oral skills, a high degree of ability to use spoken and written language, and can comprehend varying sentence structures (Pflaster, 1980). Those who are able to cope in oral programs require that only minor adjustments be made. However, children who cannot function successfully in this environment require a setting in which Total Communication is used.

Use of Total Communication in Mainstreamed Programs

Within the mainstreamed environment, students attend class where classroom presentations are interpreted for them. Throughout the day they may return to self-contained classes for instruction in English and some of the content areas. This instruction is frequently presented utilizing a form of manual communication. Approximately 65 percent of deaf students receive their education through a form of Total Communication (Jordan, Gustason, & Rosen, 1979). These situations provide children with every viable channel of communication, thus enhancing their development. Students are exposed to a mode of communication that they can comprehend while residing at home with their family. This, coupled with being in a school where their special educational needs are met, may provide them with a definite advantage over the other school settings (Schlesinger & Meadow, 1972, p. 118).

Unfortunately, there are some negative aspects within the realm of the public school setting. Three of them deserve special attention. Deaf students attending public school settings may be viewed as oddities by their hearing peers and thus be excluded from school-related activities. Second, they may be placed in a program that fosters an oral approach so that they struggle to comprehend classroom assignments. Third, due to the very nature of how language is acquired and developed, these students may experience significant deficiencies in the assimilation of the English Language. They may equate English ability with intelligence and therefore feel that they have an inferior command of the language. In turn, they may transfer this feeling into those of inadequacy and low self-esteem.

Exclusion from Peer Groups

Social problems as well as academic ones can evolve during the school years. How children perceive they are accepted by their peers is critical to their development as people. Due to deaf children's distorted speech and inability to communicate fluently, they may be ostracized by other children. No one can express better the hurt and humiliation deaf children feel when they are taunted by their peers than someone who has experienced it.

Ruth Peterson in "An Insight Into My Deaf World" expresses feelings that she experienced while attending public schools.

> *I first became aware of the stigma, "deaf and dumb," I believe when I started attending public schools. A series of incidents with other school children gradually showed me that I was "different" from them. They would stare at me, whisper to each other in front of me, push me, pull at my clothes . . . or talk to me just to find out how "dumb" I was. This nearly destroyed my self-confidence and made an introvert of me. . . . No one likes to be pointed out as a "freak."*
>
> *My first eleven years were not easy. I could not compete with my classmates. I was a scapegoat. I did not understand that I was in school to learn for myself.*
>
> *I must not leave out an important factor influencing my growing-up years. My step-mother wanted me to be "hearing." . . . When I was very young my mother had taken me to several clinics in an effort to test both my hearing loss and my IQ. . . .*
>
> *I did not know what was going on. Those experiences both scared me and made me feel I was a hopeless case. (Peterson, 1973)*

Not only did Mrs. Peterson feel alienated from her peers, but from the classroom situation and her stepmother as well. It is extremely difficult for any young child to feel that he is looked upon as a "freak." If children are not given the opportunity to experience success in another area, thus permitting them to compensate for those feelings, serious problems can develop.

Frank Bowe reveals a similar situation he experienced while he was a young child.

> *When I was in fourth grade, my best friend was a popular boy named Kenneth. Kenny and I were always together, in school and out. One afternoon as we were walking home with some other kids he turned and pointed to me: "You . . . freak!" I quickly replied: "No, my name is Frank." But the look on*

his face hurt, as did the ensuing laughter. I ran home to ask my mother what
the word "freak" meant. With tears in her eyes, she told me as gently as she
could. (Bowe, 1973, pp. 41–42)

Again, the impact that this type of brutal verbalization has on the child and also the parents cannot go unnoticed. Children can be very cruel to each other, especially during the early school years, and an incredible amount of damage can be done to the child. In order for children with a hearing handicap to develop successfully, they must feel good about themselves and their accomplishments. It can be difficult to establish those feelings while attending public school. It is important that children realize what their disability entails and establish some realistic goals, thus developing positive attitudes about themselves. If this is not done, children may continually struggle with their own feelings of self-worth.

Dealing with one's self-image knows no time limit. Very early in their childhood, children may begin to question their "differentness." Conversely, deaf children may not be faced with this reality until they transfer from a school for the deaf into a public high school. In order for them to incorporate their deafness into a positive self-image, they need to understand their handicap and how it affects them. By gaining this understanding they are able to generate a positive self-image, develop feelings of self-esteem, and self-confidence. Without these feelings they are lost.

Deaf teenagers in the public school setting are increasingly aware of the differences between themselves and their peers. They begin to focus their energies on being accepted and allowed entry into their preferred peer group. If they are denied entry and do not feel acceptance by their peers in the school environment, the impact may be devastating. This lack of acceptance is the second negative aspect of attending a public school. During this time especially, teenagers become cliquish and are known to be intolerant and cruel to those who are "different." Individuals exhibiting differences in skin color, cultural background, and petty aspects such as dress or mannerisms are arbitrarily used as examples, thus determining who will become part of the "in-group" and who will be designated as an outsider.

Because deaf individuals' spoken language skills may not be adequate, they may be denied entrance into group activities. Students may function fairly well academically but the entire time feel isolated from those around them. During the adolescent years the students' peer culture can provide strength and comfort to the adolescents who are a part of it. However, for these individuals who request admission into a specific peer group and are denied entrance due to group rejection, strong signs of distress may become evident (Wright, 1960). Deaf teenagers may be fully capable of achieving academically, but if the atmosphere in which they find themselves is not a comfortable one, they may lack the avenues necessary to explore their identity.

Although there are deaf individuals who experience academic success within the mainstreamed environment, rarely do they feel that they fit into the social milieu of the school. Thus, they experience feelings of loneliness, as they are denied access by their peers into group activities. This feeling of isolation projects itself in a variety of ways. Students may begin to identify themselves as helpless, inadequate persons who feel they must depend on others for solutions to their problems. Or they may avoid all school activities because of their lack of identity, thus avoiding life itself (Neyhus & Austin, 1978).

Psychologists find that deaf adolescents who are attending mainstreamed programs may project characteristics of dependence and passivity. They note that deaf students may be seemingly unable to become involved in the activities provided by the school and that they become distant from their peers. Life for them may assume the format of a day-to-day existence, void of the ability to establish long-range goals.

The Effects of Oral Communication

The method of communication used at the school is oftentimes the determining factor in parents' decisions as to where they decide to send their child. Parents may feel that the use of a signed system or sign language will prevent their child from developing normal speech and thus seek a school that projects an oral philosophy.

Although society and school settings have become more accepting of those utilizing manual communication, there are still those who are uncomfortable witnessing the display of sign systems. People unfamiliar with deafness may be frightened by those who they view as different and often enter into a "shock-withdrawal paralysis" reaction on first exposure (Schlesinger & Meadow, 1972). Parents may be leery of society's reaction to seeing their child use sign communication and being different. Therefore, they may want their deaf children to behave as if they were hearing and will refuse to let them use sign communication, viewing it as repulsive. Instead, they will seek out an oral day school where there is a heavy emphasis placed on speech. For some children the oral method is adequate: There are few, if any, adjustment problems. These children are generally skilled speech readers. With therapy their speech reaches a certain level of clarity; therefore, they are able to communicate vocally. They use their speech to capitalize on interacting with hearing classmates, with whom they become "part of the group." Unfortunately, this is not the case for all deaf children. When parents select an oral program, they may be satisfied, but the effect on the child may be less than satisfactory. Deaf students placed in oral situations may feel isolated and inferior. This is reflected in the passage below.

> *I was always alone. All never had were any real friends. All the schools i went to were schools where (they were) teaching speech. I grew up all very much all on (alone?) English was always hard for me. I never could understand. As a student I was a flop. . . . (Goodman, 1973)*

Parents who want their children to function as if they are hearing may deprive them of an avenue of communication, thus leaving them with feelings of failure, isolation, and loneliness. Parental expectations often shadow the realities of the child's development, and failure is imminent.

Keeping in mind that it is difficult for deaf people to rely on their lip-reading abilities, it is important to examine the classroom structure in the public schools. By the time students reach the junior high and high school years, they are usually subjected to a variety of different teachers. Each subject is taught by an individual who has expertise in that area. Students can no longer concentrate on one individual's lips, but must develop their skills in reading what several individuals are communicating. This in itself presents additional academic problems. Frank Bowe explains the problems and frustrations he experienced while attending public school.

> *I made it through grammar school with ever-increasing difficulty. Junior high school presented even more problems. Instead of one teacher, I now had six. Lectures were assuming increasing importance. My grades began to drop, my social life that had never been much dropped to absolute zero as I struggled to keep up with my courses. . . . One summer I took a week-long battery of intelligence tests that convinced me that what was holding me back was not stupidity but deafness. Incredible as it may seem to some of you, it had never really occurred to me that deafness was the reason for my 74's on my vocabulary tests. (Bowe, 1973, p. 43)*

The difficulty in keeping up academically is a major problem for deaf adolescents, and their perception of the problem is extremely important. If teenagers are not provided with information explaining the reasons behind the difficulties they experience in their academic subjects, then their total sense of identity may be affected.

The discrepancy in English language development between hearing and deaf individuals becomes increasingly evident at this time. Classroom participation for individuals with a hearing impairment may become difficult, if not nonexistent, and the impact both educationally and psychologically on deaf students is tremendous.

> *In group discussions where you alone are deaf, you do not exist. Because you cannot present your ideas through a medium everyone is accustomed to, you are not expected, much less asked, to contribute them. Because you are deaf, they turn deaf. . . . It has never occurred to them that communication is more than method or talk. That it is a sense of belonging, an exchange of understanding, a mutual respect for the other's humanity. (Mow, 1973)*

EFFECT OF LANGUAGE ACQUISITION AND DEVELOPMENT

Language provides the building blocks for communication systems. For those who can hear, acquiring a command of a spoken language provides them with the key to engage in verbal exchanges with others. Language development begins early in life and continues throughout the school years.

During the early years, ages six to eleven, the child's primary task in school is to begin mastering language academically, thus fostering scholastic achievement. Deaf children are at a distinct disadvantage, when compared to their hearing peers. In spite of their intellectual functioning abilities, their auditory handicap prevents them from acquiring and utilizing the same spoken language/experiential base that is so readily available to hearing children. The environment in which all children reside is replete with auditory stimuli. When this channel is severed and the information cannot be accessed, experiential spoken language deficits become apparent. Figure 4-1 illustrates the impact these environmental factors have on spoken language acquisition.

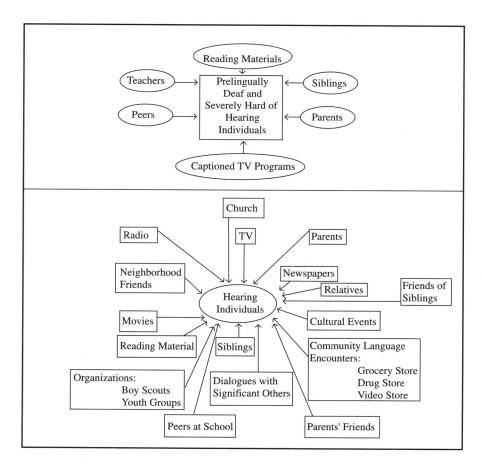

FIGURE 4-1   **Language Acquisition and Development: Impact of Environmental Factors**

The auditory handicap itself provides a barrier to deaf children acquiring a command of the English language. As a result, deaf children will remain academically behind their hearing classmates in all subjects that are heavily based on an understanding of English. The reason for this lies within the way our English language system is developed.

SPOKEN LANGUAGE DEVELOPMENT

Infants with normal hearing begin to acquire their symbol system by receiving auditory cues repeatedly in tandem with experiences that are seen, tasted, or felt. Through a repetitive process they begin to develop their skills in expressing these symbols, that is, their expressive skills. By the time a child reaches twelve years of age he has acquired skill in receiving and expressing approximately 10,974 auditory symbols. However, prelingually deaf children, those who have lost their hearing prior to the age when language patterns have been established, may reach the same age having only acquired approximately 3,256 cues (Brannon, 1968). Thus they are devoid of the symbol or language system utilized by hearing people. This does not mean that deaf children lack the concepts upon which spoken communication is based. However, they lack the written or spoken symbols to convey them, thus hampering their ability to communicate with others.

A recent survey conducted by Hart and Risley (1995) as cited in Santrock (2000) sheds additional light on the significance of language environments today. When hearing children from both middle-income professional and welfare backgrounds were examined, the children's language development reflected the following: all of the children developed normally in terms of learning to talk and acquiring all of the forms of English and basic vocabulary. However, there were enormous differences in the amount of language the children were exposed to and the level of the children's language development.

> For example, in a typical hour, the middle-income professional parents spent almost twice as much time communicating with their hearing children as the welfare parents did. The children from the middle-income professional families heard 2,100 words an hour, their child counterparts in welfare families only 600 words an hour. The researchers estimated that by 4 years of age, the average welfare family would have 13 million fewer words of cumulative language experience than the child in the average middle-income professional family. (Santrock, 2000, pp. 270–271)

The results of this study are staggering, and when applied to deaf children with their quest for developing spoken language skills, the results are significant. For even in families in which a concerted effort is made to "bombard the child with spoken English," due to the severity of the loss, and the ability of the child to speech read, only a small percentage may be received.

The public school educational setting is built around language and communication, impacting heavily on individuals learning within that environment. Young children who can express themselves well and comprehend verbal instructions usually become accepted into the system with very little difficulty. They begin to establish a solid educational foundation upon which they can build throughout the ensuing school years. Although hearing children experience some failures, their successes and accomplishments compensate for their shortcomings. Oftentimes, deaf children do not have the same opportunities for success, due to the very nature of the handicap and the way it manifests itself.

Depending on the severity of the hearing impairment, deaf children are limited in their reception and expression of speech. The ramifications of this deficit permeate the areas of social, emotional, and educational growth to cause educational retardation.

This form of educational retardation may impact significantly on children. They sense their "differentness" due to their hearing loss, and within the school setting this becomes even more acute. Academically, they may not be able to keep up with their peers and accomplish tasks at the same rate their classmates do; therefore they fall behind. In essence, they begin to feel inferior by the very nature of the situation in which they are placed.

By the time they are about twelve years old, they begin to realize that their academic work is inferior to that of their hearing peers. Although they may be working up to their fullest potential, they may be reading and comprehending at a much lower level. Studies reported on reading levels of deaf children indicate that the median reading scores of high school graduates are at a 4.5 grade equivalency level with only 10 percent of 18-year-olds being able to read at the eighth-grade level (Trybus & Karchmer, 1977). They become increasingly aware that, despite their greatest efforts, they cannot make themselves understood orally and that their written language is not comprehensible by those who attempt to read it. They may fall behind academically and interpret their shortcomings as failure.

It is possible for deaf children to succeed in the public school setting provided they receive special services such as interpreters, tutors, and notetakers and if they are given realistic expectations. Sometimes, students are placed in school settings with the idea that they will not require special help but are capable of competing and succeeding with their hearing peers. When they fail to do this, they may develop one of two different attitudes. They may either feel inferior and wish they were hearing, or they may become resentful when help is suggested, thereby refusing it. This may culminate with them denying their deafness. Students who are not prepared to handle the public school setting will usually not perform well academically and may develop feelings of inferiority.

Even though the parents are aware of their child's disability they may still be unwilling to accept it. Therefore, they deny that there is anything wrong and place them in public schools to compete as if they were "normal." When this occurs, children may perceive their parents' expectations and, as a result, feel even more pressured into succeeding. From these early school experiences, the child may begin to feel that it is "bad" or "wrong" to be deaf, and a negative self-concept may take root. By continuing to place themselves in competition only with hearing peers they begin to feel that they should not be deaf but hearing.

In deafness there is much evidence of unhealthy denial of self (Stewart, 1971). We see many hearing professionals working with deaf children who subtly and unconsciously instill in them and their families the premise that they should not be deaf but be "hearing." As Dr. Arnold Gessell, the famed pediatrician, wrote in the *Volta Review* several years ago:

> *Our aim should not be to convert the deaf child into a somewhat fictitious version of a normal hearing child, but into a well adjusted non-hearing child who is completely managing the limitations of his sensory deficit.*
>
> *The tragedy of this denial of deafness (in the oral schools) is that it lends the deaf child to think it is wrong to be deaf, that he is necessarily inferior. The implication is that if he does not try to deny his deafness he is failing to cope with it (Vernon & Makowsky, 1979).*

Mainstreamed, as well as residential school students, may arrive at their respective high schools ill-prepared to complete the required secondary school curriculum. As a result many become frustrated and drop out of school as reported by Lane, Hoffmeister, and Bahan (1996):

- approximately 29 percent of the deaf student population drop out prior to graduation
- of those who do graduate, only one in every five meet the requirements for an academic diploma; the others receive a certificate of attendance
- those attending residential schools tend to complete their programs; between 17 and 23 percent drop out, the lowest rate reported by the various types of school programs
- public schools that have integrated programs for deaf students report a 37 percent drop-out rate
- schools that restrict students to self-contained classes report a 54 percent drop out rate
- deaf students who have additional handicaps, regardless of school setting, comprise a 57 percent drop out rate
- 36 percent of those of Hispanic origin drop out
- 33 percent of Deaf females do not complete their high school education (Lane, Hoffmeister, & Bahan, 1996, p. 255)

Deaf students, from both mainstreamed and residential programs, who remain in the system may arrive at high school graduation with several similar characteristics. Both groups may lag behind their hearing peers in language development. Likewise, each group may exhibit signs of experiential/environmental deprivation due to its hearing loss. These students may have relied primarily on deaf peers as they developed their perceptions of society. Therefore, their view of the hearing world may be somewhat distorted. Throughout their youth and young adulthood, they may have relied on others to make decisions for them and upon graduation be faced with a newfound freedom.

POSTSECONDARY EDUCATIONAL SETTINGS

Individuals entering postsecondary institutions for the first time are faced with unique and challenging environments. Many experience a degree of freedom previously unknown to them, and they are not equipped to deal with the stress that accompanies their newfound independence. Throughout their initial year, they focus the majority of their energies into mastering independent living skills resulting in decreased amounts of time being devoted to their academic studies. Consequently, they encounter failure and are unable to complete their freshman year.

> . . . *The single greatest problem college students face is the problem of freedom . . . the problem of freedom and what you make of it and how well you use it will have an impact on all other aspects of your college career. (Gardner & Jewler, 1985)*

In general, typical college freshmen are faced with a myriad of challenges and frustrations. Students with disabilities encounter the same challenges; however, their frustrations are exacerbated due to their physical impairments. This is especially true for hearing impaired college students. Because their communication link with the hearing world is severed, they enter the mainstream of college life feeling inadequate and unprepared. "Hearing impairment has a profound social impact upon the individual (Thomas & Gilhome-Herbst, 1980) with social isolation as the major consequence" (Murphy & Newlon, 1987). This isolation prevents the deaf individual from interacting fully with his environment. Thus the student frequently enters the college setting environmentally deprived and lacking the skills to interact independently within the college community. This can be attributed in part to familial relationships and the constraints previously placed on the students in residential school facilities.

> . . . *Residential school life appears to be related to social immaturity as well. A number of findings indicate the parents of handicapped children generally, and deaf children specifically, are reluctant to grant them the freedom and independence that would encourage independence and consequent maturity. (Meadow, 1980)*

Deaf and hard of hearing students entering college have previously attended an assortment of multifarious secondary school settings. Some have experienced mainstreamed educational environments while residing at home. Others may have attended residential school settings since infancy, only returning home for an occasional weekend, holiday, and/or summer vacation. Many have functioned as part of the Deaf subculture while others may never have encountered another deaf individual.

In addition to their diversified educational backgrounds, their methods of communication may vary considerably. While some have been placed in an aural/oral learning environment, others have received instruction via manual communication through the channel of Total Communication, American Sign Language (ASL), or Cued Speech. Regardless of the communication mode utilized by deaf individuals, the impact on their ability to interact with the hearing world has pervasive ramifications.

Deafness is subtle and paradoxical, and it ramifies far beyond the immediate disability. It imposes few physical limitations, but its effects on social life and academic performance can be severe. It cripples neither the mind nor the body, but the ability to use our most elemental and pervasive form of communication, the human voice. Thus it strikes at the core of social life and of education. (Malone, 1986)

The ability to interact with the environment has significant implications for educational and social development. Through the discourse of daily communication, ideals are originated, values enhanced, and the persona is shaped. Because of the nature of the disability, those who cannot hear speech receive limited stimulation from their environment, restricting those factors that shape language, impart social skills, and foster educational development. Whereas the hearing individual has the advantage of input from a multiplicity of sources within his environment and can enrich his language base with relative ease, the deaf person is limited in his quest for discovering individuals with whom he can facilitate communication.

As a result, deaf college students enter the educational milieu with linguistic and communication differences, and they lack the skills to interact independently on the college campus. Although it is critical for them to learn how to access support services and be provided with independent living skill training, it is even more critical that they develop those personal social skills affording them a successful college experience (see Figure 4-2).

POSTSECONDARY PROGRAMS FOR THE HEARING IMPAIRED IN THE UNITED STATES

Until fairly recently deaf students had very limited opportunities to acquire a postsecondary education (Schildroth, 1986). If they did well academically in secondary school, they had the option of attending Gallaudet University, the only liberal arts university in the world for the deaf, or the National Technical Institute for the Deaf. Within the last several years, many postsecondary programs have been providing

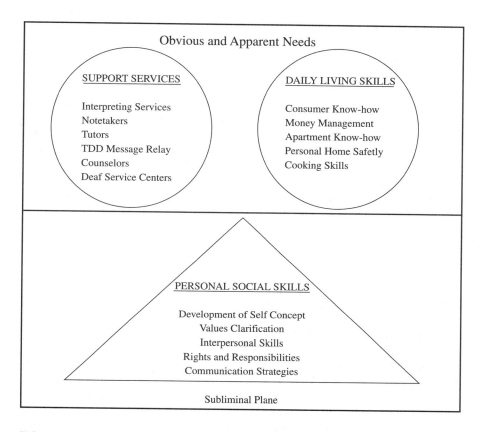

Obvious and Apparent Needs

SUPPORT SERVICES

Interpreting Services
Notetakers
Tutors
TDD Message Relay
Counselors
Deaf Service Centers

DAILY LIVING SKILLS

Consumer Know-how
Money Management
Apartment Know-how
Personal Home Safetly
Cooking Skills

PERSONAL SOCIAL SKILLS

Development of Self Concept
Values Clarification
Interpersonal Skills
Rights and Responsibilities
Communication Strategies

Subliminal Plane

FIGURE 4-2 **Development of Life Skills Within the College Environment**

services to deaf students, therefore enabling more of them to obtain a college education. Today there are approximately 150 colleges and universities providing programming for hearing impaired students (Rawlings & Karchmer, 1988). Whether the student selects a college with an exclusive deaf enrollment or one in which he will be mainstreamed with hearing students will determine the various challenges he will encounter.

Generally speaking, the deaf college student will enter college functioning at a lower achievement level. His potential may be average or above but his attainment lower. This educational lag will encumber the deaf college student's progress through school.

The most salient characteristic of low-achieving deaf persons is the over-whelming majority with normal potential. . . . They represent a failure of

> *education and other services and are testimony to a waste of human re-*
> *sources. It is obvious that the deaf person faces the world with an educa-*
> *tional handicap that is a greater disability than his deafness. (Vernon, 1970,*
> *p. 258)*

Oftentimes the educational handicap is interpreted by the deaf individual to mean "dumb" or "stupid." He or she may feel very inadequate when interacting in the classroom and, therefore, withdraw from peers, further isolating him- or herself. On the other hand, he or she may release frustration on those around him or her, through aggression causing others to withdraw from him.

Within the confines of a hearing educational setting, the deaf individual may experience feelings of inadequacy, the stigma of being different, and his own frustrations of dealing with the new educational setting. If he is unsure of himself and what he is able to accomplish, he will not be able to look beyond himself.

SUMMARY

Education plays a critical part in our development. It provides us with the necessary tools to relate to our environment and become contributing members of society. Through education, life skills, academic expertise, and socialization, processes are mastered.

Those experiences encountered in the educational arena contribute to the total development of individuals. They prepare us to confront future challenges and generations. If we are fortunate and have the benefit of a sound educational foundation, we are able to expand our horizons and explore our full potential. However, if we are lacking the fundamentals so critical to education, we will be forced to depend on others for information and ultimately for survival.

Deaf and hard-of-hearing individuals enroll in a variety of school settings. These institutions have been established to provide the students with the necessary skills to become independent, contributing members of society. While the philosophies and techniques incorporated by the schools may vary, their ultimate goal is virtually the same.

Location of school, makeup of the student population, and the mode of communication utilized will all impact on the success or failure of the student. Although the peer group and the faculty members impact significantly, communication lies at the heart of the educational experience. If children are placed in an environment that is not conducive to their communication style, they may become frustrated and fail to be successful. However, if the communication channel is open and the exchange of information can readily occur, the avenues for learning are enhanced tremendously.

▶ 5

Modes of
Communication

Communication is at the core of our existence. Individuals thrive on their ability to convey ideas and express feelings. Concepts are formed, vocabulary expanded, values instilled, and educational horizons broadened, all through the channel of communication. For at the heart of expressing oneself lies language—the basic tool that in turn links us to our culture, home, community, and surrounding environment. By being provided with the opportunity to share our thoughts, feelings, and knowledge with others, our lives become enhanced and we are able to transmit our information base to others, thus creating a bond with previous and future generations.

When there is a flaw in the communication system and all of the links do not function properly, information may be misconstrued, perceptions can become distorted, and conveying messages becomes difficult, if not altogether impossible. The daily exchange of information through either written exposition or verbal (i.e., spoken) presentation is lost in the sea of verbiage, and breakdowns in communication occur. When this happens, both the sender and the receiver may be affected. The information is not transmitted accurately, and neither party benefits from the exchange.

What are the components of communication? What differentiates one mode of communication from another? In the event that one of the channels for communication does not function properly, what effect does it have on language development? How does deafness affect the acquisition of the English language, and what ramifications does this have for the communication process?

COMPONENTS OF THE
COMMUNICATION SYSTEM

The term "communication" can be defined as a process in which two entities enter into an exchange of information to transmit thoughts, messages, or ideas. It may take the form of spoken, written, or gestural expression and is conveyed in a variety of settings.

The foundation for communication is language—a system comprised of relatively arbitrary symbols and grammatical signals that can be modified or enhanced by members of the community (Baker & Cokely, 1980). Language serves as the basis for our expression. As a result, the way individuals project themselves, both verbally and physically, will determine how they are perceived and accepted by members of their environment. Because one's instinct is to shy away from those individuals whose mode of communication deviates from the norm, the person who is unable to participate in the fluid exchange of information may be isolated from the mainstream of current events.

Language Development and Acquisition

In the previous chapter a diagram was included that illustrates the impact environmental factors have on language acquisition. By eliminating the auditory channel and simultaneously examining the vast array of information that is assimilated through it, one can begin to comprehend the meaning of the phrase "experiential deprivation."

Individuals born with and functioning with normal hearing benefit from environmental insights as these are transmitted through the auditory process. They are provided with a philosophical base from which development can occur. However, individuals whose aural channel of communication has been severed are faced with alternative modes of exchanging information to insure that an experiential base can be established.

As one reviews the literature on language development, insights can be gained from a historical perspective into the modes and methods of communication utilized with hearing impaired students. Parents, educators, and professionals have been trying to determine which method would generate the greatest exchange of information and enhance the deaf individual's linguistic skills.

Initially, the battle raged throughout the country between the oralists (those who believe in the use of speech, amplification, voice, and lip-reading skills [Meadow, 1980]) and the manualists (those who support the philosophy of incorporating a visual sign system to enhance communication), as to which method would produce the most advantageous results (Benderly, 1980). Although this controversy is still unresolved today, additional communication systems have surfaced.

By examining the early philosophies and roots of each system, greater insights can be gained into the decision-making process that parents and professionals engage in as they determine which language mode is thought to be the most appropriate for this population. By examining a visual communication versus an aural/oral communication system as each relates to cultural and sociological issues, insights into deafness and its impact on human development can be ascertained.

Sign Systems: Their History, Structure, and Role in the Deaf Community

From a historical perspective, one can find a form of sign communication being utilized as early as A.D. 530. It is believed that an order of Benedictine monks living in Italy had taken vows of silence, and in turn created a form of sign language so that they could communicate their daily needs (Gannon, 1981).

Through the centuries additional sign systems were developed for a variety of communication purposes and were used throughout the world. Each country developed its own system based on the country's individual needs; as natives from one country came in contact with those residing in another, signs were shared and systems modified (Baker & Cokely, 1980, p. 48).

HISTORY OF AMERICAN SIGN LANGUAGE

American Sign Language (also referred to as ASL or Ameslan) is a visual gestural language that was created by and for deaf individuals living in the United States. It has become the language of between 250,000 and 500,000 Americans of all ages (Baker & Cokely, 1980, p. 47). Although this system is utilized in the United States and referred to as American Sign, approximately 60 percent of all of its signs are of French origin (Vernon & Andrews, 1990). By examining the early beginnings of sign language usage in this country, one is able to trace the language back to France.

As early as the mid-1700s there are written accounts of deaf individuals living in the eastern United States communicating with hearing individuals through some form of a sign system (Vernon & Andrews, 1990, p. 72).

One community that merits special consideration is comprised of the individuals who resided on Martha's Vineyard between the late 1600s and the early 1900s. Studies by Groce (1981, 1985) indicate that a large population of deaf individuals migrated from the Kentish region of England and conversed through Old Kentish Sign Language (Moores, 1996; Levitan, 1993). The signs used by this population is presumed to have influenced the early development of American Sign Language.

However, when one reviews the history of American Sign Language (ASL) in this country, its most notable roots are traced to Thomas Hopkins Gallaudet and Laurent Clerc. In volumes pertaining to deaf education, one can read accounts of the story of Gallaudet's travels throughout Europe and his attempt to secure instructional methods and bring them to America, thus providing deaf individuals with a channel through which they could access a quality education (Scouten, 1984).

Thomas Gallaudet was a graduate of Yale University enrolled in a ministerial program. During the early 1800s, he became acquainted with his neighbor, Dr. Mason

Cogswell, whose daughter, Alice, was deaf. Gallaudet found communicating with her intriguing and sought to discover methods that would enable her to master the technique required to incorporate English reading and writing skills into her communication system.

Cogswell became so impressed with Gallaudet's efforts that he initiated a fundraising campaign, hoping to generate enough funds to send him to Europe where he would acquire teaching techniques appropriate for the Deaf community. Cogswell's goal was for Gallaudet to work with the masters in Europe and then return to the United States where he would establish a school for the deaf.

Funds were successfully generated and Gallaudet sailed to Great Britain, his goal being to learn the "oral method." When he arrived in England, he soon discovered that the British were reluctant to share their instructional methods with him. As a result he traveled to Paris where he encountered a group of deaf individuals and their instructor. He found the French to be more open and willing to share their communication methods. By working with Jean Massieu and Laurent Clerc (a deaf instructor), he was able to master the sign system that had been invented by Abbé de L'Epee. When the time arrived for Gallaudet to return to Connecticut, he had convinced Clerc to accompany him to the United States. There, the two of them were instrumental in establishing the first school for the deaf in America. On the voyage back to the United States, Gallaudet mastered de l'Epee's sign system and Clerc acquired the English language.

On April 15, 1817, based on funds secured from the State of Connecticut and other groups who supported this unique population, Gallaudet and Clerc established the Institute for Deaf Mutes, later renamed the American Asylum at Hartford for the Education and Instruction of Deaf and Dumb. The school was established to meet the needs of eighty-nine deaf individuals who were residing in Connecticut at that time. Today, the school is still in existence and is presently called the American School for the Deaf.

American Sign Language and English

American Sign Language is a language in its own right and can be viewed as a separate communication system complete with its own vocabulary and syntax. One of the most striking differences between ASL and English is that English is an aural/oral language that was developed within a community of hearing and speaking individuals, while ASL, on the other hand, is a visual/gestural language comprised of its own vocabulary and syntax. This language has been developed within a community that relies on its sight and body movements for communication.

In ASL "signs may represent more general concepts, with the refined nature of the concept derived from context and non-manual signals" (Schein & Stewart, 1995). It is important to note that signs are hand-movement configurations that convey meaning. These signs, coupled with facial expressions and body posture, determine the sign's meaning.

One cannot derive the entire meaning from a signed message from the hands alone. Rather, the listener must be attentive to nonmanual expressions, such as raised eyebrows, puffed cheeks, and eye glances. These facial expressions contain significant linguistic signals; although these signals are frequently incorporated together with signs, they can also be produced independently of any hand movement.

It is important to note that these nonmanual signals differ from the facial expressions and body postures that accompany speech. Although there are some similarities, the nonmanual markers in ASL serve a grammatical function that distinguishes them from the role that similar behaviors play in spoken languages (Schein & Stewart, p. 44).

Within the English language, parts of speech, verb changes, and word order are incorporated to facilitate communication. Likewise, within the area of ASL certain characteristics are unique to the language system. ASL incorporates tense indicators, classifiers, verbs utilizing directionality, placement of pronouns, and reduplication of signs to convey meaning (Wilbur, 1979).

As a result ASL becomes an interactive language. It is dependent on both the location of the signer and the recipient of the information. It relies on their eye contact, their use of signing space, the "linguistic signals" projected by their bodies, and their facial expressions. These features, coupled with the syntactical structure of the language, help distinguish it from English.

American Sign as It Compares to Production of Speech

When one expresses oneself through oral languages, specific words can be identified and comprehended by their sounds as they are articulated by the sender. Consonant and vowel sounds are blended together, thereby enabling the listener to comprehend the message as it is transmitted. Each word is characterized by these consonantal and vocalic segments, and is selected with the purpose of conveying the speaker's intentions. Through scientific research over the past several thousand years, our knowledge of the spoken-language system has been developed and refined.

However, research on American Sign Language is relatively new. In the early sixties, William Stokoe began studying the formation of ASL in order to determine if the signs themselves could be viewed as having independent parts. He determined that their formation could be identified by examining three aspects of each sign. He described the three components in the following way:

1. *handshape* or *dez* (designator)
   how the fingers are extended
2. *location* or *tab* (tabulation)
   where on the body or in space the sign is made
3. *movement* or *sig* (signation)
   how the hand or hands move—up, down, circular, etc. (Baker & Battison, 1980)

He further developed a system for categorizing the signs by symbols and determined that there are:

> 19 basic symbols for handshapes,
> 12 basic symbols for locations, and
> 24 basic symbols for movement.
> (Baker & Battison, 1980, p. 39)

Based on his research it was determined that signs could be identified by dez, tab, and sig, just as spoken words are identified by phonemes (i.e., speech sounds). It was further illustrated that ASL could be expressed in a written format by transferring each part into its respective sign symbol.

Although ASL can be illustrated in this format, the symbols are incorporated to represent components of signs, but they cannot be read in the same fashion as one reads printed English. Table 5-1 illustrates the transcription symbols developed by Stokoe.

The Morphological Process: Comparing Signs to Speech

Morphological processing refers to studying how a word or a sign is changed in order to express different meanings. ASL differs dramatically from English and other spoken languages in its mechanisms for modifying its lexical units (signs). In spoken languages the most widespread morphological device for modification is what is termed "affixation," meaning the addition of sound segments at the beginning, middle, or at the end of the word. Other techniques to achieve inflection include changing the vowels or consonants, repeating part or all of a word, and/or alterations in one's tone of voice or the emphasis that is placed on a phrase (Baker & Battison, 1980).

When exploring the rich vocabulary of ASL, it becomes apparent that there are several grammatical devices to ensure that inflection occurs. Through recent research it has become apparent that ASL shares inflective linguistic properties with languages such as Navajo, Greek, and Russian that are not common to English or Chinese. Thus, ASL been termed one of the "inflective languages of the world."

> *In ASL there appears to be a strong resistance to sequential segmentation as an inflectional device and hence a resistance to the morphological device frequently used by English and a great many other spoken languages: affixation. ASL signs are made by moving the hands in space; the language uses dimensions of space and movement for its grammatical processes. Rather than adding parts to signs that are like spoken language affixes,*

TABLE 5-1   **Stokoe's Transcription Symbols**

Tab symbols

1. Ø zero, the neutral place where the hands move, in contrast with all places below
2. ○ face or whole head
3. ⌒ forehead or brow, upper face
4. ⊔ mid-face, the eye and nose region
5. ⌄ chin, lower face
6. ꝫ cheek, temple, ear, side-face
7. π neck
8. [] trunk, body from shoulders to hips
9. \ upper arm
10. ✓ elbow, forearm
11. *a* wrist, arm in supinated position (on its back)
12. *v* wrist, arm in pronated position (face down)

Dez symbols, some also used as tab

13. A Compact hand, fist; maybe like 'a', 's', or 't' of manual alphabet
14. B flat hand
15. 5 spread hand; fingers and thumb spread like '5' of manual numeration
16. C curved hand; may be like 'c' or more open
17. E contracted hand; like 'e' or more clawlike
18. F "three-ring" hand; from spread hand, thumb and index finger touch or cross
19. G index hand; like 'g' or sometimes like 'd'; index finger points from fist
20. H index and second finger, side by side, extended
21. ɪ "pinkie" hand; little finger extended from compact hand
22. K like G except that thumb touches middle phalanx of second finger; like 'k' and 'p' of manual alphabet
23. L angle hand; thumb, index finger in right angle, other fingers usually bent into palm
24. 3 "cock" hand; thumb and first two fingers spread, like '3' of manual numeration
25. O tapered hand; fingers curved and squeezed together over thumb; may be like 'o' of manual alphabet

26. ʀ "warding off" hand; second finger crossed over index finger, like 'r' of manual alphabet
27. V "victory" hand; index and second fingers extended and spread apart
28. w three-finger hand; thumb and little finger touch, others extended spread
29. x hook hand; index finger bent in hook from first, thumb tip may touch fingertip
30. Y "horns" hand; thumb and little finger spread out extended from fist; or index finger and little finger extended, parallel
31. ȣ (allocheric variant of Y); second finger bent in from spread hand, thumb may touch fingertip

Sig symbols

32. ^ upward movement ⎫
33. v downward movement ⎬ vertical
34. ɴ up-and-down movement ⎭ action
35. > rightward movement ⎫
36. < leftward movement ⎬ sideways action
37. z side to side movement ⎭
38. ⟂ movement toward signer ⎫
39. ⟂ movement away from signer ⎬ horizontal
40. ɪ to-and-fro movement ⎭ action
41. *a* supinating rotation (palm up) ⎫
42. *v* pronating rotation (palm down) ⎬ rotary
43. ω twisting movement ⎭ action
44. ŋ nodding or bending action
45. ▢ opening action (final dez configuration shown in brackets)
46. ▣ closing action (final dez configuration shown in brackets)
47. ʅ wiggling action of fingers
48. ↻ circular action
49.)(convergent action, approach ⎫
50. × contactual action, touch ⎪
51. ⊓ linking action, grasp ⎬ interaction
52. † crossing action ⎪
53. ⊙ entering action ⎪
54. ÷ divergent action, separate ⎪
55. ·· interchanging action ⎭

KEY

Tab = location
Dez = handshape
Sig = movement

(© National Association of the Deaf. Reprinted with permission.)

most inflections or modifications in ASL involve spatial and temporal patterns which are overlaid on the movement of basic signs. (Baker & Cokely, 1980, p. 58)

Although many of the semantic distinctions that are expressed in ASL are commonly expressed in many spoken languages, quite frequently they are not found in the English language. Upon examining inflectional patterns of ASL they can be categorized into five separate grammatical entities: Referential Indexing, Reciprocity, Grammatical Number, Distributional Aspects, and Temporal Aspect and Focus (Baker & Battison, 1980).

Referential Indexing
This refers to the structured use of space whereby principal characters in a sentence or phrase can be identified by utilizing space and moving the ASL sign in the direction of the spatial target point. See Figure 5-1.

Reciprocity
Reciprocal inflection operates on verbs that indicate mutual relations or actions. To create this meaning the verb sign is doubled: It is made with two hands rather than one in simultaneous movement, and the hands are either directed or oriented toward or away from each other. This form of inflection indicates that some form of action will transpire between the two individuals involved in the dialogue. See Figure 5-2.

Grammatical Number
Changes in the verb form occur when one is indicating if the inflection is intended for more than one subject.

Dual Inflection.   This infers that there are two recipients or agents, and that the action is intended for "both of them."

Trial Form.   This infers three recipients or agents.

Multiple Inflection.   This general form is utilized when the object or subject receiving the action of the verb is a number that is greater than three.

Distributional Aspects
In addition to focusing on grammatical number, several inflections also focus on differentiating the actions of the verb, thus drawing these distinctions:

1. if the act itself is presented as an indivisible whole or as several separate actions.
2. if the actions occur at distinct points in time.
3. if the actions occur in a specific order.
4. if the relationship of the actions of the individuals involved in each situation can be identified as an activity that occurs for each one, only specific ones, certain groups, or just anyone.

When examining the distributional aspects of inflection, one can focus on Exhaustive Inflection, Allocative Determinate Inflection, and Allocative Indeterminate Inflection.

Exhaustive Inflection.   This refers to those actions that are distributed to *each* individual member of a particular group; that is, to do something to each of them, or when actions are viewed as a single event.

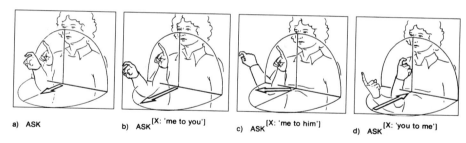

a) ASK   b) ASK [X: 'me to you']   c) ASK [X: 'me to him']   d) ASK [X: 'you to me']

FIGURE 5-1   **Referential Indexing on the Sign "Ask"**

(© National Association of the Deaf, 1980. Reprinted with permission.)

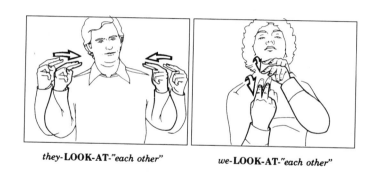

they-**LOOK-AT**-*"each other"*   *we*-**LOOK-AT**-*"each other"*

FIGURE 5-2   **Reciprocal Inflections of the Sign "Look At"**

(From *American Sign Language: A Teacher's Resource Text on Grammar and Culture,* Copyright 1980 by Baker & Cokely, T. J. Publishers. Reproduced with permission.)

Allocative Determinate Inflection.   This form of inflection refers to those actions that are distributed to specific individuals at distinct points in time; that is, something is done to certain ones at different times. See Figure 5-3.

Allocative Indeterminate Inflection.   This refers to actions that are distributed to unspecified individuals over time; that is, to do something to anyone at different times.

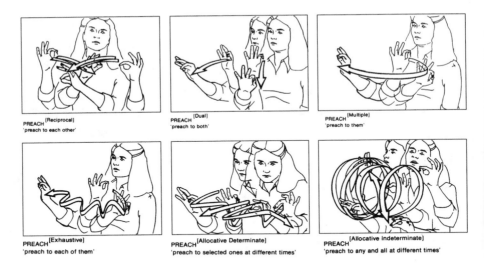

PREACH [Reciprocal]
'preach to each other'

PREACH [Dual]
'preach to both'

PREACH [Multiple]
'preach to them'

PREACH [Exhaustive]
'preach to each of them'

PREACH [Allocative Determinate]
'preach to selected ones at different times'

PREACH [Allocative Indeterminate]
'preach to any and all at different times'

FIGURE 5-3 **Inflection for Reciprocity, Number, and Distributional Aspect**

(© National Association of the Deaf, 1980. Reprinted with permission.)

Temporal Aspect and Focus
Verb signs are also inflected for "temporal aspect" and "temporal focus." One can view signs being executed to convey a wide array of inflectional forms that express meanings such as "uninterruptedly," "overtime," "regularly," "for a long time," "over and over again," "from time to time," "characteristically," and so on.

For example, depending on how the verb "look at" is signed, it can be interpreted to say the following:

> to stare at uninterruptedly
> to gaze at over a period of time
> to watch regularly
> to look at for a long time
> to look at again and again (Baker & Battison, 1980, p. 64). See Figure 5-4.

Manner and Degree
Signs can be moved along lines, in circles, arcs, or in vertical or horizontal planes, thus expressing distinctions between such concepts as mental preoccupation, accomplishing a task with ease, or being able to do something "readily."

Inflections for temporal aspect rely heavily on *temporal* patterning, so that the signs change their dynamic qualities, such as rate, tension, evenness, duration, and manner of movement.

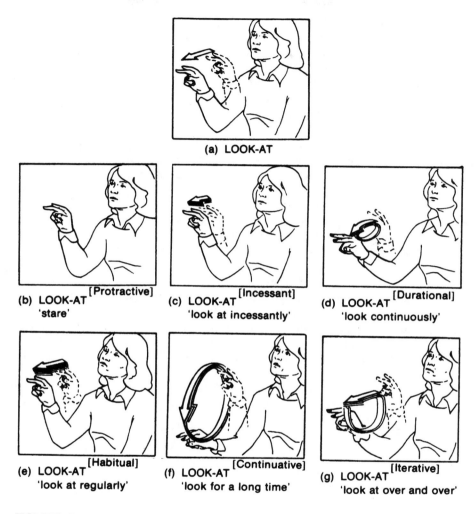

(a) LOOK-AT

(b) LOOK-AT[Protractive]
'stare'

(c) LOOK-AT[Incessant]
'look at incessantly'

(d) LOOK-AT[Durational]
'look continuously'

(e) LOOK-AT[Habitual]
'look at regularly'

(f) LOOK-AT[Continuative]
'look for a long time'

(g) LOOK-AT[Iterative]
'look at over and over'

FIGURE 5-4 **Inflections for Temporal Aspect**

(© National Association of the Deaf, 1980. Reprinted with permission.)

Derivational Processes

ASL can be further distinguished as an independent language system by examining the derivational processes that occur in the lexical roots of its language base. Basic verbs can be changed into nouns or adjectives; adjectives can be transformed into verbs, nouns, and so forth.

Research conducted by Supalla and Newport in 1978 described 100 activity verbs and their formationally related concrete nouns. They illustrated how those noun-verb pairs differ systematically in the way they are produced, specifically pertaining to frequency of repetition and the manner of their final movement. Within the noun-verb pairs, the related nouns are produced with restrained repeated movements that are abbreviated.

In addition, certain nouns can form predicates by altering their movement. Through this derivational process selected nouns can assimilate the characteristics of verbs or adjectives based on the movement that is incorporated into the communicative process. In this derived form, the movement of the sign is made once and is fast and tense with a restrained beginning. This process changes a noun to a predicate thereby indicating "to act like _____" or "to appear like _____" (Baker & Battison, 1980, p. 68). See Figure 5-5.

There are other morphological processes that seem to operate when a sign adopts a figurative or extended meaning. When examining the language there appear to be additional pairs of well-established signs that seem to be derivationally related in which one sign of the pair is a good candidate for metaphorical or figurative extension of the other and differs from it primarily in quality of movement. This can be illustrated by the hands becoming lax, tense, or accelerated as the meaning is conveyed. Concepts such as "hungry" can be altered to mean "horny" or "feel" can become "hunch," depending on the nature of the sign and the way in which it is expressed (Baker & Battison, 1980, p. 68). However, it is important to note that figurative extensions of meaning are usually accompanied by minimal changes in movement.

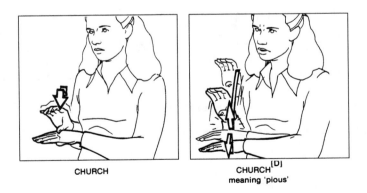

CHURCH   CHURCH[D]
                      meaning 'pious'

FIGURE 5-5   **The Sign "Church" and a Derived Form**

(© National Association of the Deaf, 1980. Reprinted with permission.)

Nonmanual Aspects of American Sign Language

There are a few signs that are comprised entirely of facial and other nonmanual movements. Other signs incorporate movements in the signer's eyes, face, head, and body to generate adjectives, adverbs, and pronouns. In addition to being utilized in the formation of signs themselves, continuing research on the role of eye, face, head, and body movements has shown that they are even more important at the level of the whole sentence (Wilbur, 1987). These nonmanual behaviors are important for binding signs together into clauses and sentences, thus indicating what type of clause or sentence the signer is using.

Specific grammatical signals in ASL are utilized for questions, negated statements, asserted statements, negated questions, and questions about assertions. Within simple sentences there do not appear to be any special nonmanual signals; however, there are thirteen different types of sentences in ASL that utilize nonmanual signals and indicators. These nonmanual signals assist in conveying the structure and meaning of the sentence and are the key to the syntactical structure of American Sign Language. Sentences such as those that involve rhetorical questions and "yes/no" questions all incorporate different nonmanual behaviors (Baker & Cokely, 1980, p. 123).

Nonmanual behaviors may be as simple as a raise of the eyebrows, or as complex as a brow raise, head tilt, and constant eye gaze on the addressee, combined with variances in sign production. However subtle or complex these cues are, they play an integral part in the delivery of the message. Figure 5-6 illustrates the use of nonmanual signals. A question is changed into a rhetorical statement by raising the lowered eyebrows.

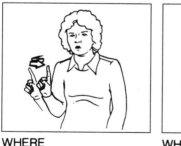 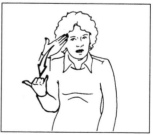

WHERE   WHY

FIGURE 5-6 **The Sign "Where" with Accompanying Facial Expressions**

(Sign illustrations from *A Basic Course in American Sign Language* by Humphries, Padden, & O'Rourke. Courtesy of T.J. Publishers, Inc., 817 Silver Spring Ave., Silver Spring, MD 20910)

Formation of Plurals and Tense Indicators

Within the structure of American Sign, the speaker has several options when he or she elects to change a noun from a singular to a plural. Jones and Mohr (cited in Lane & Grosjean, 1980) concentrated on the expression of noun plurals and have commented on several ways in which these nouns can be produced. They state that:

1. nearly all nouns can form the plural with the quantifier MANY;
2. modifications for noun plurals include changing the number of hands used to make the sign; and
3. use of reduplication and continuous movement while adding a horizontal sweeping motion (Lane & Grosjean, 1980). See Figure 5-7.

Within this rich language system are specific techniques for establishing and changing tense patterns. Although the English language indicates time and tense through verb usage, American Sign does not. ASL allows for the time or tense to be established at the initiation of the conversation and does not require mention of it again until the tense changes. In order to establish tense, one incorporates a "time line." Frishberg and Gough (1973, cited in Lane & Grosjean, 1980) describe this line as passing along the side of the body from behind the head to a distance no greater than the full extent of the arm in front of the body, passing just below the ear.

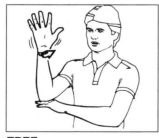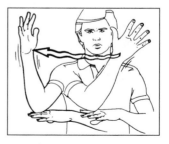

TREE

FIGURE 5-7   **Use of Reduplication: Changing a Noun from Singular to Plural**

(Sign illustrations from *A Basic Course in American Sign Language* by Humphries, Padden, & O'Rourke. Courtesy of T.J. Publishers, Inc., 817 Silver Spring Ave., Silver Spring, MD 20910)

- *Present tense* is indicated by the space immediately in front of the speaker.
- *Near future tense* can be communicated by extending the hands slightly more forward; by extending the hands out a greater distance from the body, one can achieve the concept of *distant future.*
- To communicate *past tense,* the signs are delivered toward the back of the body. *Near past* is signed in the space above the shoulder just about in line with the ear, and *distant past* can be indicated by signing back over the shoulder.

If the speaker does not indicate a time frame at the onset of the conversation, one assumes that the information being expressed pertains to present tense. See Figure 5-8 for an illustration of the time line.

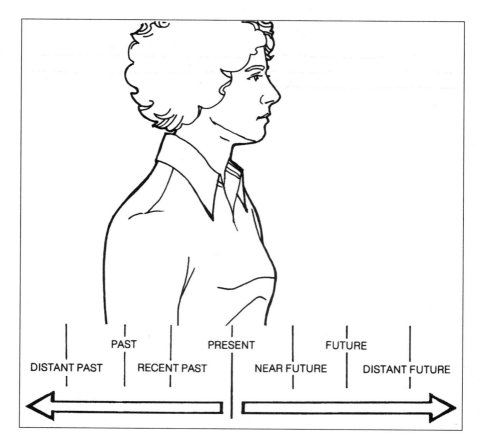

FIGURE 5-8 **Time Line Used in ASL to Indicate Tense**

(Courtesy of Baker & Cokely, 1980. Reprinted with permission.)

CONTACT SIGNING (CS)—A LANGUAGE BRIDGING THE GAP

Because language serves as our communication link with our environment, members must be able to adapt to the mode being utilized in order to express their ideas. When deaf individuals fluent in ASL encounter hearing individuals who are skilled in English, a common ground of communication must be established. As in other foreign languages, when two variant groups seek to interact with each other, a system of language exchange must be developed. The system in foreign languages is referred to as a pidgin.

A pidgin is a language that develops when individuals who are not familiar with the other's language attempt to communicate with each other. It is not a native language but one that typically combines certain vocabulary items and grammatical structures from the native languages of each group.

When establishing a midground for communication between those who converse in ASL and those who rely on a form of signed English, a Pidgin Signed English or Contact Signing can be employed. When this occurs the communication mode can assimilate strong characteristics of ASL or reflect a more English base. This provides deaf and hearing individuals with the opportunity to share their messages, with each other.

CS becomes the middle ground for communication between deaf individuals whose native language is ASL and hearing individuals who are familiar with ASL, but not fluent in it. By placing CS on a continuum, one is able to see how it interrelates with the other language bases. See Table 5-2.

Although home signs appear on one end of the continuum and variations of signed English systems occur at the opposite end, one must not lose sight of the fact

TABLE 5-2 An Overview of American Sign Language as It Relates to the English Language

			English Language Sign System used to represent English
Home Signs	American Sign Language (ASL)	Contact Signing	Signed English
Gestures			Signing Essential English (SEE I)
Minimal Language Skills			Signing Essential English (SEE II)
			Linguistics Of Visual English (L.O.V.E.)
			Manually Coded English (MCE)

that there are only two discrete language systems being presented—the other communication modes are overlaps of each system and are describable in terms of current variation theory in linguistics.

The hearing person's command of ASL and the situation in which communication occurs may determine to what extent ASL is utilized when conversing with deaf individuals. Professionals in the educational arena often prefer to utilize a more English-based signing system, similar to PSE. Those who work within social service agencies and religious settings (depending on their sign backgrounds and how they acquired the language) may gravitate toward a more formal ASL format. Figure 5-9 illustrates those factors that influence the use of CS. One's command of the language and the environment in which the conversation takes place will influence the style of communication that is employed. See Figure 5-9.

In general, individuals who utilize ASL are members of the Deaf community, and they share in the culture that belongs to deaf people. Hearing individuals interacting with those who are deaf tend to communicate in a pidgin style reflective of their understanding and acceptance of American Sign Language.

As previously emphasized, ASL has been developed by deaf people for communication within the Deaf community. It is used for social exchanges of information and with few exceptions is not used in the area of education. The educational arenas are dominated by a majority of hearing people who are generally not fluent in ASL and therefore resort to a more English format when expressing themselves via signing (Allen & Woodward, 1986).

Because the main focus of education is to provide children with the acquisition of spoken and written English, very little emphasis or instruction, if any, in American Sign Language is provided. Although the school may adopt a manual communication philosophy, it is generally housed within the confines of a signed English base.

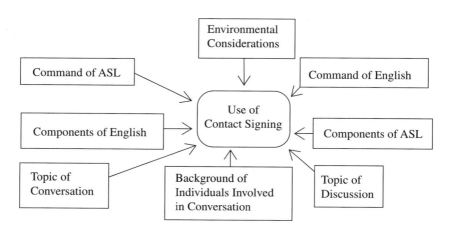

FIGURE 5-9 **Factors That Influence the Use of Contact Signing**

MANUALLY CODED ENGLISH SYSTEMS

Individuals working closely with the Deaf community (more specifically, those involved in the educational domain), have searched for a way to bridge the communication gap between the hearing and Deaf populations. Because so few hearing people sign, and written expression is utilized to exchange information, professionals have attempted to devise special signed systems, thus enhancing the English base of those who are hearing impaired.

Signed English

Because American Sign Language (ASL) is a foreign language, it is not possible to speak English while simultaneously signing in ASL. As a result many parents are opposed to their children learning this language. To remedy the language differences, signed English was developed to provide a sign system in which words could be signed in the same order as they appear in an English sentence (Bornstein et al., 1983).

Signed English incorporates two types of visual representations, sign words, and fourteen sign markers. Within this system, a sign word can be used alone or in conjunction with a sign marker. These markers with the exception of one (the one that stands for "opposite of") always appear at the end of the sign word.

Sign markers are incorporated to reflect changes in verb form, number, possession, and so forth (Bornstein et al., 1983, p. 12). See Figure 5-10.

In the event a signer wishes to change from present to past tense, as in "cook" to "cooked," the sign word is signed first followed by the regular past tense marker. In addition, singular nouns can become plural by adding the "s" marker as in "cat" and "cats." See Figure 5-11.

Seeing Essential English (SEE I)

In the 1960s, David Anthony, a deaf man himself, devised a system whereby English could be presented visually to deaf children the way hearing children hear it. Within this system, Anthony proposed that every English word would have a sign. He further developed a method incorporating signs for parts of words and suggested that signs should be delivered in the spoken word order. In essence, he developed signs for morphemes.

Linguistics of Visual English (L.O.V.E.)

A spin-off of the group utilizing SEE I was a system developed by Dennis Wampler. His philosophy centered around the idea that signs should be presented in the symbols that Stokoe had developed as opposed to descriptions or drawings of the signs. To accomplish this, he developed the Linguistics Of Visual English system. His philosophy also stated that a word should be signed the same way regardless of its content.

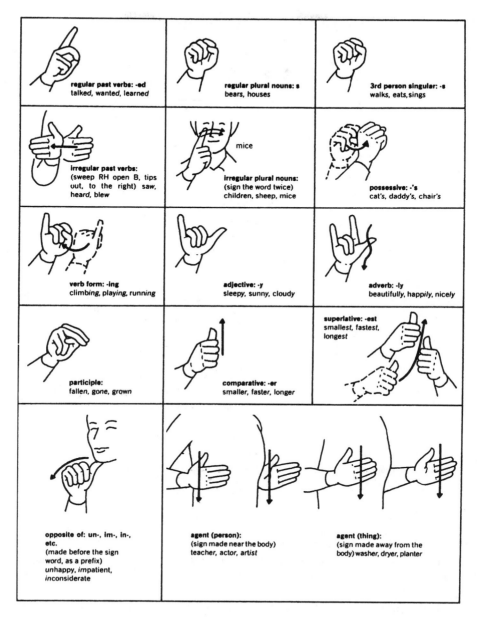

FIGURE 5-10 **Signed English Markers**

(Reprinted by permission of the publisher, from Bornstein, Saulnier, Hamilton, editors, *The Comprehensive Signed English Dictionary* (1983): 13,81. Washington, DC: Gallaudet University Press.)

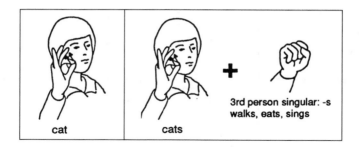

FIGURE 5-11   **Changing the Sign "Cat" to "Cats"**
Using the Sign Marker

(Reprinted by permission of the publisher, from Bornstein, Saulnier, Hamilton, editors, *The Comprehensive Signed English Dictionary* (1983): 13,81. Washington, DC: Gallaudet University Press.)

Although this system was developed in 1972, it is not used widely today. This is due, in part, to the fact that there is a lack of materials that can be easily accessed (Baker & Cokely, 1980, p. 66).

Signing Exact English (SEE II)

In the early stages of developing SEE I, a group of individuals worked together with David Anthony. However, because of some philosophical differences the group divided. Later, three of the members worked together to develop a signed system with one basic objective in mind: They wanted to ease the basic acquisition of English by deaf children. This system, developed by Gerilee Gustason, Donna Pfetzing, and Esther Zawolkow, introduced initialized signs into the sign system and also added signs where none were previously available. The result is referred to as "Signing Exact English," or SEE II.

ROCHESTER METHOD

A much older system that dates back to 1919 and was introduced by Zenus F. Westervelt, then superintendent at the Rochester School for the Deaf, is referred to as the Rochester Method.

It was originally called "The Great Innovation," a system that is based on fingerspelling spoken or written English words. Fingerspelling, also referred to as dactylology, is a procedure whereby one handshape is incorporated for each letter in the alphabet. There are twenty-six handshapes that correspond to the twenty-six letters in the alphabet. See Figure 5-12.

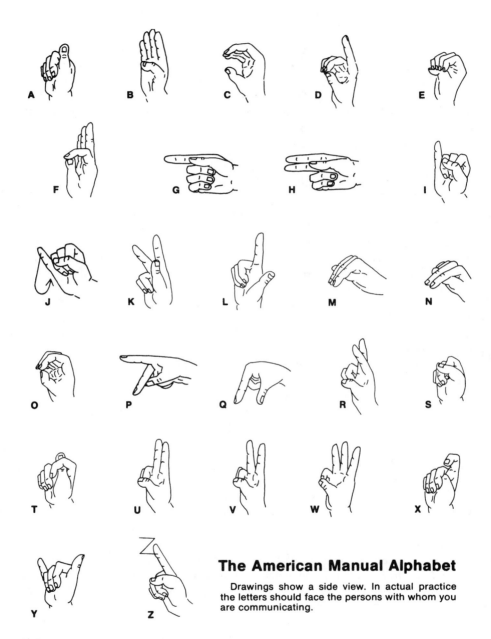

The American Manual Alphabet

Drawings show a side view. In actual practice the letters should face the persons with whom you are communicating.

FIGURE 5-12 **The American Manual Alphabet**

(From *The Joy of Signing,* Dr. Lottie L. Riekehof. Copyright 1978 by Gospel Publishing House. Used with permission.)

Fingerspelling is a manual representation of the language that is spoken. Therefore, it has no separate syntax, morphology, phonology, or semantics; rather, it is dependent on the linguistic structure of the language it is representing (Wilbur, 1987, p. 270). As words are formed and messages are conveyed, they are spelled out in much the same way as one would spell words incorporating Braille or a Morse Code system.

Although the original system did not incorporate a signed vocabulary system but relied exclusively on fingerspelling, it has been modified to meet the communication needs of individual students and is in use at the school today.

TOTAL COMMUNICATION

Throughout the 1960s when new systems were being developed and school boards were trying to determine which method to adapt to their program, another term surfaced. It quickly became a catchphrase in the professional community. The phrase that received a great deal of attention was referred to as "total communication." The individual who initially proposed this system was Roy Holcomb who later became known as the "Father of Total Communication."

This philosophy was initially embraced by the Maryland School for the Deaf and by 1976 the members of the Conference of Executives of American Schools for the Deaf provided this term with an official definition: "Total Communication is a philosophy requiring the incorporation of appropriate aural, manual, and oral modes of communication in order to insure effective communication with and among hearing impaired persons" (Gannon, 1981, p. 369).

By 1976, two-thirds of the schools for the deaf had incorporated this philosophy for instructional purposes. However, the form of manual communication and the extent to which it is utilized still varies in the United States today.

ORAL COMMUNICATION

When one traces the formal beginnings of education of deaf students in the United States, it becomes apparent that throughout the early years the vast majority of the schools embraced the manual philosophy. Only two schools in the 1800s are known to have incorporated oral philosophical methods.

Although periodic attempts were made to teach articulation and speechreading, most of the efforts were focused on the hard-of-hearing. Throughout the early years two movements surfaced. One favored combining the oral method with the manual mode; the other stressed an oral-only approach.

Due to the heavy emphasis placed on manual education, some parents and educators felt that no effort was made, or only a minimal attempt was sustained, to teach articulation in the schools. As a result they formed a group that influenced the establishment of the pure oral schools in this country.

Alexander Graham Bell, who has been identified as the father of American oralism, was highly instrumental in the early establishment of oral schools in the United

States. The foundation for establishing these schools was based on Bell's philosophy in which he stated:

> *In many of our schools the principle is adopted that no word shall be presented in writing until after the child can read it from the mouth. That is what is meant by the pure oral method in our country. (Scouten, 1984)*

Because some parents and educators felt that it was essential for deaf children to learn to lip-read and to speak, they formed a coalition to outlaw manual communication in the schools. As a result, when the Second International Congress on Education of the Deaf was held in Milan, Italy, in 1880, those individuals attending who were supporters of oral education voted to restrict the use of sign language within the deaf education environment. This meeting was a landmark event that helped change the course of deaf education in this country.

Based on this conference, some schools became exclusively oral while others incorporated a "combined approach." That is, they continued to use manual communication, while at the same time they added a curriculum incorporating the instruction of speech and speechreading. Although the emphasis on oralism was placed in the primary division, those schools embracing the combined approach continued to use sign and fingerspelling at the upper grade levels.

Individuals supporting oralism felt the need for the hearing impaired population to be able to acquire speech and speech-reading skills and felt by succeeding in this area, they would be able to transfer their knowledge into written expositions. By preparing them to function accurately in these three modes, it was determined that a smooth system for communication would transpire.

CUED SPEECH

Cued speech, developed by R. Orin Cornett, is based on the hypothesis that several of the speech sounds in our spoken language look similar when produced on the lips. By providing the hearing impaired person with a visual indicator of what sound is being produced, fuller comprehension can be achieved. The purpose of this system is to overcome the limitations of pure oral/aural methods without deviating from or compromising any of the objectives that are inherent in the oral philosophy.

Cued speech consists of eight configurations and four positions of one (either) hand; these are used in synchronization with speech to produce, with the hands and lips in unison, different patterns representative of each syllable of the English language as it is perceived visually. Because different hand configurations are employed for different sounds, speech that might otherwise look alike on the lips can be differentiated through the assistive indicator provided by the cue.

In Cornett's system, there are 36 cues for the 44 phonemes of English. The vowel cues are represented by hand configuration. To achieve various vowel-consonant pairs, consonant hand configurations can be combined at the location where the vowel is placed. Although some of the handshapes are similar to those used in ASL, cues serve a very different purpose. Whereas ASL is a separate language, cues are only incorporated to enhance speechreading (Wilbur, 1987, p. 273). Cued speech is not intended to be viewed as a language system, but rather a communication tool devised to enhance speechreading and accurate production of speech sounds.

The chart on page 131 illustrates the handshape and the position for the various vowel and consonant sounds. It should be noted that the T Group cue is also used for an isolated vowel (those that occur without a preceding consonant). See Figure 5-13.

WRITTEN FORMS OF COMMUNICATION: LANGUAGE-TEACHING SYSTEMS

Within the realm of education of the deaf, the topic of communication generally conjures up thoughts of the oral/manual controversy. However, that is only one dimension of communication. The written aspect is one of vital importance when discussing communication strategies employed by deaf and hearing individuals. For regardless of what channel of communication is utilized in the school setting, the end result is information sharing with the "hearing world." Frequently the parties involved will enter into a written exchange of information.

The Barry Five Slate System

One of the early attempts to provide structure to prelingually deaf students' English writing skills can be attributed to Miss Katherine B. Barry, a teacher at the Colorado School for the Deaf in 1893. Ms. Barry's system originally consisted of the use of five separate columns, beginning on the left and including basic sentence elements: subject, verb, object, preposition, and object of the preposition. A sixth column was added later to accommodate the adverbial elements that, depending on the structure of the sentence, might shift its position. This procedure was soon adopted by several of the schools for the deaf in America.

Wing's Symbols

In the mid-1870s, George Wing, a hearing impaired teacher at the Minnesota School for the Deaf, was also exploring techniques that would help prelingually deaf students to master the essential elements of the English sentence.

In 1884, he wrote out his language system under the title "Function Symbols," which outlines the general plan. The symbols he devised to assist the students in developing cohesive English sentences were subsequently known as "Wing Symbols." Figure 5-14 outlines these symbols.

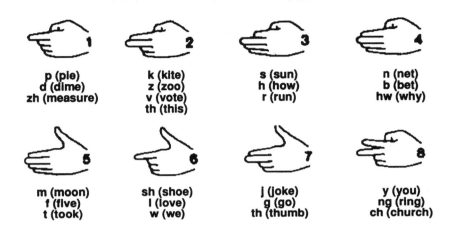

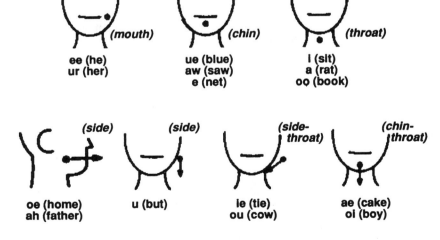

FIGURE 5-13 **Handshapes Used in Cued Speech**

(Reprinted with permission from *Cued Speech Instructional Manual* by Mary Elsie Daisey.)

Essentials, indicated by Letters:

Subject, ... s.
Verb, intransitive . . . . V⊃
Verb, transitive active . . . . V⎺
Verb, transitive passive . . . . ⎺V
Object, ... o.
Complement, ... c.

Modifying Forms, indicated by Numbers:

Appositive, ... 1.
Possessive, ... 2.
Adjective, ... 3.
Preposition Phrase, ... 4.
Adverb and Adverbial Phrase, ... 5.
Infinitive, ... 6.

Special Symbols:

Auxiliary, ... +
Conjunction, ... ⊃⊂
Ellipsis, ... *

Modifications: The object and complement of the infinitive and participle are distinguished from those of the finite verb by lines over the symbols (ō. c̄). Intransitive, active, and passive infinitives and participles may be distinguished by forward and backward strokes over the symbols, imitating like modifications in the verb symbol.

The above are all the symbols necessary to indicate the office of every word, phrase and clause in any English sentence. No additional symbols should be used until Grammar is taken up as a regular study. With advanced classes studying the rules of grammar a few further modifications may be introduced, e.g.

Nominative Absolute, Ⓢ; Nominative Independent, ⬛S.

Mr. Wing then provides his "four essential forms of declarative sentences," using his symbols to distinguish them.

   s V⊃
John walked.
   s V⊃ c
John was angry. (An angry boy.)
   s V⎺   o
John struck a dog.
   s ___⎺V
John was bitten.

Following "are some elliptical constructions which may be considered as combinations of these forms," e.g.,

  s V⎺   o c s ⎺ ⎺V c
He made the dog angry. He was made angry.

FIGURE 5-14 **Wing Symbols and Their Use in Sentences**

(From *Turning Points in the Education of Deaf People*, E. L. Scouten. Copyright 1984 by Interstate Printers and Publishers. Reprinted with permission.)

Prior to Wing's system, educators felt that students had to memorize information in order to understand it. Wing disagreed with this philosophy and set out to establish an alternative method. It was based on the premise that the essentials of a sentence could be taught and students could be instructed in how to vary word order. This provided the teacher with an instrument that could be incorporated for use in the classroom.

Throughout this system, the basics of writing are taught and students have the opportunity to make corrections. Although some of the previous language systems have become defunct, these symbols continue to be used today in a few of the schools for the deaf.

Straight Language System—The Fitzgerald Key

Edith Fitzgerald, a deaf woman, produced her work, *Straight Language for the Deaf,* in 1926. As an instructor of English in a school for the deaf, she was interested in developing a sequenced approach to the teaching of English. Her system was based on three premises: first, that the teacher must be acutely aware of the child's mental picture, thus providing him or her with language to make the picture clear; second, because the hearing sense is impaired, the child must be provided a substitute channel to permit expression of thought; and third, that deaf children could not be taught English with the same method by which a foreigner would assimilate English.

In her attempt to bring form and order to the English language, Ms. Fitzgerald utilized certain key words that appeared across the blackboard. These six key words were used in various combinations and were designed to help the children generate various sentence patterns. In addition, Ms. Fitzgerald developed arbitrary symbols to represent the eight parts of speech plus the infinitive. Figure 5-15 represents the symbols designated by Ms. Fitzgerald (Scouten, 1984, p. 267).

The six key words were intended to assist the students with proper placement of words and also to provide them with the opportunity for self-correcting instruction. Figure 5-16 illustrates the placement of the key words.

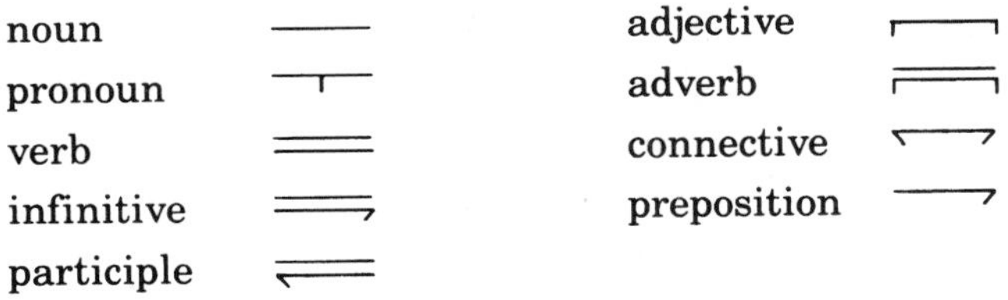

noun	——	adjective	⌐——
pronoun	—⊤—	adverb	⌐==
verb	====	connective	⌄——⌄
infinitive	==→	preposition	——⌄
participle	⇐==		

FIGURE 5-15 **Symbols Utilized with the Fitzgerald Key**

(From *Turning Points in the Education of Deaf People,* E. L. Scouten. Copyright 1984 by Interstate Printers and Publishers.)

FIGURE 5-16 Illustration of Placement of Key Words Using the Fitzgerald Key

Whose: / Who: / What:	What: / ( ) / Whom:	Whose:	What:	Whom:	Where:	For . . . : / With: . . . : / How:	Why:	How far: / How often: / How long: / How much:	When:
I see	=								
I saw	a top.								
I have	a ball.								
Emmitto has	a tie.								
Mary has on	brown eyes.								
I like		Ruth's	cap.						
James likes	bananas.								
I do not care for	bananas,								too.
Bonnie does not care for	honey,								either.
Mr. Murphy and	honey,								
Mr. Scott are	kind.								
Joan is	a good baby.								
Miss Scaright was	my teacher								last year.
It was	I.								
Miss Holt's									
coat is					in the closet.				
Betsy lives					in Dallas.				
The study hall looked	pretty								
The sun shone									
It is raining.									
It is lightninged									Friday night.
and									
thundered									all day yesterday.
It is	very windy.								last night.
it became	cloudy.								About ten o'clock
It snowed									for a long time this morning.

(From *Turning Points in the Education of Deaf People*, E. L. Scouten. Copyright 1984 by Interstate Printers and Publishers.)

This system became very popular for use within the schools for the deaf, both manual and oral, and was used extensively from 1927 through the early 1970s. At one point in time, the Fitzgerald Key was used in three-fourths of the schools for the deaf (Gannon, 1981, p. 170).

WRITTEN COMMUNICATION SAMPLES—A LOOK AT DEAF ADULTS TODAY

Within the United States today, the majority of schools for the deaf and institutions providing programming for hearing impaired students embrace the philosophy of Total Communication. Educators continue to search for techniques that will serve to enhance the production of written language for students studying under their tutelage. The challenge of selecting the most meaningful instructional method is still at the forefront of education of the deaf. As educators seek to discover the most beneficial method for instruction, students continue to proceed through the system striving to develop their communication skills. Although many of them develop the ability to express themselves fluently in American Sign Language, they find that they still experience difficulties when expressing themselves by utilizing the written English format. By examining a random sampling of writing samples of freshmen college students enrolled in vocational programs, one can gain some insight into written language patterns expressed by young deaf adults.

Writing Sample #1

> I'm happy my friend help with me. I think still help my friend and other people all. I and my friend play the pool and Baseball. My friend more fun with me. I alway take to my friend go the trip. I'm happy about my friend give to me for fun play and trip Prounble. I help with people and my friend abuoy around with people. I favor help and care me friend. my friend thank me for I alot help my friend all. I hope my friend fine Now. my friend run in my apt well I said can help you well my friend said alot provblem ok. well Now hilp with me friend. my friend happy Now clan relex yourself.

Writing Sample #2

> I really like {} college. The reason that is good for me. Also they have many student that I know. That school is good for me and keep my mind up and keep busy. they have good education in {}. Maybe I will try for A.A. class next year. Now I am taking M.B.T. class this year. Also that M.B.T. is good for in the future. that M.B.T. is the best pay and it is hard work. There is many different jobs in the U.S.A. I am not sure what I want like plumbing, electric, or building. I hope that I an succeful in the future. Also I want my family proud of me what I am doing this.

Writing Sample #3

I like dicide a topic to write about. I like main {} College. I will be to happy make good Education. I want to more Learn Englist, Read, I want to keep my brain, I don't need to forget my word. I want to show you Prove, I can do it Anything. I can to made a good future And a good my Life. I must to be on time in class. I don't playing Around in class. I can to Learn Either {}.

Writing Sample #4

Last family Saturday good tims I will enjoy plan fun thing diffened kind of trips betweent fell out area found in Tallahassee and Crawford for coundry just visit at slave less car. I want promise hold soon buy for car four door frist cheaking body look good try ask you Boss it or Back again not worry about think so plan next one week. This friday try again maybe Back come here. I hope will again make get can it.

Writing Sample #5

I want see my friend. I will walk go my friend's house. I knock to door. She walk open door. She happy see him. She let in my house. She said you want a drink. He said fine. She give he used drink. She said Love my favorite music. He said too mee. She and he are dance to music. He said you want with me go to movie. She said find. He open car for her. She said Thank you! She and he look funny to movie. Then she's house. He said bye and I Love You. She too -me! She is dial talk him. He is Ring call." He oh see her! She and he are long talk to call. She said Please Stop call ok. He said fine. He said her want go to boat. She said want with you! She is happy with you! She and he enjoy to boat and funny week!

Writing Sample #6

My name is {}. I born in {}, Ala when I was little girl. So my all family is Deaf but one is hearing.

Well my mom put me in school in Alabama School for the Deaf in Talladega, al. When I was six years olds so I stay there at the same school until I grow up now so I think I still at this school for 19 years

Well I really like this school to learn about good Educated.

Well my brother {} {} have been go to college in {} {} {} college so two years ago he have been graduate from this college so now I am the last baby in this family so I am going to college in {} {} that whole my brother go there before me.

Well, I am the lucky deaf family is my mom name is {} and I have two brother that are deaf is {} and {} but I have other one sister is hearing that she know how to use sign language real good to talk with my family then they said anything so I real enjoy be with my family.

So Well I have to close for now so that all I want to tell you.

SUMMARY

The controversy over the best system of communication to use with deaf individuals raged from the eighteenth century into the twentieth. The controversy split families, broke up marriages, and led to divorces. It embittered deaf children as well as deaf adults, leaving lifelong scars (Gannon, 1981, p. 361).

During the 1960s, the use of sign language became acceptable again, and schools embraced the concept of "Total Communication." The mode for transmitting language symbols became secondary to the concern with providing deaf individuals with the ability to develop their reasoning processes. It became apparent that "the symbol system is not the language, the symbol system is simply the bearer of tidings" (Schowe, 1979, p. 123). The real question became: What "tidings" are being transmitted? Professionals began to focus on communication systems and to question which techniques possessed enough versatility to provide for the transmission of information. Gannon addressed this point very eloquently when he stated:

> *The ear no more than the eye is the unique window of the soul, and no less. Each one, the eye and the ear can be developed by the aid of a truly synthesizing imagination, combining all the senses or available senses to give insight about a living human person and his world. (Gannon, 1981, p. 123)*

▶ 6

The Art of Reading

Reading is a form of communicating that evolves in infancy and unfolds gradually throughout one's lifetime. Through this dynamic and intricate process, we discover new information, entertain ourselves and others, and find solutions to life's problems. How do we learn to read? Why do some children find reading more enjoyable than others? What impact does deafness have on the reading process? How can parents instill a love of reading in their children?

LEARNING TO READ

Our initial exposure to text generally occurs during early childhood when parents begin labeling pictures with words. From this rudimentary inception spoken sounds are equated with a set of visual symbols, and the beginning of literacy emerges. Based on these early social interactions, the child's knowledge of the world expands, and the foundation for reading is established.

There is an abundance of research citing the combination of interrelated skills required for reading comprehension to develop (Andrews & Mason, 1991; Baron, 1992; Berk, 1998; Bouvet, 1990; Kelly, 1990; Owens, 1996). Most agree that these skills must occur simultaneously in order to accomplish this task. According to Berk (1998), reading involves using all aspects of our information processing system. In essence, this requires:

- perceiving single letters and letter combinations
- translating them into speech sounds
- holding chunks of text in working memory while interpreting what it means, and then
- combining the meanings of various parts of the text into an understandable whole. (Berk, 1998, p. 296)

Although researchers are not exactly sure how children acquire all of these abilities, they are in agreement that it is essential that they be able to recognize letters as symbols, thus enabling them to attach meaning to them. Making this connection requires a two-step process. First, the sounds a letter makes must be paired with the written "squiggles," and an understanding that the squiggles represent letters must occur. Second, the child must be able to attribute meaning to the letters. In essence:

> *Becoming literate requires a whole collection of skills: visual ability to distinguish easily between letters like b, d, and p; cognitive ability to relate the shape of a letter to its name and to the sound it stands for, and patience to work through the linear decoding process (Berk, 1998, p. 200).*

From these early associations, reading expands to envelope "more than isolated knowledge of phonetics, grammar and comprehension skills, [its goal becomes] to construct meaning from printed text" (Conway, 1990, p. 140). Thus, the reading process can be viewed as hinging on how the individual's experiential, linguistic, and cognitive knowledge interact with the printed material placed before him (Conway, 1990, p. 140).

According to Chall (1983), children progress through six phases while learning to read. He identifies the first one as the prereading phase, reporting that it is associated with early childhood, birth through age five. The phases continue throughout the school years and culminate with adulthood. Throughout each one, specific skills are introduced and must be mastered for reading comprehension to occur. By successful completion of the tasks, readers are equipped with a variety of literary tools required for ease in understanding written materials.

Prereading Phase (Birth to Age 5)

During this initial phase parents introduce books to their children. They begin by pointing to pictures and naming the objects for them. This is followed by a narrative whereby youngsters are introduced to how stories are structured.

At this time children are also exposed to print in their environment. This is accomplished through trips to the grocery store, drug store, and frequenting fast-food restaurants. In addition, most are entertained by television programming such as *Sesame Street* and *Barney,* by which their visual and auditory channels are bombarded with sounds and letters.

By the time children are three years old, parents begin reading stories to them, and through this repetition they start to recognize some of the words found in books. Thus, by age four, most youngsters can identify their names in print as well as a few words that they have memorized (Dickinson, Wolf, & Stotsky, 1993). Furthermore, at this time "approximately 80% recognize the word 'stop' and they all probably know McDonalds Golden 'M' " (Goodman, 1986).

Phase One (Ages 5 through 7)

As children progress through the second grade they continue concentrating on decoding single words found in simple stories. At this time they are relying on their oral language and their metalinguistic skills to comprehend the text placed before them. Metalinguistic skills enable the child to divide words into syllables, pronounce written words accurately, and understand what words mean out of context.

> *About half of kindergarteners and 90% of first graders are able to segment words into syllables. By the end of the first grade about 70% of the children can segment by phoneme (Liberman, Shankweiler, Fisher, & Carel, 1974).*

By the time children are 7 or 8, they must be aware of word boundaries, where one word ends and another begins, in order to become successful readers. Furthermore, these elementary students are characterized as having acquired "the graphemic, syllabic, and word knowledge they need to become competent readers" (Owens, 1996, p. 392). These skills, in turn, enable them to focus their attention on the visual configuration of words that assists them with word recognition skills.

Phase Two (Ages 8 and 9)

As children enter the third and fourth grades, they begin to analyze unknown words. This is done by examining words in context while also being attentive to the orthographic patterns of the words. Through the process of sounding out words, inspecting surrounding text, and scrutinizing accompanying pictures, graphs, and charts, they are able to decipher meaning.

Phase Three (Ages 10 through 14)

A major shift occurs in the reading process during the fourth through the eighth grade. At this time, decoding skills become entrenched, and the child is able to focus his or her attention on comprehending the written materials at hand. Throughout these school years, children develop their abilities to scan written materials while gleaning important information.

Phase Four (Ages 15 through 18)

As adolescents enter secondary school, they are able to incorporate higher level reading skills. During this time they draw on their ability to make inferences and examine varying perspectives and viewpoints found in the literature.

Phase Five (Ages 18 and above)

With all of their lower level reading skills firmly intact, adults are able to read a variety of materials and comprehend the meaning found within. This is due in part to their ability to integrate what they read into their existing knowledge base. By employing their critical reading skills, they can decipher the meaning of new words, grasp the hidden message of phrases by "reading between the lines," and gain new insights and inferences.

How does one move through these phases to become a competent reader? What strategies must be learned before one can successfully complete one stage and enter the next? What approach is most instrumental in ensuring reading success?

There are three major approaches to teaching reading: a phonetics approach or Bottom Up Approach, a whole language or Top Down Approach, and an Interactive Approach. Each of these theories purports specific techniques that are designed to develop and enhance the reading process.

Bottom Up Models

Bottom Up Models can be traced to the early work of Gough (1972) and later the influence of others such as LaBerge and Samuels (1974), as cited in Paul (1998). These models stress the importance of lower level perceptual and phonemic processing and their influence on higher cognitive functioning (Owens, 1996, p. 388). Using this approach readers analyze letters, decode syllables, and are then able to focus on the meaning of the text. Within this approach reading instruction emphasizes phonetics and the basic rules for translating written symbols into sounds (Santrock, 1999). Initially, simplified reading materials are utilized until phonological rules are mastered. Once this is accomplished, children are presented with more advanced books and poems.

When this model is incorporated, identification of letters and words is stressed with comprehension receiving very little attention. Based on a hierarchial philosophy, the reader must first be able to master sounds before he or she can advance to the next level, which is comprehension. Therefore, meaning is extracted through the use of decoding skills.

Throughout the first three grades, emphasis is placed on phonetics, with the assumption that once word recognition is automatic, the child can focus on higher level comprehension tasks. According to this theory, children experience difficulty reading because they lack the ability to make the connection between English speech sounds and printed letters. Therefore, printed texts remains abstract until the mastery of phonemic patterns occurs.

Top Down Models

Top Down Models, known as problem-solving models, focus on the cognitive task of deriving meaning from what lies in the reader's head. According to this theory, the individual forms hypotheses and makes assumptions about what he or she is reading based on his or her knowledge, the content of the material, and the syntactic structures that are presented (Owens, 1996, p. 388). Based on this theory, the reader comprehends "the largest units (meaning) and proceeds downward to the smallest units (letters and words)" (Paul, 1998, p. 35).

This model is couched in the philosophy that children do not need to be taught reading. Rather, they just require being exposed to reading and writing activities for them to develop ease in accomplishing both tasks. Instructional techniques associated with Top Down Models are identified as Whole Language or Language Experience Approaches. When incorporated, the goal is to provide children with constant exposure to text in its complete form. It stresses that reading instruction should parallel the child's natural language learning and that materials presented should be "whole and meaningful" (Santrock, 2000, p. 292). By presenting them with literature on a daily basis, instructors help children to appreciate the "communicative function of written language" (Berk, 1998, p. 297). Therefore, the child will be motivated to discover the necessary skills required to master the printed word.

Interactive Models

Interactive models reflect the principles found in several theories; however, all place an emphasis on the notion of parallel processing (Paul, 1998, p. 41). This concept is considered to be more accurate in explaining how both beginning and mature readers ascertain information.

The framework for Interactive Models lies in the premise that beginning readers are "text driven" while mature reading, is for the most part, "reader driven." When embracing this philosophy, the instructor recognizes the need for implementing both the Bottom Up and the Top Down Models simultaneously within the classroom setting. Paul (1998) describes this:

> reading is an interactive process involving the text, reader, and the reading context. The reader's goal is to construct a model of what the text means by using information from the text and the information in his or her head by considering the context of reading. (p. 41)

Using this type of model, both word identification and comprehension are stressed. Emphasis is placed on understanding the association between sounds and letters through the teaching of phonetics. By promoting this at an early age, it is postulated that these skills can then be incorporated into the Top Down Model in which comprehension is stressed.

Furthermore, this approach stresses that instruction should capitalize on the prior experiences of the reader. Within the classroom setting, questions are asked, and the use of "semantic maps" are incorporated. Semantic maps involve a series of questions through which one can demonstrate vocabulary and key points contained in a story. This enables the reader to organize information and store important points in his or her memory.

In essence, by incorporating this approach, readers are presented with a balance between word identification and comprehension skills while using their previous experiences to comprehend meaning embedded in the text (Paul, 1998, pp. 45–47).

Regardless of the approach that is applied, the ultimate goal is to equip the child and later the adult with the ability to construct meaning from printed text. Individuals must be able to extract information from their personal experiences and relate it to their linguistic and cognitive knowledge bases. When this interaction occurs, perceptions can be formed, and comprehension can be facilitated.

For some, learning to read is an exciting, challenging, and enjoyable adventure. Once the connection between words and meaning is formed these children's worlds are expanded and their horizons are broadened. They thoroughly enjoy having someone read to them and later relish selecting their own materials.

However, not all children and adults share this passion for reading. For some, it becomes an arduous task, filled with struggles and frustration that renders very few, if any, rewards. When this occurs, reading becomes a chore associated with a negative connotation, soon to be discarded once the school years are completed.

Volumes have been devoted to explaining why some children become successful readers while others do not. These texts generally agree that the potential for reading success lies in the ability children have to equate their oral language skills with their metalinguistic competencies. These skills "enable the child to decontextualize and segment linguistic material" (Owens, 1996, p. 292). Thus, reading can be facilitated.

What happens when sounds are not received through audition? What impact, if any, does this have on the reading process? Do some deaf children, regardless of their hearing loss derive the same amount of pleasure from reading as their hearing contemporaries?

THE IMPACT OF DEAFNESS ON READING DEVELOPMENT

Reading can become one of the most essential skills a deaf individual possess in his or her tool box. In a world where oral communication can become thwarted and fluency in sign language is limited to a small percentage of the hearing population, one must resort to reading and writing in order to engage in interactive communication. What role does deafness play in the development of reading skills? As deaf children progress through the various phases of reading, what do they accomplish?

Impact of Deafness During the Prereading Stage

Deaf children, who are born into families of deaf parents, experience language and reading in much the same fashion as hearing children with hearing parents. From the onset, mothers converse with their deaf infants with the same ease in communication that is shared between their hearing counterparts. They continually sign to their children, in much the same manner as hearing mothers talk to their infants, initially not caring if they are understood. Whether they are changing a diaper or conversing with another adult, the child is privy to observing signed communication. This, in turn, provides the early basis for language development. In the months that follow, they observe their children signing and assist them in accurate sign production. This parallels the practice followed by hearing mothers who listen to their children's early expressions of speech sounds and later mold and modify these vocalizations into articulate speech. This affords both groups of children with the opportunity to be observed and have their speech or signs corrected, therefore, enabling them to produce a recognizable form of their language (Bouvet, 1990).

Studies conducted by Andrews and Zmijiewski (1997) indicate that deaf parents who actively read to their children are instrumental in fostering literacy. From this early age their children are exposed to books and reading. These parents secure the attention of their children, point to illustrations found within the book, connect the pictures and later the words to signs, and relate the content of the story to the child's life experiences. Through a combination of mime, gestures, sign, and fingerspelling the child begins to develop vocabulary, cultivate concepts, and grasp the meaning of printed materials.

By twelve months of age hearing children generally produce their first words, and between 18 and 24 months they acquire a rudimentary syntax. They are able to combine two-word sentences and add word endings indicating tense and number. The same holds true for deaf infants. By 12 months they are producing one word signs. They also begin entering the two-word stage between 18 and 24 months (Meier, 1991). Studies conducted by Bonvillian and his colleagues have reported that signing children of deaf parents had acquired a ten-sign vocabulary by a mean age of 13.2 months, approximately two months earlier than the hearing infants reported in a study by Nelson (Meier, 1991, p. 65).

By age three the child is capable of developing a link between fingerspelled letters and the orthographical system of print that can be used as a means of encoding written words (Padden, 1990). Throughout this process, the mother questions the child about the story. This provides her with an interactive tool to assess her child's understanding of the words found within the book. By reading and questioning their children, they provide them with exposure to language, information, and a broad array of experiences. Through these early interactions children develop a foundation upon which later reading experiences will be based.

However, most deaf children are born to hearing parents. They reside in homes where communication can become challenging and oftentimes overwhelming. Under these circumstances, reading may revolve around speech or incorporate minimal signs and therefore it becomes less than meaningful for the child. Parents may elect to use oral communication with their children. If this channel becomes ineffective, they may feel they are ill-equipped and abandon the task altogether. Bouvet's (1990) insights on deafness as a "shared handicap" are very poignant; the implications for reading, significant.

This eagerness to "make" the deaf speak at any cost can also be explained by a fact we might not want to acknowledge: deafness is a shared *handicap. Deafness is different . . . from blindness or paralysis. One doesn't become blind with the blind or paralyzed with the paralyzed. We can see for the blind to guide them, and walk for the paralyzed, but we can't speak for the deaf . . . The deaf child is not like a blind person who is seen though he cannot see; the deaf person not only can't hear, but is not heard . . . which puts—deaf and hearing alike—in the* same *predicament. (p. 86)*

When deafness is diagnosed in a child, it is the mother who "loses" her speech. The knowledge that her child is deaf squelches her anticipation of the infant's speech and makes her feel that she can no longer connect with her baby—her words won't get through. Consequently, she herself becomes communicationally handicapped, unable to speak naturally to her child. (p. 108)

When these feelings emerge, prereading tasks may take a "back burner" to fundamental communication strategies, thus stifling the progression of reading readiness. As a result, these children often arrive at school with a weakened language base, limited meaningful incidental learning experiences, and marginal fluency in either English or sign language.

Impact of Deafness During Phase One

During the first three years of formal education, children are bombarded with language. From the early recognition of vocabulary words to the comprehension of basal readers, they are expected to work through the maze of printed text as they decipher an array of syntactical structures.

Deaf children of deaf parents generally arrive at school with ASL in tow, only to discover that their native language is not acceptable or understood (Lane et al., 1996). Although they possess a wealth of experiences and have been exposed to storytelling, their channel for literary expression becomes thwarted. It is as though they have landed on foreign soil that embodies a totally different set of expectations.

Deaf children of hearing parents repeatedly arrive with limited, if any, English skills and, oftentimes, even fewer sign skills. This, coupled with their fragmented background knowledge, gleaned from books and incidental information, does not prepare them for what lies ahead. Often raised in homes where the focus is on spoken communication, the child is presented with words from which they can derive some meaning. However, when these same words are "strung together" in a sentence, they find that they are unable to extract meaning from them. These youngsters also find themselves at a disadvantage when they enter the door of the classroom.

Reading curricula are based on the premise that children arrive at school with English language intact. Therefore, when both of these groups embark on their educational journey, they are met with preexisting expectations that they are ill equipped to meet. Like all children, they must possess the necessary literary knowledge required to decipher words and sentence structures. This information is needed for devising predictive and general application strategies for making text intelligible. Furthermore, they must have a general "working knowledge" of the world around them. This is imperative for deriving meaning from printed materials, thus enabling them to restructure this information into a form that they can understand (Lane et al., 1996, p. 284). If these preliminary skills are not intact, they may find their early school years devoted to mastering these tasks before they can become active, instead of passive, readers.

Impact of Deafness During Phase Two

Children in third and fourth grade analyze unknown words, pay attention to words in context, and look for clues in pictures and graphs. Their ability to read more complex sentences increases as new materials are placed before them. They become sensitive to the orthographic structure of new words and rely on their phonological skills to sound them out. In essence, they incorporate skills from both the Bottom Up and the Top Down Models.

Do deaf children incorporate these same strategies as they progress through the school system? Research indicates that while some prelingually and profoundly deaf individuals who are skilled readers find phonological recoding beneficial, the majority of those with average reading abilities do not (Kelly, 1993). Hanson and Fowler (1987) indicate that students exposed to intensive oral communication and speechreading may acquire a sound-based strategy for reading. However, Hanson (1991) emphasizes that the phonological information these individual's receive may not be comparable to that held by hearing readers. Due to the fact that this information is received visually instead of auditorily, it may be distorted and, therefore, contribute to spelling deficiencies.

Other Bottom Up methods include the ability to use orthographic strategies. These readers rely on sight reading to recognize words. When this skill is employed, alphabetic information about the words is stored in memory. Then the task of reading becomes one of "automatic" word recognition rather than a decoding task (Grushkin, 1998). When Quinn (1980) studied orally trained, severely to profoundly deaf and hearing subjects, she discovered that her more skilled deaf readers tended to pay attention to English orthography. Kelly's (1993) research further supported these findings. He hypothesized that although these advanced readers incorporate some phonological strategies, they are also attentive to the "conventions of English orthography" and that they maintain a more complete record of grammar during their reading. This has also been determined to be true of hearing readers (Grushkin, 1998, p. 187). These youngsters incorporate a variety of reading strategies that include phonological encoding and recoding, use of orthographic techniques, and contextual clues. Through a combination of these techniques they are able to remain on par with their fellow hearing classmates.

However, one must not lose sight of the fact that the students in the aforementioned paragraphs are above average in their ability to incorporate these skills, and they have the potential to remain on task as they complete each grade level. For the average deaf reader, the challenge of incorporating techniques found in the Bottom Up Model can be less than satisfactory.

Kelly (1993) found that average readers were not able to draw on phonological recoding when asked to demonstrate verbatim recall of sentences that had just been read. Furthermore, studies conducted by Hanson and Fowler (1987), Kelly (1993), and Moores, Kluwin, Johnson, Cox, Blennerhassett, Kelly, Ewoldt, Sweet, and Fields (1987) indicate that these readers struggle with lexical and syntactic knowledge. Furthermore, when they attempt to draw from a phonological code, they process sentences inaccurately or inefficiently, thus taxing their working memories and preventing effective comprehension (Kelly, 1995, p. 3). Because of these deficits, average deaf readers may find they have a difficult time comprehending English.

In essence, when they arrive at second or third grade with impoverished vocabularies, limited word attack skills, and poor strategies for drawing from contextual clues, they may find an insurmountable barrier to mastering reading. This, in turn, affects their ability to access other academic subjects that require a strong literacy base. As they complete this phase, they begin to lag behind their hearing classmates as they struggle to master new vocabulary and uncover meanings found within complex sentences.

Impact of Deafness During Phase Three

From fifth through ninth grade, students become deluged with an abundance of written materials. At this point they are subjected to everything from history to science, and basic mathematical concepts expand to include more technical domains where the fundamentals of algebra and geometry are tackled. At each of these junctures, students find themselves forced to rely on their mastery of English to enable them to grasp and decipher the content found in each of their subjects.

There are very few deaf students between the ages of ten and fourteen who arrive at the ninth-grade level with a mastery of English. As a result they are denied easy access into these courses. Studies indicate that their vocabulary scores remain low, and their ability to extract meaning from paragraphs is less than satisfactory.

Paul and Quigley (1994) researched the syntactic development of prelingually, profoundly deaf children by examining their results on the Word Meaning subtest of the Stanford Achievement Test. Their findings indicated that 10–12-year-olds scored at a 2.5 grade level; 13–15-year-olds scored at a 2.9 grade level, and 16–18-year-olds scored at a 3.6 grade level. These scores reflect similar results of previous studies conducted with school-age deaf children. By examining the increase in scores during the study, the researchers concluded that this population only gained 1.1 grade level throughout the nine-year period (Paul, 1998, p. 72).

Additional studies have been conducted that focus on deaf students' abilities to: select the correct definition when multimeaning words are presented (Letourneau, 1972); use the cloze procedure when determining the correct vocabulary word to put in each place when fill-in-the-blank sentences are provided for students to determine the correct meaning (LaSasso & Davey, 1987); and determine how they handle function words (words like *of, but,* and *by*) when attempting to comprehend paragraphs (Lane et al., p. 285).

Results from all of these studies indicate that there is a strong relationship between low vocabulary scores and low reading scores (Paul, 1998, p. 72.). These studies further reflect that deaf school-age children experience difficulty with selecting accurate definitions for multi-meaning words, and that they struggle with syntax as they attempt to integrate information found in words, phrases, and sentences (Paul, 1998, p. 81). Without an adequate understanding of vocabulary and syntax they are unable to effectively draw inferences from the material. Faced with this dilemma, they are characterized as learners who experience difficulties with both the Bottom Up and the Top Down Models of reading. They may lack the basic vocabulary required to rely on contextual cues, and their experiential base may be limited, thus prohibiting full comprehension.

As they continue through the educational system, the reading demands become more rigorous, leaving them in a plethora of words, where they are unable to glean critical information from meaningless trivia. With each advancing grade, the gap between hearing and deaf students widens as those who cannot hear attempt to rise to the demands established by the academic community.

Impact of Deafness During Phase Four

By the time students enter high school, they are reading for content as they gloss over incidental details. Scanning becomes a crucial tool as they determine what is and what is not critical information. Skilled readers, who are deaf, may enter this era prepared to accomplish this task. They complete reading assignments with little regard for the process it entails. However, this is not the case for all readers who are deaf. At this level, the majority are still paying attention to the details of reading and are focusing on reading for the sake of reading, not for deriving content (Lane et al., 1996, p. 286). Many are still struggling with limited vocabularies and a weakened grammatical base, thus, presenting insurmountable barriers to comprehension.

The reading levels for this population remain low, with those experiencing severe to profound losses struggling the most. Their ability to use the cloze procedure remains at a fourth-grade level and their mean vocabulary word scores at a 4.5 grade level (Moores, 1996, p. 226; Paul, 1998, p. 72). They complete their high school education equipped with minimal reading strategies.

Impact of Deafness During Phase Five

Literacy provides one of the essential keys that unlocks the door to higher education. One must possess a certain proficiency level to be granted admission and frequently hearing and deaf readers alike find they are in need of remediation. While some enter vocational schools and community colleges where they enroll in developmental classes, others forego formal training and enter the workforce. The route they take has a bearing on the reading material they will encounter.

The majority of college-age deaf students find themselves required to enroll in developmental reading classes. For some, remediation is accomplished in one semester; for others, repeated attempts are needed to master the material. Once beyond this stage, many continue to take advantage of support services as they are bombarded with the material contained in college texts.

STRATEGIES FOR ENHANCING READING THROUGH A MULTISENSORY APPROACH

Reading is recognized as a basic life skill, a cornerstone upon which academic success is built. Without it, formal learning is stymied and job opportunities are limited. The ability to read affects our personal, social, and vocational goals and is instrumental in influencing our views of ourselves and the world around us.

Throughout the history of deaf education, professionals have studied, researched, and developed classroom strategies for deaf readers. While some have focused on an oral approach, others have attempted to incorporate sign supported speech (SSS), also referred to as simultaneous communication, into the curriculum.

The oral approach is based on the philosophy that these children can comprehend written materials by utilizing their residual hearing and their speech reading skills. Classroom teachers view them as "hearing children" who experience varying degrees of hearing loss. Although most emphasize the value of amplification and speech reading, they see very little need for any additional modifications. These children are exposed to reading in much the same way as hearing children. Fortunately, for some, this approach is successful. However, for the majority, it is not.

Teachers, who rely on simultaneous communication, teach reading by signing stories in English word order while they speak. This provides the child with a word to sign representation of the text. The philosophy underlying this approach is that by providing sentences in this manner, children will "absorb syntactic, semantic, phonological, and pragmatic rules encoded in the underlying structure of language, beneath word-level meaning (LaBue, 1995). This is built on the assumption that deaf children arrive at school with the grammatical rules of English embedded in their communication system. For some, this is the case; they enter kindergarten equipped to respond to English signs when they are presented in English word order. In essence, "they understand those signs as if they were hearing English" (LeBue, p. 195). Although some students arrive at school possessing a Signed English base, many more do not.

When this method of communication is used, it is assumed that the rules of one language (English) will be conveyed through another language (Sign). Unfortunately, language does not work that way. These students receive a smattering of English through a contrived sign system, rendering them ill prepared to handle reading assignments.

Although both approaches are found to be beneficial for a few students, many others struggle, thus falling short of prescribed academic expectations. These students reach a reading plateau where they remain, even though they are routinely passed along through the educational system. Their low achievement scores continue to plague teachers and administrators as they search for solutions to solve the problem.

Recently, some educators have begun looking to the Deaf community for assistance. Recognizing the superior reading abilities, as evidenced in the test scores, of deaf children of deaf parents, these professionals have begun making a concerted effort to discover how they read to their children. Over the past several years, these inquiries have resulted in a number of articles being published. One, in particular, merits discussion. In the article "Principles for Reading to Deaf Children," David Schleper (1999) explores fifteen principles deemed necessary for reading success. Each of these principles is discussed below.

Principle 1. American Sign Language is used by deaf readers to translate stories.

ASL is the native language used by members of the Deaf community. Upon reviewing the literature, Lartz and Lestina (1995), Mather (1989), Schick and Gale (1995), Whitesell (1991), and Schleper (1999) notes that mothers and fathers, who are deaf, read to their children through ASL, not English. They use their language to make the stories come alive and hold the child's interest. When young children are first exposed to books, very little, if any, attention, is paid to English word order. Rather, emphasis is placed on the characters as they are identified and brought to life. By creating this early interest in books, the stage is set for future learning to occur.

Principle 2. Both ASL and English are visible to the deaf child as books are being read.

Andrews has written numerous articles (Andrews & Akamatsu, 1993; Andrews & Mason, 1986; Andrews & Zmijewski, 1997), regarding the importance of exposing deaf children to English and ASL while reading books. While keeping the printed text visible, parents sign the story, thus permitting the child visual exposure to both languages. Furthermore, deaf parents have been observed on a routine basis, pointing to text, signing the content, and then pointing to the words in the story again. From the onset children begin to relate signed concepts with printed words, thus fostering a connection between the two languages.

Principle 3. Deaf readers feel free to expand sentences found in stories.

Sensitive to experiential differences and the need to draw upon information found in illustrations, deaf adults use this opportunity to enlighten their young readers. Additional background information is provided, and the underlying theme of the book is conveyed by elaborating on the text. No attempt is made to render a word by word message; rather, the emphasis is placed on conveying the meaning of the story.

Principle 4. Stories are read repeatedly on a "storytelling" to "story reading" continuum.

Hearing and deaf children alike enjoy having the same stories read and reread. By exposing them to this form of repetition, their vocabulary, sequencing, and memory skills improve (Trelease, 1995). Through this repeated exposure, children become comfortable with the story; they begin to ask questions and their comprehension improves.

Schleper (1995) indicates that when a story is initially read, a great deal of elaboration may be required. However, with each successive reading, there is less expansion, as the signing becomes closer to the actual text. As this transpires, the ASL interpretation moves along the continuum to become a more direct representation of English text.

Later, this same process can be incorporated into the classroom. As children have stories read and reread to them, they develop background knowledge, enhance their vocabulary, and become familiar with the basic structure of the language.

Principle 5. Deaf children lead; deaf readers follow.

Children are far more receptive to reading when they are able to select books that they find interesting. Initially, children should be allowed to "set the pace." Although adults may emphasize specific pictures or draw the child into designated dialogues, the child should be permitted to turn the pages at will, spending as much time on individual pictures as he or she wants. With young children, the text is frequently ignored as the story is related through the illustrations.

While deaf parents may be comfortable adhering to the their child's time frame, teachers occasionally are not. Caught in the constraints of the curriculum, they struggle to get their students to adhere to their lead, only to realize that it is counterproductive.

Principle 6. Deaf readers take implied meaning and make it explicit.

Deaf readers "read between the lines" and structure their storytelling to incorporate implied meanings. By directly explaining what certain passages mean, the main idea of the story can be clearly relayed. This is an especially useful technique when stories contain morals that are embedded in the text. Intuition, coupled with personal experiences, enable deaf readers, through sign, to clarify the "true meaning" of the story.

Principle 7. Deaf readers use spatial signs to convey meaning.

Frequently, deaf readers incorporate sign/movement into a text, thus clarifying meaning while adding interest. A classifier representing a car might be placed on the car in the text where it is moved down the road; a rabbit might be shown hopping across a field, or a dog might be shown chasing a cat. Sometimes signs are made on the child's body, while other times they are expressed in their traditional locations. By varying sign placement children seem to connect with the story being presented.

Principle 8. Deaf readers make adjustments in their signing style to bring the characters to life.

Just as hearing readers alter the tone, intensity, and pitch of their voices to reflect the personality of the character, deaf readers likewise adjust their signing styles. Through facial expression, sign size, and intensity of sign movement, characteristics such as timidity, boldness, aggression, and compassion can be conveyed.

Principle 9. Events that occur in stories are connected to the real world.

Deaf parents capitalize on situations presented in stories by relating them to events in the child's environment. By drawing these relationships, children begin to realize that words found in books represent actions and feelings that they may have personally experienced or observed in the behavior of others.

Principle 10. Attention maintenance strategies are employed while reading books.

Eye contact, light shoulder or leg tapping, and gentle nudges are all used by deaf readers to encourage the child to pay attention. These communication strategies are part of ASL and are used in conversations as well as storytelling.

Principle 11. Eye gaze is used to encourage participation.

Eye gaze is an important component of ASL. While signing, it is incorporated to indicate whether one, or several, individuals are being addressed. Through eye gaze, children are alerted to the fact that the message or the question is intended for them.

Principle 12. Role play is utilized to extend concepts.

The use of mime, gestures, and role play can be instrumental in enhancing comprehension. When young deaf children experience difficulty following the story, deaf readers will role play the troublesome spots. Through this technique, clarity can be achieved and interest is maintained.

Principle 13. Sign variations are used to represent repetitive English phrases.

Children's books frequently contain repetitive phrases. While hearing parents may alter their intonation, pausing, and intensity while repeating these expressions, deaf readers may alter them completely. By exposing deaf children to different sign presentations, they are able to observe how repetitive phrases can be signed in a variety of different ways. This technique is beneficial for broadening sign/text representations as well as for expanding English word meanings.

Principle 14. A positive and reinforcing environment is established for deaf readers.

In order to promote involvement in any activity, it must be viewed as an enjoyable experience. Deaf parents, who are interested in promoting active reading on the part of their children, strive to make it fun. They use positive reinforcement to encourage active involvement while eliciting a warm, nurturing environment. By making these early experiences positive, the foundation for future reading success is laid.

Principle 15. Deaf children are expected to become literate.

Of all of the principles, perhaps this one is the most critical, for it provides the thread that weaves all of the other principles together. Based on the premise that when we expect our deaf children to read, they will, these deaf parents consciously strive to achieve this goal. Many of them love to read, recognize the value of early reading experiences, and want their children to adopt these same values and beliefs.

APPLYING THE PRINCIPLES TO THE CLASSROOM

It is critical that we enhance the quality of our reading instruction to ensure that deaf students are provided with the tools required to engage in this task. Regardless of the mode of communication selected, it is vital that a connection between printed words and their representative meaning is formed.

Andrews, Winograd, and DeVille (1996) have proposed that prereading instruction be implemented to assist congenitally deaf children with accessibility to English texts. They also recommend that teachers employ an ASL summary technique. This technique entails a six-step process designed to help students with reading comprehension.

In a study conducted by Andrews and her two colleagues (1996), prelingually deaf children, with severe to profound losses, ages 11 and 12, were presented with fables. The purpose of the study was to determine whether sign language summaries of the fables, when presented, would be effective.

Within the study, two groups were studied. One group was presented with the ASL summaries prior to reading the fable. The other group read the fable without being exposed to the technique. In essence, the ASL summary technique is "designed to build background knowledge in the reader, activate old background knowledge, and focus the reader's attention on information in the text before he reads the actual text" (Andrews, Winograd, & DeVille, 1996, p. 31). The six steps involved in this technique are as follows:

Step 1. The teacher gives a SUMMARY of a short fable in ASL.

Step 2. The student independently READS the fable.

Step 3. The student individually RETELLS all he or she can remember about the text.

Step 4. The student TELLS the MORAL LESSON of the fable to the teacher.

Step 5. The teacher and the student DISCUSS the student's retelling and moral-lesson response.

Step 6. The teacher FILLS IN semantic and conceptual gaps. (Andrews et al., 1996, pp. 31–32)

The results of the study indicated that the students exposed to the six-step process showed greatly improved skills in "retelling" the fables and in comprehending the moral lessons found within the reading selections. The steps, themselves, merit further discussion.

Students exposed to this summary technique are given the opportunity to integrate skills found in both the Bottom Up and the Top Down Models. In the initial step the teacher signs a summary of the story. This provides the children with background information as they begin to read. As the children read the story independently (Step 2), they ask for sign clarification of words they find in print. This provides them with an opportunity to connect the two languages.

As they move through the remaining steps, they rely on their recall and understanding to reiterate the story. Through a series of questions, the students learn to make inferences, thus expanding their general knowledge base.

The authors state that this approach is not limited to fables, but can be applied to reading other narratives, including short stories and novels. The key to its success lies in providing students with a language-rich environment whereby they can reap the benefits of learning to read.

SUMMARY

Reading is a complex process that evolves in early childhood and continues well into adulthood. It requires language mastery and the ability to process information. We relate what we read to our background experiences as we generate ideas, form insights and opinions, and gather information.

Numerous volumes have been written regarding the reading process. Theories, models, and approaches have all been explored as researchers and educators alike attempt to unlock the secret to reading success.

Teaching reading to deaf children poses a special challenge to parents and educators. Due to the ramification of deafness, instructional techniques must be modified to meet the needs of this unique population. Many of these successful modifications stem from the strategies developed by deaf parents, strategies they engage in while reading to their deaf children.

Deaf parents have been very instrumental in demonstrating that deaf children are not only able readers, but they can develop into very capable readers who possess a true love for literature. When interactive communication is accessible, and language instructors are prepared to adapt their methods of instruction, the stage is set for deaf children to master reading, thus giving them one more tool to use as they strive toward academic success.

7

Cognition and Intellectual Functioning

The complexity of the human mind has perpetually eluded and fascinated those intrigued with human development. For centuries scientists and psychologists have probed the mechanism of our intellectual functioning and abilities, attempting to determine how we *process* or *acquire* information and ideas (cognition) and how we reason, perceive, or understand knowledge provided by experiences (intelligence). This area of study has changed significantly since the early nineteenth century. Beginning with theorists such as Franz Joseph Gall, who attributed head shape to intelligence, this quest for understanding has progressed into the twentieth century with contemporary theorists, such as Howard Gardner, espousing the theory that we possess multiple intelligences (Gardner, 1983). Through the years, extensive research has been conducted in the area of cognition, providing us with insights into the development of our intellectual capabilities. Related to these investigations has been the examination of and establishment of intelligence testing. Although the two areas are related, each involves a distinct set of activities, different goals and procedures, and separate terminology. In the area of cognitive development the recent focus of attention has been placed on stage theories. Psychologists have attempted to compare experiences individuals undergo as they advance from childhood to adulthood. The origin of intelligence testing, by comparison, has evolved out of efforts to ascertain and quantify individual differences. These tests are administered providing scores that are indicative of the individuals' aptitudes in several areas of intellectual functioning. The areas of intelligence that are tested include the ability to deal with abstractions, to learn, and to solve problems (Sternberg & Detterman, 1986). Although these tests may prove beneficial in predicting academic achievement, they remain the subject of controversy, being viewed as limited in scope and biased in favor of middle class whites (Scarr, 1981).

The issues and theories surrounding cognition and intelligence are complex and are continually providing the scientist with provocative and challenging dimensions to explore. In the field of deafness these topics are of particular interest to those involved in the study of human development. By examining theories relative to cognitive growth and intellectual functioning and reviewing the research conducted with deaf individuals, insights can be gained into the thought processes of this specific population.

THEORIES OF COGNITIVE DEVELOPMENT

Theories of cognitive development provide a framework for studying the mental activities individuals engage in at various stages in their development. They focus on those internal methods that are employed when decisions and choices are made and plans are developed (Dworetzky, 1987). Within these theories, particular attention is bestowed upon those issues pertaining to hereditary factors, linguistic abilities, and the development of social skills.

Three psychologists, Jean Piaget, Jerome Bruner, and Lev Vygotsky, have all worked extensively in the field of cognitive development. Their theories deserve special consideration. Jean Piaget is probably the most noted for his testing of children and his stages of cognitive development. He has analyzed the internal mental structures of children as they respond to their environment. Jerome Bruner also views children as growing through the various stages of cognitive development. However, he feels that the interaction between significant others in the environment as well as the ability to process internally and store a symbol system is critical to growth. A third view of cognitive development can be attributed to Lev Vygotsky. His philosophy has also emphasized the importance of the social environment of the child. He feels that a person's culture is responsible for selecting the segments of information that they consider important; therefore, children's cognitive growth has its origins in the culture prior to the development of their psychological processes.

By examining these theories further, insight can be gained into the process of cognitive development experienced by children through adulthood.

Piaget's Theory of Cognitive Development

Basic to Piaget's theory of development is the tenet that cognitive growth is facilitated by two general factors: heredity and environmental experience. Heredity accounts for the basic nature of the physical structures and the ability to organize experiences and adapt them to the environment. This is accomplished through assimilation, accommodation, and equilibrium. He refers to experience as environmental interactions with the world and classifies them according to three experiences: physical, mental, and social (Biehler & Snowman, 1986).

Piaget's theory is based on the premise that children develop progressively more complex intellectual capabilities through the process of seeking an equilibrium between what they presently perceive, know, and understand, and what they see in any new phenomenon, experience, or problem (Gage & Berliner, 1988, p. 119). When individuals are confronted with new information, one of two events takes place. If they are able to incorporate their newfound information, their equilibrium is not disturbed. However, if they cannot absorb it, some intellectual work is needed to restore the equilibrium.

This intellectual process, affording them the opportunity to adapt this new information to their present knowledge base, is comprised of two processes: assimilation and accommodation. Although they are distinct processes, they occur simultaneously.

Assimilation occurs when individuals transform what they perceive so that it can be categorized into their existing cognitive structures. In cognition these structures refer to the representation or acquisition of a concept (Gage & Berliner, 1988). When information is received that they are not familiar with, such as a description of a rare tropical bird, their perception would change to fit an existing cognitive structure. The visual description of the bird would be transformed into the category of "birds" as part of the mental picture. Once the mental picture is perceived and the basic concept is changed to fit those cognitive structures previously in place, accommodation occurs. In this way, the person's perception of birds would be modified to include the image of a new bird with unique or unusual characteristics (Gage & Berliner, 1988, p. 119). It can be difficult to differentiate between the two processes. Assimilation and accommodation work in tandem with each other and become an integral part in the developmental process. Through this process ideas and concepts are assimilated and accommodated and a state of disequilibrium occurs. By creating a state of disequilibrium, the stimulus is provided enabling concepts to change through the accommodation process. This promotes intellectual growth and development. These processes also provide people with the ability to maintain a sense of equilibrium between themselves and their environment.

Thus, as individuals are challenged with new experiences and ideas and are forced to interpret, construe, or structure the nature of the reality to fit their own cognitive structure, they are engaging in the process of assimilation. In turn, accommodation is utilized as their ideas are adjusted, a memory is recalled, or a similarity or analogy is conjured up to facilitate a sense of reality. These two processes have a lasting effect on cognitive structures.

As individuals adapt to experiences they encounter, their cognitive organizations and structures gradually change as they go through the developmental process. In respect to an individual's organizational abilities (beginning with childhood), Piaget further states that as individuals interact with their environment, they are able to organize specific patterns of behavior or thoughts into schemata. These schemes can be behavioral or cognitive in nature. However, when children encounter new experiences that do not comply with an existing schema, they must adapt the information to their existing reference point. In order to achieve this, they must employ the process of adaptation. Piaget feels that individuals accomplish this by engaging in two subprocesses: assimilation and accommodation. As children are forced into making "everything fit," new schemata are created, and individuals are permitted the freedom to organize information at a higher level, thus fostering adaptability and stimulating learning.

Piaget believes that children are continually thinking and learning. In his perception, children are constantly and actively experiencing new knowledge and information and are reconciling it with their present knowledge base. As children continue to develop, problems they encounter become more complex and abstract and are reflected in the nature of the schemata they exhibit. Piaget further believes that as children work toward and acquire better forms of knowledge, they are working toward a state of equilibrium.

According to Piaget, organization and adaptation are invariant functions. This means that these thought processes function the same way for infants, children, adolescents, and adults. However, schemes are not invariant. They undergo systematic change at particular points in time. This results in real differences between the ways in which younger and older children think and, comparatively, in the way children and adults think. He further explains and classifies the differences found in the schemata by categorizing them into four stages of cognitive development. Table 7-1 provides a synopsis of the four stages.

TABLE 7-1   **Piaget's Stages of Cognitive Development**

Stage	Age Range	Characteristics
Sensorimotor	Birth to two years	Develops schemata primarily through sense and motor activities.
Preoperational	Two to seven years	Gradually acquires ability to conserve and decenter, but not capable of operations and unable to mentally reverse actions.
Concrete	Seven to eleven years	Capable of operations, operational but solves problems by generalizing from concrete experiences. Not able to manipulate conditions mentally unless they have been experienced.
Formal operational	Eleven years and older	Able to deal with abstractions, form hypotheses, solve problems systematically, engage in mental manipulations.

Sensorimotor Stage

The first stage incorporates infants and children up to the age of two years. During this time they acquire their understanding of the environment primarily through sensory impressions and motor activities, thus giving it the name "sensorimotor stage." Because infants are unable to move around a great deal during this time, their schemata are primarily developed through exploring their own bodies and senses. By the time children reach the end of the second year, their schemes are becoming more mental in nature.

Preoperational Stage

This stage encompasses the preschooler between the ages of two and five years and extends upward to children seven years of age. At this point children are able to master symbols, such as words, thus permitting them to benefit from recalling past experiences. According to Piaget, children are able to perceive symbols from mental imitation that involves both visual images and body sensations. The schemata of this stage build on the schemata of the previous stage. Preschool children are capable of more sophisticated thought processes than infants in the sensorimotor stage. However, they are limited in their ability to use their new symbol-oriented schema. Although children are able to form many new schemata, they do not think logically. There are three primary reasons logical thought processes do not occur during this stage. Piaget refers to these impediments as perceptual centration, irreversibility, and egocentrism.

> Perceptual centration *refers to the strong tendency to focus attention on only one characteristic of an object or one aspect of an event or problem at a time.*

> Irreversibility *is defined as the inability of children to understand the logic behind mathematical reversal or reversal of physical properties.*

> Egocentrism *refers to the fact that youngsters find it difficult, if not impossible, to take another person's point of view. At this stage it is important to note that Piaget is not implying that preschoolers are mean, selfish, or conceited. Rather, they assume that others perceive things in the same way they do.*

Concrete Operational Stage

Children from age seven through eleven are exposed to formal instruction that, combined with their informal experiences and maturation, gradually permits them a greater understanding of logic-based tasks. At this point, children become less influenced by perceptual centration, irreversibility, and egocentrism. They are able to comprehend tasks such as *conservation* (matter is neither created nor destroyed, but simply changes shape or form), *class inclusion* (constructing hierarchical relationships among related classes of items), and *seriation* (arranging items in a particular order).

Primary school-age children tend to react to each situation in terms of concrete experiences. They solve problems by generalizing from one situation to another situation that is similar. However, they are inconsistent in their thought processes until the end of the elementary school years. In addition, the concrete operational child is likely to be stymied when asked to deal with a hypothetical problem. During this stage, the typical 7-year-old is not likely to be able to solve abstract problems by engaging in mental explanations.

Formal Operational Stage

This stage is characterized by the child's ability to generalize and engage in mental trial and error by thinking up hypotheses and testing them "in their heads." The term *formal* reflects the ability to respond to the *form* of a problem rather than its content, and to form hypotheses (Biehler & Snowman, 1986, p. 118). At this stage children can read analogies containing material that is different and can understand that the form of the two problems is identical. When this occurs, the same principles are incorporated that permit the formal thinker to understand and use complex language forms, including proverbs, metaphors, sarcasm, and satire.

Piagetian theory emphasizes the nature of the child's internal mental structures with little attention being given to the demands of specific tasks. As a result, other theories that incorporate an information-processing model have been developed. In the information-processing model, the nature of the task to be mastered is frequently emphasized.

Bruner's Theory of Cognitive Development

Jerome Bruner has also examined the area of cognitive development. He has focused on the way children come to represent cognitively the world into which they are born. His theory places particular emphasis on one's language base and the individual's ability to communicate and interact with the environment.

Bruner purports that infants must begin to acquire a language system through which they can establish an internal information processing and storage system, capable of describing reality. Without this language system, which represents the world, the individual can never predict, extrapolate, or hypothesize novel outcomes.

In addition, Bruner states that intellectual development does not occur unless individuals have the ability to express to others, in words or in symbols, what they have done or will do. In summary, this is the essence of self-consciousness. Bruner states that exposure to systematic interactions between a tutor and a learner is vital in order for cognitive development to occur. Within his theory, being born into a culture is not enough; rather, a designated teacher must interpret and share the culture with the child.

Bruner feels that language is the key to cognitive development. He considers language vital to the learning process, as it is through language individuals communicate their conceptions of the world to others and question how the world functions.

Bruner sees this function as increasing in importance as one ages. He states that as people become older, language is employed to mediate experiences. Thus, the ability to provide linguistic mediation ties one event to another in a causal way, links new information to that which is familiar, and allows individuals to code events. This enables them to deal with internal representations.

Bruner also notes that cognitive growth is marked by the increasing ability to grapple with several alternatives simultaneously, to perform concurrent activities, and to pay attention sequentially to various situations. When viewing these characteristics of cognitive growth, Bruner further identifies three stages of growth reflecting the way children internalize the world around them. A synopsis of these stages is found in Table 7-2.

Enactive Stage
Within this stage, children understand the environment through actions. The stage revolves around touching, holding, moving, and manipulating objects. During this time there is no imagery.

Iconic Stage
By contrast, at this level there is imagery, and information is processed accordingly. Although children continue to make decisions based on sensory impressions, visual memory is developed. At this stage decisions are not based on language and the children are "prisoners of their perceptual world" (Gage & Berliner, 1988).

Symbolic Stage
Within this stage understanding through action and perception is replaced by an understanding of the world by means of symbol systems. Logic, language, and mathematics become integral parts of the cognitive process. Individuals are now able to compute formulas, comprehend metaphors, and store and retrieve vast amounts of information.

Bruner believes that children move from the enactive through the iconic and on to the symbolic stages of representation. However, he also feels that adults are capable of functioning in all three stages and that certain individuals are dominated by one stage more than another.

TABLE 7-2   **Bruner's Stages of Cognitive Growth**

Stage	Characteristics
Enactive stage	Child understands environment through action; there is no imagery of words
Iconic stage	Information is carried by imagery. Child makes decisions based on sensory impressions, not language.
Symbolic stage	Understanding occurs through a symbol system

Feuerstein's View of Cognitive Growth

Reuven Feuerstein, an Israeli educator, shares Bruner's view that cognitive growth occurs due to mediated learning experiences. He believes that although learning takes place through incidental interactions that occur in the environment, we also benefit from mediated learning. He defines mediated learning as "learning which is assisted by an adult who focuses, sharpens, elaborates, emphasizes, provides cues, and corrects as he or she tries to get the learner to understand and solve a problem" (Gage & Berliner, 1988, p. 104).

In order for children to possess the structural ability to adjust and adapt to life situations, they must achieve a level of cognitive competence (Scarr, 1981). In this context, structure refers to the cognitive/intellectual and affective schemes that enable individuals to adapt to novel situations. Feuerstein states that construction of these schemes is affected by two modalities of learning: direct learning experiences and mediated learning experiences. Through the constant bombardment of direct stimuli, individuals respond and their behavioral repertoire is expanded. In mediated exposure, direct experience with environmental stimuli is transformed through the actions of an "experienced, intentional and active human being" (Feuerstein, 1979, p. 110).

Feuerstein's (1979, 1980) mediated learning theory, consisting of both direct and mediated learning modalities, is perceived as essential to development. Like Bruner, he contends that through mediated learning the individual is able to benefit from direct experiences, which not only enhance learning but are essential for continued direct exposure to it. Feuerstein also contends that this type of learning is a prerequisite for the child to independently and autonomously make use of environmental stimuli. By engaging in such activities, the child is able to develop an attitude toward thinking and problem solving, enabling him to organize the stimuli in the world around him. Through a repertoire of actions, the mediating agent organizes and orients the phenomenological world for the child. Appropriate learning sets are transferred to the child by the caring person, and cognitive growth occurs.

Within the framework of cultural deprivation, Feuerstein has stressed that involved in the culture itself there is a lack of "intergenerational transmission." In this respect, the culture is viewed as being established and shaped through the intergenerational transmission of ideas as opposed to the concept that the culture found in ethnic subgroups deprives its members of the ability to learn cognitively. Feuerstein states that the culture is not responsible for lags in cognitive development but rather the lack of significant mediational learning taking place within that culture.

Vygotsky's Philosophy of Cognitive Development

Lev Vygotsky, a Russian psychologist, has attributed a special role in cognitive development to the social environment of the child. His philosophy revolves around the premise that children begin learning from the people around them. He further supports the premise that the social world is the source of an individual's concepts, ideas, facts, attitudes, and skills. He feels that a person's culture provides the stimuli that individuals become aware of and pay attention to. Vygotsky states that each culture selects different segments of information that they consider important, thus creating a unique social-cultural patterning of events. Therefore, cognitive development has its origins in interactions that occur among a group of people prior to the onset of psychological development (Gage & Berliner, 1988, p. 124).

Vygotsky emphasizes the fact that social interactions between adults and children influence the child's cognitive development. Individuals' personal psychological processes are dependent on their exposure to social interactions that are, in turn, patterned by a specific culture. In order for the child to grow personally, two factors must be incorporated. First, the adult involved in the social interaction must determine the child's actual developmental level and, second, it must be determined what the child can do without adult guidance.

Vygotsky expands upon this concept by stating that children's actual developmental level can be assessed by observing their problem-solving abilities without any adult help. In addition, projections of the children's potential developmental abilities are feasible when the children are working with adults. Vygotsky defines the difference in these two levels of functioning as the zone of proximal development. He further states that for children to undergo maximum learning, the individual responsible for instruction must enhance those functions that are in the process of maturing, that is, in the zone of proximal development.

Therefore, the key to cognitive development is to discover where the children are and lead them into more complex levels of functioning. Social knowledge acquired through social interaction becomes personal or individual knowledge; as it grows, it becomes more complex. The end product is the individual who can function successfully within a particular culture or community.

All three of these theories provide insight into the realm of cognitive development. How do they relate to the deaf infant as he or she progresses through the various developmental stages? Does inability to hear have any impact on cognitive abilities or does development continue in a similar manner as it does for hearing children? Is command of an English language system critical for development to occur, or is language a separate entity that is nonrelated to cognition?

EFFECTS OF DEAFNESS ON COGNITIVE DEVELOPMENT

The influence of deafness on cognitive development has been a fascinating and thought-provoking topic of study. Research has been conducted regarding the relationship between language and thought, problems related to the attainment of concepts, perceptual-motor processes, attributes of memory function, and the deaf child's ability to participate in evaluations consisting of intelligence and academic achievement testing (Meadow, 1980).

In the area of deafness, many of the basic issues with respect to cognition and intellectual functioning continue to be debated. Professionals representing the various disciplines have discussed the influence of heredity and environment on human behavior. The question of major importance is whether the lack of a major sense—in this instance, hearing—affects the way people develop and use their intellectual skills. The degree of hearing loss influences the amount of input received from the environment. This difference in environmental stimulation has sparked a vast amount of interest among professionals (Moores, 1987). As a result, a significant amount of research has been conducted by psychologists, linguists, and psycholinguists pertaining to the effect deafness has on cognitive development. Unfortunately, much of the work has been conducted under the premise that deaf individuals deviate considerably from their hearing peers and manifest multiple deficiencies in addition to their hearing loss (Conrad, 1979). Consistently, however, throughout the years the majority of these studies have found no differences between hearing and deaf children.

There are some studies available today indicating that the condition of deafness imposes no limitation on the cognitive capabilities of individuals (Moores, 1987; Ottem, 1980; Rittenhouse & Spiro, 1979). There is no evidence to suggest that a deaf person thinks in more concrete ways than a hearing person. Those studies previously purporting that deaf individuals reached a plateau in their ability to function intellectually were based on results utilizing test instruments that were inappropriate for use in assessing deaf populations (Martin, 1985). Deaf children develop in a similar manner as hearing children and progress through the cognitive stages from simple to complex, concrete to abstract, familiar to unfamiliar, and so forth. One can examine the various theories of development previously mentioned and reflect on the ways in which this development occurs. By reviewing the research within the framework of Piaget, Bruner, Feuerstein, and Vygotsky's theories, one is able to gain some insight into the cognitive abilities of deaf individuals.

Relating Deafness to Piaget's Theory of Cognitive Development

One of the key tenets in Piaget's theory revolves around the issue of equilibrium. According to Piaget, a sense of disequilibrium must be experienced in order for cognitive growth to occur. He states that one of the primary stimuli for disequilibrium at all ages is the conversation of other children who are cognitively more advanced and thus able to challenge the learner's current beliefs (Athey, 1985).

While equilibrium itself may be presumed to function normally in deaf children, the impetus for cognitive restructuring is probably attenuated because of a diminished opportunity for external disturbances (Liben, 1978). This attenuation may be caused by three factors. First, hearing parents of deaf children may not have the communication skills necessary to engage in an extended, logical communication exchange. As a result, they may circumvent complex communication by avoiding *situations of conflict.* According to Liben, informal comments by teachers, parents, and residential counselors suggest that there is a tendency for parents to avoid frustrating the child by acceding to the child's demands (Liben, 1978, p. 208). Therefore, the deaf child may not have the benefit of being involved in "conflict situations." This results in a lack of development that may inhibit the ability to perceive others' viewpoints, thus forcing the child to maintain a socially and cognitively immature egocentric perspective.

The second factor that can be noted as contributing to the diminished opportunities for disequilibrium to occur lies in the area of peer contacts. If deaf children do not have the opportunity to engage in conversations with peers who can challenge their equilibrium, their world is likely to remain undifferentiated (Athey, 1985, p. 24). It is imperative that children have contacts with individuals who are cognitively more advanced so that current beliefs can be challenged and learning can occur.

The third area influencing cognitive development lies within the school environment. In this setting, the children must be exposed to dialogues and encounter situations that will stimulate thinking. If they receive instruction primarily through a drill/lecture format, cognitive growth will not occur as readily. Frequently, in classrooms where hearing impaired students receive instruction, communication of a "give-and-take nature" is lacking. Interaction between the teacher and the students is minimal. A study conducted by Craig and Collins, focusing on communicative patterns in classes for deaf children, found that communication was overwhelmingly dominated by teachers.

> *As was true at all age levels and in all instructional areas, the teachers at the primary level accounted for the major portion of the expressive communication. During the intervals of language-dependent instruction, teacher-generated communication accounted for almost 80% of the relevant behavior observed. Of this, 75% was actual teacher communication and 25% was student response to teacher-initiated communication. Students, on the other hand, initiated communication less than 3% of the time observed and teachers responded to these attempts less than .4%. The remaining interaction was divided between "no communication" and "confusion." (Craig & Collins, 1970, p. 82)*

Bonvillian, Charrow, and Nelson (1973) reviewed several studies of deaf children in the classrooms. They found that deaf children were not deficient in intellectual ability. However, they did experience difficulties in processing Standard English. Further, when compared to hearing children, they showed significant differences in tasks requiring word-association techniques (Bonvillian et al., p. 30). Rodda and Grove (1987) have postulated on this research, suggesting that these results might be attributed to the fact that deaf children, when compared to hearing children, have less experience in dealing with tasks involving open-ended or undirected responses. They have hypothesized that such techniques are used less frequently because communication difficulties experienced between the adult and the child encourage the adult to use questions that require pointing, monosyllabic, or very brief answers (Rodda & Grove, 1987, p. 163).

The factors listed above pertain to an exchange of ideas and information primarily through communication and interactions with significant others. It is important to note, however, that cognitive development can and does occur separately from linguistic development. Some of the most notable research in this area has been conducted by Hans Furth. In research conducted with deaf children, Furth employed Piagetian theory in order to determine if logic and intellectual functioning abilities were dependent on language. Furth concluded that logical, intelligent thinking does not need the support of language, but language is dependent on the structure of intelligence (Furth, 1966, p. 228). It is important to clarify that at the time Furth conducted his research, language, by definition, referred to a form of oral or spoken language, rather than American Sign Language.

Extensive research has been conducted with deaf individuals involving tasks pertaining to Piaget's stages of cognitive development. Although consistent results have not always been obtained, it can be concluded that the majority of deaf individuals do not experience any difficulty in learning or discovering preconceived concepts in structural situations. In addition, evidence suggests they are able to shift categories with a normal degree of flexibility. However, when engaging in multiple categorization and rule learning, their responses appear to be more ambiguous. Research suggests that, for the most part, when deaf individuals are provided with explicit directions and training, they are able to shift categorization procedures. However, a number of investigators have noted that they experience difficulties when asked to do so spontaneously and may be rigid in their responses (McAndrew, 1948; Oleron, 1953; Youniss & Furth, 1966).

Within the formal operational stage of Piagetian theory, the performance of the deaf individual becomes less clear. It has been shown that deaf adolescents and adults can be taught how to use very complex logical operational principles. However, their ability to discover these principles on their own seems to be impaired (Furth & Youniss, 1965). Obviously, deaf individuals have the ability to engage in symbolic thought. However, due to environmental constraints, they experience a degree of difficulty in spontaneously acquiring these principles (Quigley & Kretschmer, 1982).

Relating Deafness to Bruner's Theory of Cognitive Development

The importance of significant others and how they interact with children is at the crux of Bruner's theory of cognitive growth. As children progress through the developmental stages, they encounter various individuals in their environment. These people have an impact on them and influence their ability to develop their mental faculties. Because of the communication barrier frequently existing between deaf individuals and others in their environment, cognitive development may appear to be delayed. Internally, there is evidence that deaf children have the capabilities to experience cognitive growth comparable to that of their hearing peers. The outward manifestations of the process, however, may be hampered due to conditions within the environment. This becomes apparent in the academic arena where deaf students may experience difficulties. The reason for student failure to grasp subject matter may not lie in the area of cognition at all; rather, the educators may not be capitalizing on the deaf student's strengths within the learning environment (Moores, 1987, p. 165).

Ottem reviewed fifty-one cognitive studies dealing with deaf subjects and found that deaf and hearing subjects performed equally well when required to refer to one set of data. However, when the examiner administered tasks that required reference to two sets of data, the deaf students functioned more poorly. Based on these studies, Ottem speculated that the difficulty occurred because the training received by the deaf individuals focused on teaching only how to communicate single events rather than how to deal with multiple units of information (Ottem, 1980, p. 568).

If, in fact, deaf individuals do not express certain blocks of information, it may be because they have not been instructed in a particular knowledge base and provided with appropriate strategies to access the information. In this case, again, the ability for cognitive growth is present but is not being tapped by significant individuals in the deaf child's environment. Research conducted by Karchmer and Belmont (1976) supports this notion. When Karchmer and Belmont administered a test involving short-term memory to deaf and hearing students, the test results indicated that the deaf students functioned at a much lower level than the hearing students. However, once appropriate strategies were taught, it was found that deaf students could function at the same level as hearing students. This seems to support Bruner's theory that cognitive growth is stimulated by those engaged in a teaching role within the child's environment.

In addition to the role teachers and the educational classroom play in one's development, the form of the parent-child relationship also significantly influences cognitive development. Hess and Shipman (1965) examined social class differences and forms of communication within parent-child relationships. Within the family constellation they identified two major types of maternal control strategies. One was referred to as the "cognitive-rational" control strategy whereby explanations or reasons were provided for rules or demands. The second type of strategy was identified as the "imperative-normative" strategy in which rules are given without justification. Hess and Shipman's findings suggested that controls that include rationales are more conducive to cognitive development than controls that are based on authority. The implications for deaf children of hearing parents is significant. Because hearing parents frequently experience difficulties in communicating with their deaf children, they may resort to the use of imperative-normative control strategies. Thus, the environment may be minimally conducive to cognitive growth.

Relating Deafness to Feuerstein's View of Cognitive Growth

Feuerstein's theory may also provide a framework for understanding the differential cognitive development within the deaf populations. Some studies have been conducted over the past twenty years in which deaf children of deaf parents are compared to deaf children of hearing parents. Results indicate that the deaf children of deaf parents perform significantly better on measures of educational achievement (Vernon & Koh, 1970), intellectual achievement (Brill, 1969; Conrad, 1979), and social behavioral adaptations (Meadow, 1980; Schlesinger & Meadow, 1972). Studies comparing the scores of these two groups and noting the increased performance exhibited by deaf children of deaf parents tend to reinforce the importance of mediated learning in the development of cognitive competence. Keeping in mind that 90 percent of deaf children are born to hearing parents who may struggle with communicating with their deaf child, the concept of mediated learning may serve to clarify and explain the differential cognitive development within this group.

Feuerstein discusses his concept of cultural deprivation by stating that in order for individuals to adapt to the external reality of their group, they must have adequate cognitive processes and autonomous exercise of control over the cognitive system rendering it flexible and modifiable (Feuerstein, 1980, p. 3). If these processes are underdeveloped, mediated learning must intervene in order to promote structural cognitive change within the culturally deprived individual. Without the quality and quantity of communication with other deaf individuals and significant others, voids in information may occur and may be reflected in inferior test scores in the area of test measurement. In the event that deaf children do not possess the communication skills to interact with significant others, they may refrain from asking questions. Other times when explanations are given in response to their questions, they may not understand the context of the message.

Research conducted by Nass (1964) may be reflective of test results when deaf individuals experience voids in information. Nass examined the ability of deaf and hearing children to draw inferences from statements based on varying degrees of experience (i.e., "how do leaves fall off trees?", "how is it that stars shine?"). The results of Nass's study indicated that deaf children (ages 8–10) had more difficulty than their hearing peers in drawing inferences from those statements that were not of a direct, experiential nature. Nass concluded that young deaf children had less adequate reasoning abilities than their hearing peers. However, Liben has suggested that these early differences experienced by deaf children can be attributed to a limited information base, rather than a deficit in their reasoning abilities. Lack of information must be viewed as separate from reasoning abilities (Liben, 1978, p. 205).

In tandem with the need to provide adequate information is the importance of utilizing role models for the transmission of knowledge. Those behaviors necessary for the deaf child to transcend egocentricity and enter into the realm of decentered perspectives are often ignored in the deaf child's education. Due to a scarcity of role models and inadequacies in the quality and quantity of communication, these appropriate behaviors may be lacking. However, as identification between model and child is enhanced (deaf child in contact with deaf adult), the entire process is presumably strengthened. Empirical work conducted by Mischel and Mischel (1971) further demonstrates the need for individuals to be provided with culturally similar role models in order for imitation to occur and enhancement to take place. This is particularly true of deaf role models, with whom deaf children can communicate at levels not found in interactions with hearing individuals. With the avenue of communication being optimal, the exchange of information can occur freely and one's potential for learning is enhanced.

Feuerstein believes cognitive development is fostered by the interplay of those environmental experiences, either direct or mediated, that impact on the individual. Although he does not blame cultures for lags in cognitive development, he does attribute these lags to a lack in significant mediated learning experiences. Because these experiences are communicated either directly or indirectly to members of society, studies that pertain to deaf individuals' abilities to process manual communication via a Manually Coded English (MCE) system or American Sign Language (ASL) merit special consideration.

Studies pertaining to deaf individuals' ability to process information via a form of manual communication have received considerable attention throughout the past twenty years. The researcher Best compared the performance of three groups of deaf children with varying exposure to signed and spoken language as they performed a group of classification tasks. Of the three groups, the hearing children performed the most effectively. Those deaf children who had received the most exposure to both oral and manual language performed better than those deaf children who had not had the benefit of both forms of language stimulation. All of the groups were found to progress through the same stages of cognitive development, even though the hearing children appeared to progress more rapidly (Best, 1970).

A study conducted by Morariu and Bruning focused on the ability of deaf individuals to comprehend various modes of communication. This study was conducted with deaf and hearing high school students and consisted of two experiments. The first task centered around tasks involving free recall. Both hearing and deaf students were provided with passages in English and ASL syntax through visual and printed materials. Although only the hearing subjects were able to comprehend the test items, deaf individuals not previously trained in ASL exhibited a familiarity with the syntax that was not exhibited with hearing subjects. In the second part of the experiment, two meaningful passages were presented to prelingually deaf individuals in four language contexts (Signed English, Signed ASL, printed English, and printed ASL). Results showed a greater recall from ASL than from English contexts, irrespective of mode of presentations. This leads to the belief that the visual orientation of deaf individuals, regardless of their training in ASL, leads to the development of a signed-based encoding system that responds to ASL as a familiar language (Morariu & Bruning, 1985, p. 89).

A study conducted by McDaniel further supports this evidence. In a testing situation using sign language, McDaniel reported that deaf and hearing children performed comparably on visual memory tasks. His findings further suggested that there is no special deficit among the deaf for tasks involving temporal order (McDaniel, 1980, p. 17).

Additional studies have been conducted investigating the encoding strategies that are incorporated by prelingually deaf individuals when information is presented. Goldin-Meadow and Mylander examined young deaf children of hearing parents who were unable to acquire oral language naturally and who had not been exposed to a conventional manual language. They concluded that the visual information encoding system these children employed differed significantly from that developed in normally hearing individuals. Their observations further suggest that children who lack auditory input can develop communication with language-like properties without a tutor modeling or shaping the structural aspects of the communication (Goldin-Meadow & Mylander, 1983, p. 22). Further study by Treiman and Hirsh-Pasek (1983) suggests that second generation congenitally and profoundly deaf adults who are native signers of American Sign Language (ASL) encode and retrieve printed information utilizing a multiple-step process. Although their findings did not reveal that they recoded into articulation or fingerspelling, it did suggest that they recode into sign.

Deaf individuals have the ability to process printed information into their own conceptual system. Two experiments reported by Tweney, Hoeman, and Andrews (1975) support the premise that deaf and hearing subjects respond to abstract verbal materials in a very similar fashion when no demands are placed on syntactical skills. Based on two studies in which deaf and hearing adolescents were asked to sort words into categories, the adolescents' scores in both groups were about the same. In the first study common nouns and words related to sound were categorized; in the second, concrete (high imagery) and abstract (low imagery) words were included. Rodda and Grove (1987) have indicated that this study is particularly interesting as it contradicts the frequent assertion that deaf people are limited in their abilities and can only entertain concrete thoughts (Rodda & Grove, 1987, p. 163).

Studies such as these and research such as Vernon's (1967, 1968) suggest that:

- Deaf people perform as well as hearing individuals when given tasks that do not require mastery, but do require higher order cognitive skills
- There is no functional relationship between verbal (i.e., spoken) language and cognition or thought processes
- Verbal language is not the mediating symbol system of thought (Braden, 1985).

Cognitive growth and development can occur and differences can be minimized by challenging the thought processes of prelingually deaf children, providing them with an opportunity to engage in direct and mediated learning situations utilizing appropriate communication, and by providing them with an environment conducive to learning.

Relating Deafness to Vygotsky's View of Cognitive Development

Vygotsky, like Bruner, stresses the importance of adults in a child's environment. In addition, he views the social environment as impacting significantly on the individual's personal and cognitive growth. Because deafness alters perceptions of the environment and the way individuals respond to their surroundings, cognitive development may be affected.

Although Furth suggested that cognitive operations exist independently of language and that language is of minor concern when investigating cognition, other individuals have emphasized that language and its acquisition are a natural outgrowth and direct result of more general cognitive processes and operations. According to this orientation, it is the dominance of cognition over language and other behaviors that presumably explains the fact that hearing impaired individuals are able to function adequately in most situations, particularly those that do not require direct use of the core culture's language. The hearing impaired individual is then viewed as a foreigner living in a strange land who does not know the language of the host culture (Quigley & Kretschmer, 1982, p. 55).

Because deaf individuals may be viewed by society as "different," the experiences they encounter and the way hearing individuals respond to them may influence their perceptions of information and behaviors exhibited by the larger society. Frequently, information and explanations afforded deaf individuals are minimal, their social experiences may be restricted, and their opportunities for growth limited.

Evaluative processes used by psychologists have begun to respond to these issues. A praxeology has emerged that assesses the development of individuals relative to their experiential base. Although the classical descriptors, such as degree of hearing loss, age of onset, and etiology, may be useful in identifying this population, the effects of hearing loss as they relate to psychosocial development are also being analyzed. The unique relationship between reality and the individuals' interpretations of that reality has been acknowledged for a long time. By evaluating deaf individuals in light of their experiences and the beliefs they hold relative to these experiences, further insights can be gained into the mind-sets of those who are hearing impaired (Myerson, 1963).

Individuals outside the world of deafness may respond differently to those who experience this sensory deficit. As a result, a form of environmental deprivation may occur. Klein (1962) has suggested that one can make a clear distinction between the two varieties of deprivation. He states that individuals may have a specific sensory restriction or deficit and may experience a form of deprivation because they are isolated from their environment. Klein has illustrated that it is also the interpersonal isolation, not the sensory deficit alone, that disrupts the synthetic function of a child's ego or personality development. When examining the experiences deaf children encounter through the developmental process, it is important to consider the types of expectations that are communicated to the child. If parents and teachers respond to children utilizing highly directive, intrusive forms of communication, the children may develop feelings of helplessness and thus their attempts to develop independent thinking may be stymied.

Frequently, teachers and family members lower their behavioral expectations for the deaf child. They enforce social restrictions and do not provide adequate explanations for decisions and rules that directly affect the child. Oftentimes, because inadequate communication exists between the child and the parent, deaf children's outlets for venting frustrations, disappointments, and anger may be narrowed; so their emotions are often expressed in an impulsive and immature manner. During the past ten years there has been considerable interest among clinical and behavioral psychologists in identifying factors that contribute to the conceptual tempo of reflection impulsivity. Several studies have systematically examined the variations of impulse control in deaf children (Altshuler et al., 1976; Binder, 1971; Harris, 1978; Moores, Weiss, & Goodwin, 1978; O'Brien, 1987). Although most reports characterize deaf children as exhibiting poor impulse control, many of the early samples were based upon nonstandardized observations.

Two of the studies cited above merit special discussion. The testing conducted by Harris (1978) was specifically designed to determine the differences between impulse control of deaf children of hearing parents and deaf children of deaf parents. The results uniformly confirmed that deaf children of deaf parents obtained greater impulse control scores than the deaf children of hearing parents. This study would tend to support Vygotsky's theory that environmental influence has a direct bearing on cognitive development. Traditionally, deaf children of deaf parents not only exhibit greater impulse control but frequently are more socially mature. They are nurtured in the Deaf culture, providing them with the ultimate avenue for exchanges in communication to occur and socialization to develop. This further supports the premise that although language is an important vehicle for expressing oneself within the framework of communication, the quality of the information and nature of the experiences conveyed are equally as important.

O'Brien's (1987) study further supports this premise. O'Brien examined the relationship of the cognitive style of reflection-impulsivity to communication mode (oral vs. Total Communication) and age in deaf and hearing boys. Her population was too small to assess any differences between deaf children of deaf parents. Her results suggest that the deaf groups were more impulsive than the hearing children on some of the test measures. However, there were no significant differences between the oral and the Total Communication groups. Significant differences were noted between age groups indicating that as both deaf and hearing children become older, they exhibit fewer signs of impulsivity.

In conclusion, when the individual's internal mental structures function properly, when thought processes are stimulated, and when the environment is conducive to cognitive development, both deaf and hearing children will experience growth in their abilities to process information. Deafness, by itself, does not prohibit cognitive growth. However, the ramifications of this sensory deficit may create an environment of lower educational and behavioral expectations, restricted opportunities for social interactions, and a sense of community isolation. In turn, these factors may impinge on the deaf child, preventing him from developing to his fullest ability.

INTELLIGENCE TESTING

Origins

The origins of intelligence testing can be traced to Paris, France, in the early 1900s. At that time the school system appointed a commission of experts to study and recommend procedures for educating retarded children. One of the individuals was Alfred Binet, a French psychologist and expert on individual differences.

In 1905 Binet and Theophile Simon, a colleague, proposed a thirty-item scale of intelligence to measure the same mental processes that contribute to classroom attention. The processes revolved around mental abilities such as memory, attention, comprehension, discrimination, and reasoning. Binet and Simon tried to select sample bits of behavior, or critical points, that reflected mental ability (Gage & Berliner, 1988).

The first intelligence test was normed on a group of fifty nonretarded children ranging in age from three to eleven. After norms had been established, children suspected of being mentally retarded were given the test. Their performance was compared with children from the norm group of the same chronological age. Those students, performing significantly below their intellectually normal agemates, were viewed as incapable of entering the regular classroom and were assigned to a classroom for mentally retarded individuals. The scale was refined twice, the second time in 1911.

The next significant event in the development of intelligence tests occurred in 1916 when Lewis Terman of Stanford University published an extensive revision of Binet's 1911 test. The revision became known as the Stanford-Binet and remains very popular. Within this revised test, Terman expressed a child's level of performance as a global figure called an intelligence quotient (IQ). In addition, this instrument was normed on four hundred American children, ages four through nineteen, from a variety of backgrounds. The directions Terman provided for administering the items were clearer and more detailed than Binet's, thus rendering it a more reliable and useful instrument (Edwards, 1979; Seagoe, 1970). From the onset, Binet's and Simon's test items were devised to differentiate between children who could profit from normal classroom instruction and those who would require special education. In essence, they were designed to predict classroom success.

What They Measure

Early in the 1900s, when intelligence tests were beginning to be administered, the British psychologist Charles Spearman noticed that children given a battery of intelligence tests tended to rank consistently from test to test. It became evident that some children scored well on some tests but performed poorly on others. Spearman explained this pattern by saying intelligence was made up of two types of factors: a general factor (g) that affected performance on all intellectual tests and a set of specific factors (s) that affected performance only on specific intellectual tests. Although Spearman's research was done in 1904, contemporary intelligence tests are still designed to provide the examiner with specific and general measurements of intelligence.

Additional Views

Contemporary psychologists, such as David Wechsler (1974), have emphasized that "intelligence is not simply the sum of one's tested abilities" (Gage & Berliner, 1988, p. 169). According to Wechsler, intelligence is the global capacity of the individual to act purposefully, to think rationally, and to deal effectively with the environment. This definition, which is endorsed by many psychologists, further states that the tests are designed to predict the person's global capacity to perform effectively on academic tasks in a classroom environment.

Although people display intelligent behavior outside the classroom situation, to assess total intelligence would require test instruments that are extremely subjective. Two contemporary psychologists, Robert J. Sternberg (1985) and Howard Gardner (1983) felt the arena of intelligence testing should be expanded to include assessments of how well individuals can apply their intelligence to a variety of settings. They both stressed that intelligence is multifaceted and cautioned society against focusing on the results of IQ tests to the exclusion of other worthwhile behaviors.

Limitations

When examining intelligence tests and attempting to gain a perspective on their usefulness, four issues warrant special consideration. First of all, the appraisal of intelligence is limited by the fact that it cannot be directly measured. Second, one must be aware that the intelligence we test is a sample of intellectual capabilities that relate to classroom achievement better than they relate to anything else. Third, keep in mind that no intelligence score is an "absolute" measure; it is merely an estimate of how successfully a child solves certain problems as compared with his peers. Fourth, because these tests are designed to predict academic success, anything that occurs in the classroom to enhance learning can have a positive effect on intelligence test performance.

Description

One of the intelligence tests frequently administered to deaf individuals is the Wechsler Intelligence Scale for Children-Revised (WISC-R, 1974). It is one of three individual intelligence tests devised by David Wechsler that are currently in use. The

TABLE 7-3 **Weschler Intelligence Scale for Children—Revised**

List of Subtests in Order of Sequence Given

Verbal	Performance
1. Information	2. Picture Completion
3. Similarities	4. Picture Arrangement
5. Arithmetic	6. Block Design
7. Vocabulary	8. Object Assembly
9. Comprehension	10. Coding
11. Digit Span	12. Mazes

other two are the Wechsler Preschool and Primary Scale of Intelligence (1967) and the Weschsler Adult Intelligence Scale-Revised (1981).

The WISC-R can be given to children ages six through sixteen. It is comprised of twelve subtests equally divided between a verbal scale and a performance scale. Table 7-3 provides a chart indicating the names of the subtests and the sequence in which they are given.

The WISC-R yields three summary scores: a verbal IQ, a performance IQ, and a full scale IQ. The mean of the test is 100, and the standard deviation is 15. In addition, 99.72 percent of all IQ scores fall between 55 and 145 (these scores represent three standard deviations below and above the mean).

The items for each subtest range from easy to difficult, thus accommodating the six- to sixteen-year-old range and the full range of intellectual ability that can be seen at any age. The test questions are designed to reflect general knowledge and experiences common to practically all children.

INTELLECTUAL TESTING AND DEAFNESS

Several studies have been conducted with deaf individuals to determine how they function intellectually when compared with hearing individuals. In a recent report submitted by Braden (1985), patterns of cognitive skills "virtually identical" to those of hearing children were noted. By computing scores for 1,228 deaf children, Braden concluded the average performance IQ score was 96.89, only slightly lower than the hearing children's norm of 100. He attributed the small differences to the probable higher incidence of brain damage among deaf children (Martin, 1985, p. 164).

In addition, Braden's results reflected:

• virtually identical composition in deaf and hearing samples, in spite of the vast linguistic and auditory differences separating deaf and hearing children

- support for earlier work conducted by Vernon and Oettinger (1981), in which his contention was that deaf and hearing people do not differ in flexible, intelligent, nonverbal problem-solving ability
- the factor underlying intellectual functioning may in large part be organically determined
- that whatever nonverbal intelligence differences exist between deaf and hearing people, the differences are small and ancillary to general nonverbal reasoning structures. (Braden, 1985, pp. 499–500)

Braden's work supported earlier work conducted by Vernon (1968). Vernon viewed a large number of studies and concluded that children with severe to profound losses have essentially the same distribution of intelligence as the general population, even though the mean score for deaf children may be slightly below that for hearing children (Meadow, 1980, p. 47). A review by Wolff concluded that although slight differences occur, the supposed cognitive deficits alluded to in the traditional literature are usually attributed to secondary handicaps and/or problems of communication (Wolff, 1985, p. 79).

Children who are deaf due to hereditary causes are less likely to have additional handicaps than are children who are deaf from other causes (Mindel & Vernon, 1971). It has been shown that deaf children with genetic etiology show better academic achievement (Jensema, 1975) and higher nonverbal intelligence scores (Schildroth, 1976) than children deafened from nonhereditary causes (Kusche, Greenberg, & Garfield, 1983).

Examiners involved in the assessment of deaf children frequently encounter difficulties when incorporating verbal subtests. As a result, only the performance subtests of the WISC-R are generally administered. Investigators examining the test results of deaf individuals have found consistently that the highest subtest scores were earned on Object Assembly, a task that required the subject to assemble puzzle pieces into a coherent whole. It has been theorized that emphasis on visual training and perception in the activities of deaf students may foster achievement on this subtest. Agreement on the lowest scoring subtest of the WISC-R is less great. The two tests that are most frequently cited as falling farthest below the mean performance score are the Picture Arrangement Subtest and the Coding Subtest (Meadow, 1980, p. 49).

Studies comparing the intellectual development of deaf children with deaf parents with deaf children of hearing parents have received considerable attention. In a classic study, Vernon and Koh (1970) compared deaf children of deaf parents (dc/dp) to deaf children of hearing parents (dc/hp) on achievement, communication skills, and psychological adjustment. This study differed from previous studies in that all of the subjects had genetic etiologies. The subjects were matched on nonverbal intelligence scores, chronological age, and hearing loss. The hearing parents involved in the study were far better educated than the deaf parents. The groups also differed on early modes of communication (manual vs. oral). The results demonstrated that the scores of deaf children of deaf parents reflected a better overall educational achievement, including better reading skills and written language. No differences were found between the groups for speech intelligibility, speechreading, or psychological adjustment (Kusche et al., 1983, p. 459).

Several studies have been conducted comparing dc/dp with dc/hp. The majority of them have reported superior IQ scores for dc/dp (Brill, 1969; Conrad, 1979; Conrad & Weiskrantz, 1981; Schildroth, 1976; Sisco & Anderson, 1980; Vernon & Koh, 1970). In light of these studies, Kusche has proposed that the reason for these findings is not primarily due to experience but may alternatively suggest the possibility of a genetic explanation. However, she proposes that while a genetic basis may explain the IQ differences, it does not, by itself, explain superior achievement. As a result, she hypothesized that in the area of achievement, experience plays a more important role as nature interacts with nurture (Kusche et al., 1983, p. 459).

ADMINISTERING INTELLIGENCE TESTS TO DEAF INDIVIDUALS

Deaf children may experience similar difficulties as those experienced by hearing children who do not speak standard English upon entering testing situations. In many cases, the former possess minimal speech skills and have difficulty understanding what is expected of them unless the psychometrist is experienced in dealing with deaf children. As a rule, the scores of deaf children tend to be depressed if a test requires a proficiency in speech or speechreading or in knowledge of standard English (Moores, 1987, p. 155).

Most school psychologists, regardless of the orientation of their educational programs, are not prepared to test deaf children (Sullivan & Vernon, 1979). Levine (1974) found that fewer than 20 of 172 school psychologists working with deaf children were able to communicate in sign language and that 83 percent had no special preparation to work with deaf individuals. Preliminary data from a longitudinal study of public high school programs for the deaf (Moores, Kluwin, & Mertens, 1985) suggest that there continues to be a lack of school psychologists with special training in the area of deafness (Moores, 1987, p. 147).

When reviewing intelligence test scores of deaf individuals, it is essential that professionals:

- understand the purpose for which the tests were designed
- consider the language base contained in the verbal sections
- consider the manner in which the tests are administered (mode of communication of examinee and the examiner's background and training in the field of deafness).

SUMMARY

The issues and theories surrounding cognition and intelligence are complex, continuously affording the professionals involved in science and research with new areas to explore. Theorists such as Piaget, Bruner, and Vygotsky have provided stages and frameworks through which one can study cognitive development.

This area of study has been of particular interest to professionals involved in the field of deafness. Recent research has provided those working in the field with new insights into the thought processes of deaf individuals. Studies reflecting the abilities of deaf children to think abstractly and function on par intellectually have added new dimensions to the world of the deaf. Recognizing this fact, professionals must begin exploring avenues and resources that will stimulate the thought processes of deaf individuals, thus empowering them to develop to their fullest potential.

▶ 8

Moral Reasoning and Values Clarification

The fabric of our moral development is comprised of those beliefs and convictions that enable us to determine what is right or wrong. Morality is not a behavioral concept; rather, it is a philosophical tenet consisting of the intentions and reasons that sustain our actions (Windmiller, Lambert, and Truel, 1980). The role reasoning plays within the framework of moral development has been a topic of interest for philosophers, psychologists, and educators for centuries. Investigators have studied the relationship between moral reasoning and moral behavior in an attempt to gain some insight into the factors that are associated with these processes (Norcini & Snyder, 1983).

Over the past forty years, moral development has been examined within the context of learning theory, cognitive development, and affectivity (Youniss, 1981). Learning theorists purport that individuals identify with existing moral codes and thus internalize those beliefs that are currently expressed by the community. Within the realm of cognitive development, individuals are viewed as taking existing codes and constructing, transforming, and organizing the information into mental conceptions. The more contemporary theories of moral development base their roots in affectivity. This is defined through dimensions such as responsibility, empathy, and concern for others. Theorists supporting this view have established that individuals develop their sense of morality out of their concern for others. However, Youniss (1981) has proposed that affectivity need not be viewed in contrast to cognitive development but rather as working in tandem with it. In this situation, moral judgment stems from within individuals (self-reflective cognition) based on their concern for others (affectivity) (Youniss, 1981, p. 396).

As individuals develop, they examine their ideas pertaining to what is right and wrong and therefore engage in a philosophical activity. As they mature they apply their philosophy to situations they encounter. This application can be viewed as the establishment and reflection of a moral code.

DEVELOPING A MORAL CODE

Although moral philosophers have varying views about what it means to have a moral code, almost all of them will agree on three points:

1. Moral codes focus on what is good or bad for people. In addition, they pertain to those elements that promote or detract from human happiness, well-being, or satisfaction.
2. Moral discourse—viewed as moral principles, codes, judgments, or admonitions—has some bearing on behavior. Essentially, behavior may be in harmony or conflict with what is actually said.
3. Individuals may choose to behave in accordance with their beliefs and thus avoid behaviors that are in direct conflict with their moral code. If they behave in a manner contradictory to these beliefs, they may experience feelings of guilt or discomfort. These feelings arise either from social disapproval or from conflict with one's own ideals (Sieber, 1980).

There are three major theories in moral philosophy that attempt to explain what it means to embrace a moral code. The three theories can be identified as intuitionism, emotivism, and prescriptivism.

Intuitionism

Intuitionism asserts that individuals know intuitively what is moral and good. Morality and goodness are properties that are independent of all other properties; therefore they cannot be further defined. This theory believes that people "have a sense" of knowing what is right or wrong. Because the theory of intuitionism focuses on one's "sense of knowing," there is no rational basis provided for the individual in order that he might determine what is, or is not, moral (Sieber, 1980, p. 136).

Emotivism

Emotivism, which originated within the logical positivist school, proposes a radically different explanation of moral development. It has become known as the emotivist theory of morality. The logical positivists believe that a moral judgment conveys only an attitude and that this attitude is used to influence oneself or others to behave in a certain way. In addition, a moral judgment may or may not state reasons or deal in facts. It is viewed as a command and produces a predisposition to feel and behave in a specific way. In essence, then, a moral behavior is viewed as a be-havior that demonstrates obedience to a moral command (Sieber, 1980, p. 136).

Prescriptivism

Prescriptivism, summarized by Hare (1972), suggests that moral statements are meant to guide or prescribe rather than to influence behavior. The individual can un-derstand the moral code. Although the tenets contained in the information may be false, it is of a rational nature. It can also be viewed as universal whereby the same judgment would be made in any situation of a comparable nature (Sieber, 1980, pp. 136–137).

A STRUCTURAL-DEVELOPMENTAL THEORY OF MORAL DEVELOPMENT

The development of moral codes and the factors associated with moral reasoning have been researched extensively. One major theory pertaining to this domain lies in the area of cognitive development. Within this theory a structural developmental ap-proach is incorporated that focuses on the processes and reasoning abilities that evolve as individuals progress through the various stages of moral development.

Psychologists from this school of thought believe that learning takes place as in-dividuals interact with their environment. Existential knowledge determines individ-uals' ability to restructure their information base and respond to their exigencies by the assimilation of a unique conceptual framework. Therefore, the way children or adults respond to and interact with their environment will determine their self-con-cept and perceptions of the world.

The structural developmentalist believes that, based on the uniqueness of the in-dividuals' moral knowledge, individuals will develop their own sense of morality through actively structuring and restructuring their social experiences during each of several distinct developmental periods. The underlying assumption is that the per-son's own behavioral representation of moral rules and values is uniquely organized at each developmental level. As he or she progresses through these developmental periods and is confronted with various experiences, his or her moral knowledge base expands. When this occurs, individuals reorganize and restructure their thinking. This restructuring enables them to advance to the next moral stage. All children ex-perience these developmental reorganizations in the same order, that is, in invariant sequence. In their terminology, modes of organization with these properties have tra-ditionally been referred to as stages (Windmiller et al., 1980, p. 38).

When reviewing the literature pertaining to stage theories and moral develop-ment, the works of two individuals merit special consideration. Jean Piaget and Lawrence Kohlberg have both made significant contributions to the study of moral development. Through their research, morality can be examined as a process that involves distinct stages in personal development. The basic premise underlying both theories is that as children interact with their environment, they progress through unique stages, and growth occurs. Children begin to form their own concept of morality, a concept that may be independent of the philosophy reflected by adult society. Thus, the moral judgments made by children and adolescents can be placed in perspective according to their contemporary stage rather than by perceiving their decisions as a reflection of adult behavior. By superimposing a stage framework, as proposed by Piaget or Kohlberg, children's moral decisions can be considered representative of each unique stage of growth and development. This model then permits children's responses to be viewed as individual in nature rather than as imperfect versions of adult moral values. Subsequently, their responses can also be viewed as part of a developmental process that progresses along a continuum, culminating with adulthood.

Piaget's Theory of Moral Development

Piaget was intrigued with all aspects of human development. As a result, he devoted time to studying morality and how children enhance their reasoning abilities. His basic premise was founded on the idea that if he observed children playing games and noticed how they adhered to the rules, he would gain some insights into the process and sequence of moral development. After Piaget learned how to play marbles, he began spending a great deal of time observing children play and questioned them about their interpretation of the rules (Slavin, 1988). His hypothesis was that children's rule-following behavior was indicative of a respect for social rules. While observing the children's rule-following behaviors, he determined that the interpretations of the rules followed by the participants in marble games changed with age and that there were four distinct stages in which varying degrees of moral development could be observed.

Stage One

According to Piaget, the first stage begins at about age two and is one of play, rather than one of true morality. Although children engage in "symbolic play," they invent their own rules, change them at will, and assimilate the game into their own private rituals and symbolic fantasies. During this stage children express an awareness of rules, but do not understand their purpose or the need to follow them. The rules become purely "motor," which are received unconsciously as interesting examples, rather than realities that they are obliged to follow (Piaget, 1965). During this early stage, children do not differentiate the regularities involved in their individual activities (play and rituals) from "real" moral rules. They quickly incorporate particular rituals into their game independent of those established by other children. It is not until later, when they conceive of obligation, that they are able to separate moral rules from other kinds of behavioral regularity. During this time rules are evident. However, they are viewed as originating from within the children, rather than being instilled in them by older youths or peer groups.

Stage Two

Piaget found that children from around age five or six and continuing through age eight begin to acknowledge the existence of rules, although they are inconsistent in following them. He observed frequently that children playing the same game are each playing by a different set of rules. They each engage in their own game, with neither attempting to win. He also noted that children at this stage have no understanding that the rules of the game are arbitrary and can be changed. Instead they view the rules as being imposed by some higher authority and not changeable.

Piaget was fascinated by the way children follow rules. Therefore, he decided to use the interview method to obtain more systematic information about moral development. He designed pairs of stories and asked children of different stages to discuss them. He discovered that they responded to the stories based on their concepts of rules.

Because children functioning at the second stage regard rules as permanent and sacred, not subject to modification for any reason, they confuse morality with adult constraint. Piaget states that when this occurs it results in a form of moral realism. This suggests that children have a tendency to regard duty as something that is independent of the mind. They view it as being imposed upon them regardless of the circumstances in which they are involved (Piaget, 1965, p. 111). Moral realism maintains at least three features. First, duty is viewed essentially as heteronomous. Those acts or behaviors that comply with adult commands are good; those acts that do not conform are bad. Rules are not to be interpreted by the mind, only followed. Therefore, good is defined by obedience. A second tenet in moral realism demands that "the letter, rather than the spirit of the law" shall be observed. The consequences of an act are valued more than the intention behind the act. The third premise states that children evaluate acts not in accordance with their motives for engaging in them but in reference to conforming exactly to established rules (Piaget, 1965, p. 111).

This is illustrated in Piaget's story of the broken cups. When presenting six-year-olds with the scenario that a child broke eleven cups by mistake and one cup on purpose, six-year-olds typically respond that the incident involving the eleven cups would merit more severe punishment. This reflects the manifestation of the moral thought processes at this stage (Piaget, 1965, p. 125).

Stage Three

"Autonomous morality," or "morality of cooperation," arises when the children are approximately eight years of age. At this time, they begin to establish feelings of mutual respect for their peers, and they see rules as cooperative regulatory agreements that are useful for all. Heteronomous morality, or "morality based on relations of constraints," begins to decline and an autonomous morality emerges. In addition, they begin to regard rules as being manmade and realize that they are changeable agreements between equals rather than unalterable commands that are handed down by adults.

During this time social reciprocity develops. Children begin to cooperate with their peers rather than adhering to adult constraint, and this "peer cooperation" becomes their reason for obeying moral rules.

By the end of this stage, children may utilize a substantial amount of their play-time engaging in the development of rules to govern their games. A change in rules is acceptable as long as all of those involved in making the decision agree and the new rule is deemed fair by all. Some new rules are incorporated to add interest to the game, while others are viewed as worthless, reducing the amount of skill required to win while playing the game.

Piaget illustrated this point by describing how a group of 10- and 11-year-olds prepared for a snowball fight. They devised teams, elected officers, decided on rules to govern the distance snowballs could be thrown, and agreed upon a system of punishment for those who violated the rules. They seemed to delight in the fact that they could design rules reflective of the peer group and not handed down by their elders (Piaget, 1965, p. 50).

Stage Four

By the age of eleven, children become increasingly capable of grasping why rules are necessary. They begin to demonstrate certain second-order reasoning abilities and are able to construct new rules to cope with all possible situations. At this stage of development, children's thought processes begin operating on a plane of complex political and social issues, rather than simply with individuals and interpersonal relationships. They develop ideas of what is right and uphold the belief that individuals must proceed through proper legal channels if laws are to be modified (Piaget, 1965, p. 71).

Within the four stages, Piaget concluded that there are two basic types of moral reasoning and that they differ in several ways. He referred to the moral thinking of children up to the age of ten or so as "morality of constraint" or "heteronomous" (subject to external rules or laws). The thinking of children eleven or older was labeled the "morality of cooperation" or "autonomous morality."

Kohlberg's Stages of Moral Reasoning

Lawrence Kohlberg's (1969) stage theory of moral reasoning is an elaboration and refinement of Piaget's work. Kohlberg, like Piaget, studied how children and adults reasoned about rules that governed their behavior in varying situations.

In Kohlberg's original work, he studied seventy-five American males from early adolescence through adulthood. They were continually presented with hypothetical moral dilemmas, all of which were deliberately philosophical in nature (Kohlberg, 1981). Kohlberg focused his attention on how the men responded to a series of structured situations or moral dilemmas. The most famous situation, the one involving Heinz, is described below:

In Europe a woman was near death from cancer. One drug might save her,
a form of radium that a druggist in the same town had recently discovered.
The druggist was charging $2,000, ten times what the drug cost him to
make. The sick woman's husband, Heinz, went to everyone he knew to bor-
row the money, but he could only get together about half of what it cost. He
told the druggist that his wife was dying and asked him to sell it cheaper or
let him pay later. But the druggist said, "No." The husband got desperate
and broke into the man's store to steal the drug for his wife. Should the hus-
band have done that? Why? (Kohlberg, 1969, p. 379)

On the basis of the men's reasoning about the dilemmas at different ages,
Kohlberg constructed a typology of definite and universal levels of development in
moral thought. The typology contains three distinct levels of moral thinking, and
within each of these levels are two related stages. These levels and stages may be
considered separate moral philosophies, distinct views of the social-moral world
(Kohlberg, 1981, p. 16).

He defined the three levels of moral thinking as preconventional, conventional,
and postconventional. According to Kohlberg, moral development begins with preconventional thinking in which children obey in order to avoid punishment and ends
with the development of a sense of universal justice (Kohlberg, 1981, p. 16). Table
8-1 provides a synopsis of Kohlberg's Stages of Moral Reasoning.

Preconventional Level
At this level children respond to cultural rules and labels of good and bad, right or
wrong, but interpret these labels in terms of either the physical or the hedonistic consequences of action, that is, punishment, reward, or exchange of favors. These cultural rules can also be examined in terms of the physical power of those who affirm
the rules and labels. The two stages within this level can be described in the following way:

Stage 1.   Punishment and Obedience Orientation
    The physical consequences of an action determine its goodness or badness re-
gardless of the human meaning or value of the consequences. As a result, one ad-
heres to the rules for the sole purpose of avoiding punishment.

Stage 2.   The Instrumental Relativist Orientation
    This stage is identified as one in which individuals select the "right action"
based on what will satisfy their needs and occasionally the needs of others. Kohlberg
states that human relations are viewed in "marketplace" terms. Elements of fairness,
reciprocity, and equal sharing are present, but they are always interpreted in a physical, pragmatic way. This reciprocity can further be illustrated with the concept "you
scratch my back, I'll scratch yours" (Kohlberg, 1981, p. 17).

TABLE 8-1   **Kohlberg's Stages of Moral Reasoning**

When people consider moral dilemmas, it is their reasoning that is important, not their final decision, according to Lawrence Kohlberg. He theorized that people progress through three levels as they develop abilities of moral reasoning.

I. Preconventional Level

Rules are set down by others.

Stage 1. Punishment and Obedience Orientation
Physical consequences of action determine its goodness or badness.

Stage 2. Instrumental Relativist Orientation
What's right is whatever satisfies one's own needs and occasionally the needs of others. Elements of fairness and reciprocity are present, but they are mostly interpreted in a "you scratch my back, I'll scratch yours" fashion.

II. Conventional Level

Individual adopts rules, and will sometimes subordinate own needs to those of the group. Expectations of family, group, or nation seen as valuable in own right, regardless of immediate and obvious consequences.

Stage 3. "Good Boy-Nice Girl" Orientation
Good behavior is whatever pleases or helps others and is approved of by them. One earns approval by being "nice."

Stage 4. "Law and Order" Orientation
Right is doing one's duty, showing respect for authority, and maintaining the given social order for its own sake.

III. Postconventional Level

People define own values in terms of ethical principles they have chosen to follow.

Stage 5. Social Contract Orientation
What's right is defined in terms of general individual rights and in terms of standards that have been agreed upon by the whole society. In contrast to Stage 4, laws are not "frozen"—they can be changed for the good of society.

Stage 6. Universal Ethical Principle Orientation
What's right is defined by decision of conscience according to self-chosen ethical principles. These principles are abstract and ethical (such as the Golden Rule), not specific moral prescriptions (such as the Ten Commandments).

(From *Handbook of Socialization Theory and Research,* D. A. Goslin (Ed.), Chicago: Rand McNally, 1969. Reprinted with permission.)

Conventional Level

At this level individuals become aware of the expectations of their family, group, or nation, and perceive their expectations as valuable in their own right. Therefore, these individuals transcend the level of focusing on consequences and become more attentive to conformity of personal expectations with social order. Loyalty to the larger social element develops as these collective attitudes are internalized. They become an active member of their group, identify with the individual members, and become loyal to them.

Stage 3.   The Interpersonal Concordance or "Good Boy-Nice Girl" Orientation
    Within this stage good behavior is perceived as that which pleases or helps others and is approved by them. There is a great deal of conformity to stereotypical images of what is majority or "natural" behavior. Individuals earn approval by following the Golden Rule and being nice. In essence, justice is viewed as doing good within the context of interpersonal relationships.

Stage 4.   Society Maintaining Orientation
    This stage extends the concept of justice to include the entire social order. There is an orientation toward authority, fixed rules, and the maintenance of the social order. Justice or right behavior consists of assuming one's duty, showing respect for authority, becoming a good citizen, working hard, and maintaining the given social order for its own sake. Laws are followed without question, and breaking the law can never be justified. Most adults are probably at this stage (Kohlberg, 1981; Windmiller et al., 1980; Slavin, 1988).

Postconventional, Autonomous, or Principled Level
At this level, individuals make a clear effort to examine and define moral values and principles. They attempt to differentiate their views from those projected by groups of people and authority figures with whom they form associations (Kohlberg, 1981, p. 19). Here there is a realization that the laws and values of a society are somewhat arbitrary and particular to that society. This level of moral reasoning is probably attained by fewer than 25 percent of adults (Hogan & Emler, 1978). Laws are viewed as necessary within the context of preserving social order and insuring the basic rights of life and liberty.

Stage 5.   The Social Contract Orientation
    This stage was labeled as the "social contract" conception of morality. Individuals within this stage can contemplate issues such as why one should be moral. In addition, they perceive their moral responsibility as binding upon all those who claim the rights of society. Within this stage there is a clear awareness of the relativism of personal values and opinions and a corresponding emphasis on procedural rules for reaching a consensus.

Stage 6.   The Universal Ethical Principle Orientation
    This is the highest level in Kohlberg's system. At this stage individuals can view moral rules as abstract principles and are able to apply the principles to human rights. At this level, the concern for human dignity is critical, and solutions are discerned in terms of the universal rights of others and may transcend obedience to

society's codes. There is a fundamental respect for the human social order. Laws may occasionally be ignored in instances where great injustice would result from blind obedience.

Although Kohlberg originally postulated that Stages 5 and 6 were separate, his more recent works speculated that Stage 6 is not really separate from Stage 5, and he has suggested that the two be combined.

In some of Kohlberg's earlier writings, he referred to this scheme of development as a "typology," referring to the fact that about 67 percent of most people's thinking is at a single stage, regardless of the moral dilemma involved. The types are identified as "stages" because they seem to represent an invariant developmental sequence (Kohlberg, 1981, p. 20). The underlying premise of his theory is that moral thought tends to behave like all other kinds of thought. Progression through the levels and stages of moral development provokes cognitive and moral conflicts, compelling individuals to expand their moral reasoning abilities and experience growth. As this growth occurs, development may be defined in terms of qualitative reorganization of the individual's pattern of thought rather than the learning of new content. Thus, syntonic reorganization integrates within a broader perspective the insights that were achieved at lower stages (Colby & Kohlberg, 1981).

The stages in Kohlberg's theory and the individual's development are said to be synchronous. This is due to the premise of the sequence rather than the innate characteristics of each stage (Colby & Kohlberg, 1981, p. 3). Table 8-2 reflects Kohlberg's Six Stages of Development accompanied by answers graded according to his model. For each stage, actual answers have been provided that demonstrate the kinds of reasoning involved.

As with Piaget's theory of cognitive development, there is no guarantee that all children will reach the final stage of moral development. In fact, most people do not seem to develop beyond Stage 4 (Shaver & Strong, 1976). However, Kohlberg argues that children advance to a higher stage of moral development when they are exposed to moral reasoning slightly more advanced than their own.

Although the theory proposed by Kohlberg is a well-organized depiction of how moral reasoning develops, it does not correlate well with moral behavior. What people say they will do and what they actually will do are often two very different things (Kurtines & Greif, 1974). Frequently, the way a person responds depends more on the immediate situational forces than on the person's level of moral reasoning.

THE IMPACT OF DEAFNESS ON MORAL DEVELOPMENT

Linguistic, audiological, physical, psychological, and sociological factors all affect the developmental process of children who are disabled by virtue of their deafness and handicapped in their ability to communicate with others (Sam & Wright, 1988). Because language development, social growth, and the educational process are

TABLE 8-2 **Presentation of a Moral Dilemma with Answers Graded According to Kohlberg's Six Stages of Moral Development**

In Europe a woman was near death from cancer. One drug might save her, a form of radium that a druggist in the same town had recently discovered. The druggist was charging $2,000, ten times what the drug cost him to make. The sick woman's husband, Heinz, went to everyone he knew to borrow the money, but he could only get together about half of what it cost. He told the druggist that his wife was dying and asked him to sell it cheaper or let him pay later. But the druggist said "No." The husband got desperate and broke into the man's store to steal the drug for his wife. Should the husband have done that? Why?

Punishment and obedience orientation (physical consequences determine what is good or bad).

Stage 1	*Pro*	He should steal the drug. It isn't really bad to take it. It isn't like he didn't ask to pay for it first. The drug he'd take is only worth $200. He's not really taking a $2,000 drug.	*Con*	He shouldn't steal the drug. It's a big crime. He didn't get permission, he used force and broke and entered. He did a lot of damage, stealing a very expensive drug and breaking up the store, too.

Instrumental relativist orientation (what satisfies one's own needs is good).

Stage 2	*Pro*	It's all right to steal the drug because she needs it and he wants her to live. It isn't that he wants to steal, but it's the way he has to use to get the drug to save her.	*Con*	He shouldn't steal it. The druggist isn't wrong or bad, he just wants to make a profit. That's what you're in business for, to make money.

Interpersonal concordance of "good boy-good girl" orientation (what pleases or helps others is good).

Stage 3	*Pro*	He should steal the drug. He was only doing something that was natural for a good husband to do. You can't blame him for doing something out of love for his wife, you'd blame him if he didn't love his wife enough to save her.	*Con*	He shouldn't steal. If his wife dies, he can't be blamed. It isn't because he's heartless or that he doesn't love her enough to do everything that he legally can. The druggist is the selfish or heartless one.

"Law and order" orientation (maintaining the social order, doing one's duty is good).

Stage 4	*Pro*	You should steal it. If you did nothing you'd be letting your wife die; it's your responsibility if she dies. You have to take it with the idea of paying the druggist.	*Con*	It is a natural thing for Heinz to want to save his wife, but it's still always wrong to steal. He still knows he's stealing and taking a valuable drug from the man who made it.

TABLE 8-2 *Continued*

Social contract-legalistic orientation (values agreed upon by society, including individuals rights and rules for consensus, determine what is right).

Stage 5 *Pro* The law wasn't set up for these circumstances. Taking the drug in this situation isn't really right, but it's justified to do it.

Con You can't completely blame someone for stealing, but extreme circumstances don't really justify taking the law into your own hands. You can't have everyone stealing whenever they get desperate. The end may be good, but the ends don't justify the means.

Universal ethical-principle orientation (what is right in a matter of conscience in accord with universal principles).

Stage 6 *Pro* This is a situation which forces him to choose between stealing and letting his wife die. In a situation where the choice must be made, it is morally right to steal. He has to act in terms of the principle of preserving and respecting life.

Con Heinz is faced with the decision of whether to consider the other people who need the drug just as badly as his wife. Heinz ought to act not according to his particular feelings toward his wife, but considering the value of all the lives involved.

(From Dilemma and pro and con answers from Rest, 1968, as found in *Introduction to Child Development,* third edition, by John Dworetzky. St. Paul: West Publishing Co. Reprinted with permission.)

closely interdependent in the deaf child (Mindel & Vernon, 1987), many deaf people suffer from educational and social handicaps.

Deafness usually results in fewer opportunities for deaf children of hearing parents to engage in social interactions, both within and outside of the family unit. Breakdowns that occur among family members who do not share corresponding modes of communication may evoke feelings of frustration, and the deaf child may withdraw from social interactions (Rainer & Altshuler, 1966, 1971).

Intrinsic to the theories of both Piaget and Kohlberg is the premise that social interaction and communication are essential for progress through the various stages of moral development. As a person engages in moral reasoning at the conventional level, he is required to have an increased capacity for abstract thought and assimilation, allowing the individual's thinking to stretch outward into another perspective (Belenky, 1984). If the child, and later the adolescent, is prevented from becoming involved in these types of interactions, what effect will it have on his moral development? Does the sensory deficit experience in deafness impinge on his ability to transcend to the higher levels of moral reasoning as defined by Kohlberg?

ASSESSING LEVELS OF MORAL REASONING
IN DEAF AND HARD OF HEARING INDIVIDUALS

There have been very few studies conducted utilizing Kohlberg's instruments in conjunction with deaf subjects. However, results based on the limited studies merit special consideration. Two of the early attempts to assess moral reasoning abilities have been delineated in the work by DeCaro and Emerton.

DeCaro and Emerton (1978) conducted one of the first studies aimed toward assessing moral reasoning abilities in the deaf college population. In 1975, they administered Porter and Taylor's written version of Kohlberg's moral reasoning questionnaire to 252 students (the entire freshman class), at the National Technical Institute for the Deaf at Rochester Institute of Technology. They administered the same instrument in 1978 to forty-four randomly selected subjects at the same institution. The scores obtained from this instrument indicated that 80 percent of the subjects scored at the Preconventional Level, which was lower than the average college entrant (DeCaro & Emerton, 1978, p. 19). To insure that difficulties attributed to writing were not the cause of the lowered test scores, ten freshmen were randomly selected and the test was administered by an individual skilled in manual forms of communication. Each segment was videotaped and then transcribed into written English. The test scores obtained from the group benefiting from manual communication were similar to those from the group participating in the written test format.

Four years after the initial study, the ten subjects were re-interviewed using the same format. At this time, both handwritten and face-to-face interviews were compiled. The written interview versions from both 1977 and 1981 were then scored. Results indicated that in 1977, all ten students were reasoning at the Preconventional Level (Stage 2). At that time only four of them showed marked evidence of Stage 3 processing. However, when the same subjects were tested four years later, all showed a substantial amount of Stage 3 conventional moral reasoning with only four relying on thoughts characteristic of Stage 2. The gain was significant and suggests that delayed development can be overcome relatively late in one's life (DeCaro & Emerton, 1978).

Although the progress of these students' scores seems significant and encouraging, it still remains that their moral judgment scores are low when compared with their hearing counterparts. The investigators concluded that the students were at the Preconventional Level possibly because their

> *[e]xperiential bases are not sufficient to permit considerations of a wide array of different viewpoints . . . role taking abilities are not fully developed . . . [and] language deprivation has precluded assimilation of certain values. (DeCaro & Emerton, 1978, p. 19)*

When interpreting this type of information, it is critical to examine the possible causes for the depressed scores. The scores may have very little to do with the level of moral reasoning; instead, they reflect the individuals' perceptions of society. Based on Kohlberg's scheme, the interviewer only assigns a score at Stage 4 or higher if the individual indicates that he has taken the perspective of society as a whole.

Young adults who identify with the Deaf community may feel excluded from the hearing world. They may not take a "hearing" perspective when the moral dilemma is depicted as occurring within a society to which they cannot relate. Because Kohlberg's instrument is based on linguistic dialogues, the analysis of results from the Deaf community must be considered as they relate to two fundamental questions. How much does morality itself depend on a dialogue between individuals that presuppose a shared symbol system? Are deaf adolescents in fact delayed in moral development or, when Kohlberg's instrument is administrated, do their answers merely yield a poor response (Belenky, 1984, p. 164)?

Recent research has been conducted in this area in an attempt to gain further insights into the deaf population. In a study conducted by Sam and Wright (1988), Kohlberg's Moral Judgement Instrument (MJI) was administered to fifteen students who had an average hearing loss of greater than 100 dB in the better ear and had no other significant disabling conditions.

The MJI consists of questions that are designed to penetrate beyond the subject's opinions of what should or should not be done in the cases of nine moral dilemmas. The questions seek to determine the reasoning behind the choices thus reflecting the stage of reasoning that the subject is displaying.

To test deaf students, the language structure appearing in the dilemmas was modified. Simple sentences incorporating a subject-verb-object pattern were utilized with appropriate vocabulary. Although the sentence structure was simplified, the significant concepts in the original dilemmas remained intact. The participants had the opportunity to read written descriptions and view the same dilemmas, presented on videotape. They were then told to summarize the story to the best of their ability in their preferred mode of communication. Upon completing this segment, the students were asked questions. Results indicated:

1. All of the subjects showed a Stage 1 or Stage 2 orientation with only a few showing any Stage 3 reasonings.
2. Among the general findings, subjects were unable to fully handle reciprocity and equality in a contractual relationship. Many of the subjects were rigidly egocentric in their thinking. They showed no inclination to compromise, to suggest a deal, or to take another perspective. For many of the subjects self- preservation was of primary importance. They appeared to know the necessary social rules—that love for family and friends and relationships with them were important but this was not carried over into society at large.
3. Reading levels seemed to correlate with scores on the MJI. Those who were better readers scored higher. (Sam & Wright, 1988, p. 268)

Further results of this study indicated that many of the subjects knew conventional social rules, especially when they revolved around relationships with family and friends. However, they seemed to have learned the rules by rote with no real understanding of the principles behind them. As a result, they applied the rules indiscriminately and did not understand the reasoning on which they were based.

Individuals gain an understanding of rules and the reasons behind rule choice by actively participating in decision-making and rule-making experiences. It is through this type of involvement that people become aware that others have their own perspectives, needs, and desires. Through this communication exchange, alternative viewpoints are acquired, internal examination occurs, and moral reasoning develops.

Inherent in the system is a solid base for communication. Without this linguistic knowledge of English, deaf individuals may not be as adept as their hearing counterparts in their ability to understand themselves and their relationship to the hearing world. Deaf children of deaf parents and deaf children who are fluent in ASL benefit from similar interactions that occur within the Deaf community. However, when forced to interact with their hearing peers through an exchange of spoken or written English, they are at a distinct disadvantage.

According to Colby and Kohlberg (1981), peers at this age generally reason at Stages 2, 3, and 4. Results of Sam and Wright's study (1988) indicated that the deaf students were reasoning at Stages 1 and 2. This lag can be attributed to a disability that precludes the assimilation of the English language, thus restricting opportunities for social interaction. Deaf and hard of hearing individuals who reside in a hearing environment and have limited contacts with others who are fluent in American Sign Language (ASL) have few opportunities to receive interpretations and explanations of the feelings and perspectives of others. Consequently, their role-taking ability is minimized. Although this is not the only factor, it is essential in the development of moral reasoning (Selman, 1971).

Social interaction and role taking are only two factors that contribute to moral development. Lickona (1976), in reviewing the literature on moral development as conceptualized by Piaget, states that there are two additional factors that generally promote moral growth: cognitive development and liberation from the coercive constraint of adult authority. The importance of social interactions and cognitive development have been discussed previously. The area of parental discipline as it relates to moral development merits consideration.

LIBERATION FROM ADULT CONSTRAINTS: IMPACT OF PARENTAL DISCIPLINE TECHNIQUES

Parents are usually the most important authorities in the lives of children. The discipline methods they employ and the techniques they utilize have an overall effect on the child's moral development. Because of this it is important to review the research that has been conducted on this topic.

Hoffman (1977) and Saltstein, D'amon, and Belenkey (1972) investigated the relationship between parental discipline and their children's maturity of moral judgment. They determined that discipline could be viewed within three distinct categories.

1. Power Assertion (exercise of physical power over the child)
2. Love Withdrawal of Affection (expressing anger and withholding affection)
3. Induction (disciplining the child by pointing out the consequences of the child's behavior)

Their findings concluded that there was a strong correlation between internalization of moral values and parental use of induction as a disciplinary technique. Parents who incorporate this type of discipline point out to the child the harmful consequences of the child's behavior and encourage discussions about the range of motivations and the issues that are involved.

In contrast, Baumrind (1980) has indicated that those children who are raised in homes and disciplined with power assertive techniques, such as physical punishments and withdrawal of privileges, are found to base their morality on the fear of external punishments.

Parenting techniques, methods of discipline, and moral development were the subjects of a study conducted by Holstein (1968). He studied families involved in actually discussing hypothetical moral dilemmas. The results of his study indicated that parents who engaged in dialogues with their offspring pertaining to the issues involved in the dilemma produced the most advanced children on Kohlberg's scale of moral reasoning. Those parents who required conformity and demanded that their children parrot their opinions produced offspring who were less morally mature when evaluated by Kohlberg's scale.

In Kohlberg's terminology, Conventional Level students characterized their families as harmonious, with few parent-child conflicts. They depicted their parents as using clear rules, supported by rewards and punishments, rather than encouraging discussion and debates around differences in values. These studies further suggest that important factors fostered in moral development lie in the parents' willingness to engage in rational and productive discussions with their children about moral conflicts.

THE USE OF DISCIPLINE AND THE METHODS OF COMMUNICATION

The family domain has provided researchers with a wealth of information. Extensive studies have been conducted regarding parenting techniques including methods of discipline and modes of communication (Chess, 1975; Collins, 1969; Goss, 1970; Mindel & Vernon, 1987; Schlesinger & Meadow, 1972). These findings, which have been summarized by Belenky, are reflective of studies conducted with deaf children of hearing parents. Within the area of discipline the investigators found:

1. Parents elected to use a form of power assertive discipline when interacting with their deaf children that was not as apparent with their hearing children.
2. Mothers of deaf children tended to be more controlling, didactic, and intrusive.
3. They were less likely to delegate decision-making responsibilities to the child.
4. Physical punishments and restraints were more likely to be viewed as effective.
5. The adult constraint that is embodied early in one's development remains an important factor in the lives of deaf children. As a result, it may account for the delay found in the development of moral reasoning (Belenky, 1984, p. 168).

Children who rely on manual communication to express their ideas may find they have severely limited access to language and social discourse if sign is not available in the home. Deaf students attending mainstreamed programs rely on their families for their social and moral development. If their hearing parents do not sign and the children are unable to produce understandable speech, comprehend much of the spoken language, read, and write, they may experience an unprecedented degree of social isolation.

This in turn has direct bearing on their moral development. As previously stated, if social participation is an important precipitator of moral reasoning, it would follow that development would be delayed in those who do not have access to an efficient language and who are excluded from the give-and-take of an ongoing dialogue (Belenky, 1984, p. 171).

Schlesinger and Meadow (1972) found deaf children of deaf parents to have higher ratings on their measures of responsibility, maturity, and independence. Harris (1978), in one of the few studies exploring the relationship between the age of exposure to manual communication and subsequent development, found that deaf children of deaf parents obtained significantly greater impulse control scores than deaf children of hearing parents. His results also indicated that the younger the deaf children were exposed to manual communication, the more reflective they were in completing test items. One of the conclusions drawn by Harris was that use of manual communication during infancy may help deaf children develop cognitive and syntactic structures thus helping them to modulate their impulses more constructively (Harris, 1978, p. 62). Impulse control can be viewed as an important index of moral maturity in that one's immediate needs and wishes become secondary to the achievement of long-term goals.

Although the debate continues over whether the access to sign actually accounts for these striking differences, there are studies that suggest that acquisition of a language system is a significant contributor for many aspects of development. Research conducted by Belenky (1984) further supports the theory that a language system is critical to the individual's development. She has found that hearing adolescents and adults who grew up in environments with markedly limited opportunities for dialogues may have developmental patterns similar to those of the deaf child having a prelingual, profound loss.

These deaf individuals are frequently discouraged from participating in or contributing to ongoing dialogues in school, home, and social situations. As a result, lags in cognitive as well as moral development are evident. In order for growth to occur in both areas, a climate must be provided whereby free exchange of ideas can take place, reasons can be challenged, and judgments defended via a channel of mutual communication (Holstein, 1968; Kohlberg, 1976).

ADDITIONAL INSIGHTS INTO DEAFNESS AND MORAL DEVELOPMENT

Studies pertaining to topics surrounding moral development and involving deaf subjects have traditionally depicted deaf individuals in a negative manner. Nass (1964) found nine-year-old congenitally deaf youngsters to be approximately two years behind their hearing peers in making the transition from consequence-oriented reasoning to that involving motive intent-based moral reasoning. Hoemann (1972) found poorer performance by deaf than hearing eight- to eleven-year-olds on tasks requiring referential communication and perspective-taking. In addition, deaf and hard of hearing children are consistently characterized as more impulsive and/or egocentric than their hearing counterparts (Altshuler, 1963, 1974; Harris, 1978; Hefferman, 1955; Hoemann, 1972; Meadow, 1980; O'Brien, 1987).

Although many of these studies have emphasized lags in the development of deaf individuals, the findings must be examined in light of the following information:

1. Most of the research was conducted on children and adolescents and does not take into consideration the delays in cognitive development.
2. When adults are studied they are frequently from clinical populations in which one might expect to find a disproportionate amount of psychological problems.
3. Very few studies have been designed and conducted specifically for use within the Deaf subculture, taking environmental differences into consideration.

However, in accordance with Levine (1981), when one examines those deaf adults who are separate from the clinical population, the group as a whole is remarkably resilient and successful in coping with adult demands despite the difficult childhoods experienced. Furth (1974) and DeCaro and Emerton's (1978) research also depicts these adults as highly gregarious, active, responsible members interacting with each other in a closely knit, stable community of the Deaf. It further suggests that even though moral development may be delayed, it is not truncated.

SOCIAL LEARNING AND VALUES CLARIFICATION

According to McKinney (1980), when considering the layperson's view of moral order, the concept of "values" plays a major role. Moral judgment and consequent moral behavior are presumed to be based on some "interior units of character" that must be cultivated in order to grow and develop. Thus, churches urge parents to promote correct moral values in their children. Likewise, the secular press often attributes destruction of the social order to a decline in "values." These values include the deterioration of those ideals surrounding democracy, family life, and the American dream; all are perceived as important beliefs to be cherished (McKinney, 1980, p. 201).

How can the term "values" be defined? What differentiates beliefs and attitudes from them? What assumptions can be made about human values? Is there a difference between those that are cherished in the hearing community as compared with the ones found in the Deaf subculture?

A Definition of Values

If moral behavior is based on moral judgment, then moral judgment, in turn, is based on some internalized schemata, or cognitive units, whose properties can be studied. These cognitive units are referred to as "values," and it is in this way that values are related to the development of moral behavior. They provide the social framework within which judgments are made (McKinney, 1980, p. 204).

Values as They Differ from Attitudes, Beliefs, and Interests

Values, if viewed as cognitive units, are used in the assessment of behavior along the dimensions of what is considered to be "good or bad," "appropriate or inappropriate," and "right or wrong." They are concerned with what ought to be, rather than what is. By using this definition of values, one can begin to distinguish them from ideals that people hold.

Ideals do not always imply that people have a choice; values, on the other hand, do. The culture or environment in which a person grows up may hold certain ideals, but these only become individually held values when a person uses those ideals as a personal way of making choices.

Values can also be differentiated from beliefs. A person may hold a belief that something is "true or false," "correct or incorrect." But the term "value" can also be incorporated to imply a different type of judgment. When used in this manner, the implication is that some object or behavior is either "good or bad," "desirable or undesirable," "right or wrong" in the sense that it is personally acceptable or unacceptable. The element of this *approval* is what distinguishes values from beliefs, and that element of *selection* is what distinguishes values from culturally bound ideals.

An "attitude" is another psychological concept that is sometimes confused with a value. Attitudes are generally more specific, while values are more global and may underlie a whole set of attitudes. Although the term "attitude" may be defined as a response to an opinion, a "value" refers to a whole complex of such sets.

Values can further be distinguished from interests. Interests are not as enduring as values and may change easily. Values are more related to the core of individuals' definitions of themselves (McKinney, 1980, pp. 203–204).

To say that people have a value is to say that they have an enduring prescriptive or proscriptive belief that a specific mode of behavior or end-state of existence is preferred to an opposite mode of behavior or end-state. This belief transcends attitudes toward objects and situations; it is a standard that guides and determines action, attitudes toward objects, situations and ideology, and provides the foundation for judgments and justifications as individuals compare themselves with others.

It may be suggested that the enduring quality of values arises mainly from the fact that they are initially taught and learned in isolation from other values in an absolute all-or-none manner. It is the isolated and thus the absolute learning of values that more or less guarantees their stability (Rokeach, 1973).

The Acquisition of Values

Values are acquired through the learning process, and like all learning they are procured gradually. After a value is learned, it becomes integrated into an organized system wherein each value is prioritized with respect to other values.

Based on this premise, individuals can be conceived as being capable of reordering various situations that occur within their culture. Over time, the overall value system remains relatively stable, reflecting the individual's unique personality within his culture and society. At the same time it remains flexible, allowing for incorporation of new personal experiences to be integrated into their value system.

As children mature and become more complex, they are increasingly likely to encounter situations in which several values may compete with one another, requiring a weighing of one value against another. When this occurs, a decision must be made as to which value is more important. As individuals develop, occasional conflicts in their values may occur. Individuals may be forced to decide whether it is better to seek success or remain an honest person; they may have to choose between acting obediently or responding independently.

Values may be acquired that are social, as well as "nonsocial," or private in nature (for example, cleanliness, achievement, and independence). McKinney has suggested that "values for an individual are neither entirely objective nor entirely subjective, but like perception, lie on the interface between external reality and internal commitment" (McKinney, 1975, p. 806). They become part of the framework that allows for choices and judgments to be made.

Assumptions About the Nature of Human Values

Rokeach based his writing on five assumptions about the nature of human values. He states:

1. the total number of values that a person possesses is relatively small
2. all men everywhere possess the same values to different degrees
3. values are organized into value systems
4. the antecedents of human values can be traced to culture, society, and its institutions and personality
5. the consequences of human values will be manifested in virtually all phenomena that social scientists might consider worth investigating and understanding (Rokeach, 1973, p. 3)

These assumptions provide the foundation for other tenets of his philosophy. Within his value systems, moral values have an interpersonal focus that, when violated, arouse pangs of conscience or feelings of guilt. Rokeach separates these values from other instrumental values, which are referred to as competence or "self-actualization" values.

He has defined self-actualization values as having a personal rather than an interpersonal focus and has viewed them separately from those concerned with morality. He felt that violation of this type of value led to feelings of shame about personal inadequacy rather than to feelings of shame about wrongdoing. Thus, behaving honestly and responsibly leads to the feeling that one is behaving morally whereas behaving logically, intelligently, or imaginatively leads to the feeling that one is behaving competently (Rokeach, 1973, p. 8).

Rokeach (1973) has postulated that values provide the individual with the ability to rationalize, in the psychoanalytic sense, beliefs, attitudes, and actions that would otherwise be personally and socially unacceptable. When an atmosphere is created that fosters growth in the area of personal feelings related to morality and competence, self-esteem can be enhanced.

Clarifying Values

If, in fact, one's values can be traced to personality, culture, and society, how does the individual become aware of his values? What type of environment and dialogue are conducive to facilitating value awareness and clarification?

Although the basic premise of values clarification is that everyone has an individual set of values, it is further advocated that children can, and should, learn: 1) to be more aware of their own values and have their values in turn relate to the decisions that they make; 2) to make their values consistent and to place them in hierarchical order for decision-making purposes; 3) to become more aware of the divergencies between their value hierarchies and those of others; and 4) to learn to develop a tolerance for such divergencies (Kohlberg, 1981, p. 11). In other words, students must be provided with strategies that will enable them to recognize their values and incorporate them to their fullest, while simultaneously developing a tolerance for those who embrace a different value system.

To foster this type of development, exercises in values clarification have been designed to serve as a catalyst for value identification and clarification. The chief proponent of values clarification is Sidney B. Simon. His emphasis is placed on the philosophy that there are no right or wrong answers to questions of morality. In this approach, students are asked questions or presented with dilemmas and expected to respond individually or in small groups. The procedure is intended to help students define their own values and to make them aware of others' values. In the process, students proceed through seven steps: prizing one's beliefs and behaviors (steps 1 & 2), choosing one's beliefs and behaviors (steps 3, 4, & 5), and acting on one's beliefs (steps 6 & 7) (Benninga, 1988, p. 416). To enable the student to become more keenly aware of his values, a series of activities, many of which are paper and pencil exercises, are administered. The exercises are "value free," and one answer is as acceptable as any other. The clarification of values is left up to the individual student.

Although exercises of this nature may serve to put the student in touch with his values, critics of this approach claim that because of its controversial content, values clarification often offends community standards. In addition, critics believe this approach undermines accepted values, induces no search for consensus, fails to stress truth and right behavior, and does not distinguish between morality as a generalizable system of norms and morality as a system based on personal preference or whim (Benninga, 1988, p. 417).

Values, according to McClelland (1982), are principles that guide the individual or society to make choices. He further explains that a person's values are based on reasoning that is more or less socially and morally mature, depending on the development achieved by that person. Inherent in his philosophy is the interaction of individuals' value systems as they relate to society. Thrower (1971) examined role-taking tasks with three groups of children. Adolescents residing in foster homes, disturbed families, and orphanages were evaluated to determine their level of moral reasoning. Results indicated that adolescents raised in institutional settings had remained at the earliest stages of moral reasoning. The remaining groups were closer to their age-appropriate levels of development. Thrower indicated that within the orphanage, children engaged in limited communication between themselves and the staff. Thrower's findings support the premise that social interaction is critical to moral development.

Social interactions and exchanges with viable role models influence moral development and assimilation of values. Based on this premise, what effect does deafness and the ramifications of social isolation have on the deaf individual's value system?

DEAFNESS, SOCIAL LEARNING, AND VALUES CLARIFICATION

Prelingual profoundly deaf students invariably cannot communicate easily with their hearing peers (particularly from adolescence onward). Therefore, they are in a state of *marginality*. Marginality, in turn, prevents both enculturization and socialization (Rodda & Grove, 1987, p. 87). Deaf individuals, due to the difficulties they encounter with communication, may find that they are unable to benefit from the opportunity to engage in verbally mediated social and interpersonal activities. They may become frustrated both with their attempts to express themselves and with their inability to understand others to the point that they will withdraw from social situations. In turn, deaf individuals may opt to avoid those situations that set the stage for misunderstanding or conflict to occur.

Observational studies of deaf children's spontaneous social interaction (Heider, 1948; Liben, 1978; Meadow, 1971) indicate that deaf children do elect to avoid conflict to a greater extent than their hearing peers. According to Liben (1978, p. 208), "Informal comments by teachers, parents, and residential counselors" indicate that parents of deaf children may also circumvent complex communication by avoiding situations of conflict. Mugny, dePaolis, and Carugati (1984) have suggested that whenever children opt to avoid cognitive or social conflict by simply yielding, obeying, or conforming to the other individual's point of view, no progress in the areas of moral development will be made. Based on Mugny and collegues' (1984) hypothesis that children must confront conflict cognitively to stimulate progress, Peterson and Peterson (1989) conducted a study in which they initially predicted that no progress in profoundly deaf or hearing children would occur in those who avoided conflict via conformity but anticipated gains in justice reasoning among those who challenged the adult's viewpoint.

These deaf and hearing subjects viewed a silent videotaped story depicting two children interacting with an adult authority figure. The children in the story were instructed to perform a work task. At this point, the viewer watched the children share equally in the task. After viewing the children simultaneously working together on their task, the adult figure returned and the video paused on a shot of chocolate bars in the man's hand. The examiner then showed the subjects pictures of the boy and girl and instructed them to "give the boy as much chocolate as he deserves, and the girl as much as she deserves." Depending on the answer, the subjects were then asked, "Why did you give more to the girl/more to the boy/the same to each?"

As the tape began again, the adult was shown rewarding the boy with more candy than the girl for the same amount of work. At the end of the scenario, those involved in the test situation were asked, "Was the father right to give more chocolate to the boy?" After replying, the subjects were allowed to allocate the candy again and explain the reasons behind their answers.

The results from this study are fascinating. Compared with the hearing students in the sample, the deaf subjects were less likely to disagree with the reward allocation suggested by the adult, and also less likely to make cognitive progress when they did encounter conflict. A problem with the scoring of the deaf children's reasoning was the relatively large number of deaf children (28 percent) who, despite repeated promptings, refused to offer any coherent rationale for their reward or allocation decisions. This suggests that identical levels of overt contradiction do not always create the same levels of internalized cognitive conflict or conflict-resolution in the deaf as in the hearing (Peterson & Peterson, 1989, p. 281).

One can speculate that the deaf child simply ignores all but the most salient contradictions. Persistently frustrated efforts to communicate with the hearing, speaking world could lead to the view that much of one's social life is intrinsically incomprehensible. Communication failure or misunderstanding can also be attributed to the fact that deaf children develop a stronger motivation to avoid conflict, or stronger defenses against noticing the various ambiguities and contradictions inherent in many social situations. Liben (1978) has suggested that the typically overprotective childrearing strategies of the hearing parents of deaf children also could result in their becoming less aware of the existence of multiple viewpoints or cognitive contradictions.

Although deaf adolescents may avoid social interactions within the hearing community, peer cooperation within the Deaf culture remains active. It seems plausible that deaf children's understanding of peer relationships develop at the same rate as that of hearing children. Contact with peers who share their communication mode provides deaf students with the opportunity to socially interact with peers who negotiate and bargain with each other for arranging mutually beneficial agreements (Rest, 1983, p. 596). This is believed to create a reasonable imbalance in the child's cognitive structures, thereby encouraging growth (Brice, 1985).

SUMMARY

The essence of moral decision is the exercise of choice and the willingness to accept responsibility for that choice (Gilligan, 1982). To the point that deaf individuals perceive themselves as having no choice in the much larger hearing society they may withdraw from social interactions, thus restricting their opportunity to engage in the exchange of ideas and benefit from the diverging viewpoints of others.

Research pertaining to deafness and moral development is very scant. There are even fewer studies pertaining to values and values clarification. From the research that has been conducted, it has been established that most deaf people are socially competent. However, it has also been illustrated that they are not privy to the same environmental stimuli essential for moral enhancement.

The present results reinforce the need identified by Brice (1985) for more effective interventions to encourage deaf children to exchange thoughts, feelings, and explanations for another's behavior in their everyday social interactions with peers, parents, teachers, and other adult authorities. It is also possible that deaf children may need either more or different conflict situations than their hearing peers to further trigger cognitive growth (Peterson & Peterson, 1989).

Studies that have been conducted have only begun to scratch the surface in the area of moral development. Further research of this kind needs to be conducted with deaf subjects, using a much wider array of cognitive problems and conflict-generating tasks or experiences.

▶ 9

The Deafened Adult

The aging process is as unique as the individuals who experience it. Through one's lifetime, situations are encountered, educational and vocational choices are made, and older adults emerge exhibiting diverse behaviors reflective of a culmination of years of experiences. The rate and extent of the aging process varies considerably from one individual to the next; however, some characteristics are manifested by all who enter the domain of the senior citizen. Outward signs of aging include changes in body build, skin texture, gait, and level of agility. In addition, one's voice can be described as sounding "old," "senile," or "senescent." Research indicates that throughout the aging process one's vision, audition, and other sensory and perceptual processes reflect significant decrements (Corso, 1971). Most individuals demonstrate a decline in perceptual skills in new learning, rote memory (Gilbert & Levee, 1971), and long-term memory tasks (Smith, 1975; Meyerson, 1976).

Each day in the United States, there is a net gain of nearly 1,000 persons 65 and over contributing to the more than 25 million older adults residing among the younger and middle age generations (Carter, 1982). Although research indicates that intelligence does not decline as one ages, it does show clearly that older adults generally require more time to complete tasks involving learning. When placed in test situations that impose time constraints (speed), they do not perform as well as younger people (Kimmel, 1980).

It is well established that with advancing age many persons exhibit alterations in the auditory process that may hamper their ability to engage in day-to-day conversations. Their ability to comprehend speech sounds may be affected, restricting them to selective conversational situations.

Hearing loss associated with the aging process becomes evident in most individuals by the age of 50. By age 65, over half of all men and a third of all women suffer significant hearing losses (Carter, 1982). What are some of the characteristics of this unique population? What are the causes of hearing loss in older adults and what are the psychological effects of hearing loss on the individual as he or she progresses through the later years of life?

CHARACTERISTICS OF OLDER ADULTS

When discussing the topic of aging, this population can generally be viewed in respect to three different dimensions. Topics can be related to those issues revolving around biological, psychological, or sociological aging issues.

Biological Aging

The arena of biological aging describes the state of individuals' organ systems as indicators of their potential life span. This area also incorporates the chronological age of the individual.

Since the adoption of the Social Security Act in 1935, a widely accepted chronological definition is that anyone who has reached the age of 65 automatically becomes a member in the sector of the population referred to as "the aging." The process of aging is slow in nature and causes continuous changes in individuals from birth to death. One can further identify "the aging" population by those who are "young old," ages 55–75, to those who are "old old," ages 75 and up (Neugarten, 1975).

Psychological or Behavioral Aging

Psychological or behavioral aging includes intelligence, memory, and learning together with exploring one's feelings, emotions, and motivations. Information pertaining to how individuals adjust to the aging process, as well as their hearing loss, can be viewed under the heading of psychological concerns.

Social Aging

Social aging includes those issues pertaining to older adults' roles in society and the way in which their views and values compare with the other members of the group or society. Another topic includes those environmental factors that contribute to stress and accelerate the physiological changes of aging.

To gain insights into the world of the deafened adult, it is imperative to view the aging process from all three perspectives: biological, psychological, and sociological. Understanding the concerns and issues involved within each area facilitates the development of strategies that promote effective communication with the deafened adult population.

The deafened adult population, in this context, refers to those individuals who have lost their hearing due to the aging process. Throughout their lifetimes they have developed speech and language patterns through their ability to hear. However, as they become older, many discover that their hearing has deteriorated and that they can no longer benefit from information transmitted through the auditory channel.

PHYSIOLOGICAL CHANGES DUE TO THE AGING PROCESS

As previously stated, those individuals who have achieved membership into the generation of the older adult have undergone physiological changes, many of which have manifested themselves in outward appearances. However, perhaps the most devastating change, due to the aging process, lies in the area of hearing impairment.

Hearing loss is common, affecting one out of eleven, or a total of 21 million people in the general population. Its incidence increases sharply with age, affecting approximately 30 percent of the adult population over the age of 65 (Wax, 1987). Age changes in hearing ability are often characterized as progressive, irreversible, and detrimental, preventing successful communication in the later years of life. By examining the age-related effects on the anatomy and physiology of the auditory system, one can make certain global predictions about auditory function in the elderly.

Outer Ear

There are two major changes that occur in the outer ear that are directly related to the aging process. The first change involves the physical characteristics of the pinna. Studies by Tsai, Chou, and Cheng (1958) reported that changes in the size, shape, and flexibility of the pinna occur as one ages. However, it has not been determined whether these changes have a significant effect on auditory localization.

The second change, according to Magladery (1959), indicated that atrophy in the supporting walls of the auditory canal is associated with the aging process. When atrophy of the skin lining of the canal occurs, it interferes with the expulsion of cerumen (ear wax). This in turn creates an excessive accumulation of wax that results in a conductive hearing loss (Corso, 1971). In addition, older individuals appear to have a higher frequency of collapsed auditory canals, thus interfering with the transmission of auditory signals (Schow et al., 1978; Schow & Nerbonne, 1980).

Middle Ear

A variety of age-related structural changes occur in the middle ear; however, the functional significance of these changes remains unclear. Those changes that may affect middle ear functioning include the following: thinning and calcification of the ossicular joints (Etholm & Belal, 1974), calcification of the tympanic ring in which the eardrum is mounted, and replacement of elastic tissues in the eardrum with collagenous tissue (Etholm & Belal, 1974). These impairments indicate a decline in the elasticity of the eardrum, which affects the conduction of sound.

Inner Ear

Although some types of hearing problems experienced by the elderly may be attributed to outer and middle ear dysfunction, the primary cause of loss of hearing in this population is due to degeneration of hair cells in the organ of Corti and/or to disturbance of the inner ear metabolism (Corso, 1971; Schuknecht, 1974).

Hair cell loss with age has been well documented. Degeneration occurs within the supporting structures housed in the inner ear, as well as in the hair cells themselves. This decrease can be observed as early as the end of the second decade and appears to increase gradually with the aging process (Harford & Dodds, 1982). The pattern of loss for inner and outer hair cells is different in that the inner hair cells tend to show only a basal degeneration compared with the more widespread loss experienced by the outer hair cells.

Additional studies have reported other effects of the aging process on the inner ear cavity. Schuknecht (1974) noted the occurrence of pronounced acellularity in the spiral ligament, the basilar membrane's attachment to the cochlear wall. In addition, there is reduced flexibility of the basilar membrane, thickening of the tectorial membrane and accumulation of restrictive adhesions in the inner ears of older individuals (Hansen & Riske-Nielsen, 1965).

Age-related anatomical changes in the mechanical structures, sensory cells, neural supply, and support structures of the inner ear all contribute to the hearing loss experienced by the older deafened adult population. In light of these anatomical and physiological changes, one can examine the types of difficulties encountered by this population in respect to the aging process.

Presbycusis

Hearing loss in older individuals is referred to as presbycusis. It is a type of sensorineural hearing loss that occurs with the aging process. In the United States, presbycusis is generally taken for granted among older people. However, it has been documented that it is nonexistent in some primitive societies. This lack of appearance in some cultures can be attributed to the general diet and health of the specific population, as well as the relatively low noise level present in certain societies. There have been numerous studies conducted pertaining to presbycusis. Traditionally, it was thought that this dysfunction affected the inner ear structure only. However, more recent research indicates that it affects all portions of the auditory system. Broad-based studies focusing on presbycusis indicate that changes occur in the physical characteristics of the entire ear structure. This results in changes in the middle ear tissue that may affect the flexibility of the ligaments connected with the ossicles and the eardrum. In addition, changes occur within the basilar membrane and the tectorial membrane as they lose some of their elasticity. Neurons and hair cells degenerate and cannot be replaced. When these changes occur and the hair cells inside the inner ear are destroyed, sound can no longer be picked up properly. This type of loss becomes permanent because hair cells are unable to grow back. Although the ability to hear high frequency sounds diminishes over a lifetime, it becomes more obvious as the aging process continues. This results, on the average, in a cumulative loss in hearing of 20 decibels between the ages of 65 and 85.

Extensive research has been done in this area. However, in the discussion of presbycusis, the research conducted by Schuknecht (1974) merits special recognition. During his investigation throughout the fifties and sixties, he identified and described four types of presbycusis. A description of these types is included in Table 9-1. (Schow et al., 1978)

The individual whose hearing loss is attributed to presbycusis may be affected by those physical changes that occur in any of the four areas. In addition, any given individual may simultaneously experience more than one type of presbycusis during his lifetime. The four types reflect different patterns of structural and functional losses. In addition, the type of dysfunction one exhibits will influence the unique pattern of loss that is experienced. One cannot assume that presbycusis is reflective of only one pattern of hearing loss; rather, the pattern is as unique as the older person who experiences it.

It is critical to note that the hearing process is as complex as the aging process. Researchers are only a little closer today in fully understanding the acoustic process as it relates to the aging cycle. However, one aspect of this process that has received considerable attention is the component involving speech, language, and communication. By examining the effect this type of loss has on the individual, one is able to more fully comprehend the characteristics of the deafened adult.

Diseases and Illnesses Related to Deafness

In addition to presbycusis, hearing losses in older adults may be attributed to several causes. Permanent losses can be caused by any disease or condition that restricts blood flow to the inner ear, such as stroke or injury.

TABLE 9-1   **Four Types of Presbycusis**

Sensory Presbycusis is characterized by atrophy of the Organ of Corti and the auditory nerve in the basal portion of the cochlea.

Neural Presbycusis is associated with a loss of nerve fibers or cells in the auditory pathway of the central nervous system.

Metabolic Presbycusis refers to those defects in biochemical or bio-physical processes involved in the transducer mechanism of the cochlea.

Mechanical Presbycusis relates to the motion properties of the cochlear duct.

In addition, the senior citizen can experience other disabling hearing disorders such as noise-induced losses, otosclerosis, otitis media, Eustachian tube malfunction, sudden deafness, and Ménière's disease (Mathog et al., 1974).

Older adults who experience any of the illnesses or diseases above may find that their hearing ability decreases significantly. Although presbycusis is one of, if not the major, sensory changes associated with aging in the human body, all of the causes outlined above influence one's ability to hear and respond to environmental sounds. The degree of loss will further influence older adults as they engage in daily communication and socialization.

COMMUNICATION ISSUES RELEVANT TO THE DEAFENED ADULT

When older people lose their hearing and can no longer hear background sounds, they may begin to feel removed from the ongoing world. According to Ramsdell (1970), hearing loss occurs on three levels.

Primitive or Basic Level: This level pertains to those sounds in the environment that allow people to feel "connected" to what is happening around them. It provides individuals with a sense of being alive and alert to their surroundings. When hearing becomes impaired at this level, individuals may experience dull, empty, or isolated feelings.

Signal or Warning Level: Hearing provides individuals with information related to crises that occur in their surroundings. Sounds such as police sirens, emergency vehicles, horns of approaching cars, and cries from babies are all included in this category. When a loss is incurred on this level, individuals may develop a fear of becoming involved in accidents or becoming the victim of personal misfortune(s). This tends to increase hearing impaired persons' feelings of insecurity about themselves and their relationship to their environment.

Social or Symbolic Level: On this level we use our hearing to receive and understand language that is spoken around us. When individuals experience a loss on this level, they are prevented from engaging in relatively comfortable, daily exchanges of information. Conversations between family and friends become strained, and misunderstandings frequently occur. This by far can be the most unsettling of the three levels.

It is crucial to the integrity of older people that the lines of communication remain open, thus providing for viable exchanges of information. When a barrier to communication arises and one forfeits the luxury of communication, an erosion in feelings of self-worth occurs that may contribute to the dehumanization of the elderly.

As with all segments of our society (children, youth, and adults), the elderly develop inherent individual differences that will determine the frequency with which they choose to become involved in conversations. Individuals' personalities, educational background, intellectual functioning ability, and past vocational experiences all contribute, to some extent, to the frequency and types of interactions in which they will participate.

Although these individual differences must be taken into consideration, there are some areas of communication that remain vital to the lives of all of these senior citizens. These areas range from the fundamental need for situations requiring interpersonal relationships to those larger group encounters that require the ability to converse with more than one individual.

Within the older adult population, one's hearing loss generally occurs gradually over an extended period of time. Individuals may experience a significant loss and may be oblivious to their disability. Although they may not sustain a loss until they become older, their speech production may still be affected. In addition, they may find there are specific speech sounds that appear to be muffled when others are addressing them. As they enter into conversations, they may perceive others to be mumbling when speaking; in fact, their own inability to hear forms this perception.

Components of Speech: Understanding the Spoken Word

Aging individuals appear to understand speech when it is slow and relatively simple; however, when the rate of speech is increased or when there is background noise, they may become lost. There also are some speech sounds that are easier for individuals with impaired hearing to comprehend. For example, vowels are strong, low frequency sounds that travel across distances well, turn corners readily, and penetrate background noise more easily. In contrast, consonants are weaker, high frequency sounds. They fade quickly with distance, do not turn corners easily, and tend to disappear in noise. It is interesting to note that there are four times as many consonants as vowels. As a result, for one whose hearing is impaired, reception of speech sounds becomes difficult. At a loudness level where vowels are heard clearly, soft consonants such as "s," "sh," "t," or "f" may not be heard at all. Others such as "p" or "t" may sound alike and be confused. This is all compounded by the fact that some individuals have strong voices, while others have weak ones (Combs, 1988).

In addition to being faced with the auditory difficulty in receiving speech sounds, senior citizens may experience problems processing the information once it is received. Throughout the aging process, elderly persons are particularly susceptible to neurological degeneration and diseases that interrupt normal language functioning and the peripheral execution of speech events. Due to the normal aging process, neurological disease, or a combination of these two, the aging person experiences difficulties in engaging in spoken communication (Oyer, 1976). These reductions in intellectual functioning may be the result of three factors: 1) deteriorative changes in the central nervous system—one experiences approximately an 11 percent decrease in brain weight between 25 and 96 years of age; 2) a loss of motivation to perform specific tasks; and 3) a lack of adaptability to perform certain skills.

This reduction in intellectual functioning ability has a direct correlation to the older adult's ability to function in the speech and language area. Studies conducted by Jerger and Hayes (1977) and more recently by Shirinian and Arnst (1982) recognize and describe the age-related effects within the area of oral communication. These authors offered several findings. When hearing tests were administered to senior citizens, their ability to respond to central tones remained in the normal range. However, when the central speech tests were administered at a high speech intensity, these same individuals showed marked deterioration with age. This phenomenon, referred to as "rollover," has been documented as an eighth nerve and central auditory pathway dysfunction (Jerger, 1960). Shirinian and Arnst (1982) confirmed the presence of the "central aging effect" on word and sentence performance in elderly subjects with normal pure-tone audiograms.

Additional studies by Hinchcliffe (1962) have summarized the effects of the age-related changes in hearing ability and the ramifications in connection with the communication process. The changes he notes can be summarized as follows:

1. impairment of pure-tone thresholds, particularly for high frequency tones
2. impairment of frequency discrimination
3. impairment of auditory temporal discrimination and sound localization ability
4. impairment of speech discrimination ability
5. decreased ability to understand distorted speech
6. decreased ability to recall long sentences (p. 332)

The increased difficulty in speech reception and word discrimination experienced by the elderly can create breakdowns in the communication process and create stressful situations. Those wanting to communicate with the older adult may find it is very difficult to engage in any exchange of information and, therefore, unintentionally isolate the elderly person. This has negative implications for all of those who are involved.

A PSYCHOSOCIAL PERSPECTIVE OF DEAFNESS THROUGHOUT THE SENIOR YEARS

The way in which one accepts deafness in the later years of life differs radically from that experienced by the prelingually deaf. The newborn or young infant has no understanding of a "different" auditory ability. However, those who experience deafness later in life undergo the traumatic experience of adjusting to a loss of something they once valued and cherished.

Frequently, the loss experienced by the senior citizen is a gradual one; thus, there may be an extended period of time during which the person denies that it exists. This extended period of denial in deafened adults delays the acquisition of new skills (Levine, 1981). In addition, people who are experiencing a progressive loss may be unable to share their feelings with others, thus preventing the dissipation of stressful feelings. As a result, progressively deafened adults may cling to and become increasingly disturbed about the residual hearing that keeps diminishing rather than face the current hearing loss or the prospect of continuing loss (Pintner, Eisenson, & Stanton, 1941).

Acceptance of the finality of acquired loss occurs more readily when loss is sudden rather than progressive (Glass, 1985). Those who experience a sudden and profound loss are more inclined to make a more rapid decision about rehabilitative services, surgical techniques, and communication modes than do the progressively deafened adults.

Responding to the Initial Diagnosis of Deafness

Studies conducted with deafened adults indicate that although many suspected they had some degree of loss, when confronted with the actual diagnosis, over 50 percent of them responded with accompanying emotions. While over half of the respondents surveyed by Martin and colleagues (1989) expected the diagnosis, most experienced additional emotions including sadness, worry, fear, and disappointment. Anger, surprise, and shock were described by 15 to 22 percent of the respondents. In addition, the correlation between the severity of the hearing loss and the reaction of fear was significant.

It is critical that senior citizens undergoing diagnosis for a hearing loss receive the services of an understanding and compassionate professional. Deafened individuals writing about their personal experiences regarding the initial diagnosis complained that they were the victims of insensitive, uninformed professionals. As a result, many left the testing situation with a complexity of feelings that included shock, denial, grief, depression, and shame. They believed these feelings often went unacknowledged by the professional involved (Martin et al., 1989). Quite often, deafened adults feel that the professionals do not understand the difference between deafened adults and prelingually deaf persons. Therefore, they leave the diagnostic arena with many fears and several unanswered questions.

Psychological Effects of Hearing Loss

Severe hearing loss experienced by older adults may affect them psychologically. Many will deny that they have a loss because they fear that by admitting it they are confirming the conception that they will be unable to perform certain personal and social tasks. Additional psychological effects include the following feelings.

Uncertainty
Very frequently, deafened adults appear to walk a very fine line between hearing and not hearing. Sounds and noises either become too loud or too soft, and older people will be unsure about what has been said. This creates feelings of uncertainty about what others are thinking and how others perceive them. The previous comfort level of communicating with others diminishes and early signs of withdrawal occur.

Frustration
Coupled with uncertainty are increased feelings of frustration as they seek to understand the events and communication surrounding them. Deafened adults remember the quality of life they once experienced and may become very frustrated with that which is diminishing around them.

Anger
As uncertainty and frustration are enhanced, anger becomes apparent. Elderly people may be angry at themselves for getting older, angry because their hearing is diminishing and communication has become increasingly difficult, and angry at the professionals who do not seem to comprehend the global effects of the disability.

Stress
As they worry about their degenerative hearing and the ramifications it entails, the amount of worry and stress increases. They realize that they are losing the facility to interact freely with friends and relatives. While attempting to engage in conversations, they experience an increased level of stress as they strain to hear and understand the verbal exchange directed at or around them.

Effect of Hearing Loss Involved in the Transmission of Information

As older individuals acquire a hearing loss, many misunderstand what is being said. They may respond to this lack of understanding in several ways. First, those who cannot hear may try to guess the content of the message. However, frequently they guess wrong, embarrassment occurs, and there is a breakdown in communication. Second, the speaker may sense that the person with a hearing loss is not understanding and may repeat the message. This may cause the deafened person to feel embarrassed or insulted because the speaker is repeating him- or herself. Third, older persons may feel that others are losing patience with their lack of understanding and will therefore withdraw from the situation and occasionally remove themselves physically from their environment.

Communication Within the Family Unit

This breakdown in communication occurs quite frequently in family situations. According to Oyer (1976), about one-third of the senior citizen population lives with adult children. As a result, important familial communications occur on a routine basis. When older adults experience a hearing disability, the channel of communication may become quite strained and occasionally break down completely. It is important to note that as senior citizens attempt to engage in conversations with family members, their hearing loss, as well as the topic of conversation, may contribute to a potentially stressful situation. Due to the "generation gap," older adults' view of themselves as a unique part of the family unit, and the way other members in the family perceive them, will influence the degree of interpersonal communication that occurs within their domicile.

Coping with a hearing loss always means dealing with attitudes—deafened adults' attitudes toward themselves and the attitudes others have toward them. The attitude toward individuals with hearing loss is decidedly different from that toward those who do not experience the disability. Frequently, they are ignored and, gradually, they become estranged from their family and associates. They may feel they are social outcasts and begin to withdraw from their family and their social environment. They may claim they have no friends, feel lonely, and generally experience dissatisfaction with life because of the communication problems associated with their loss.

Hearing loss can create feelings of emotional isolation. One may begin to feel isolated not only from family members but from those living outside of their home. Upon interviewing senior citizens with significant hearing losses, Thomas and Gilhome-Herbst (1980) determined that 40 percent of them felt that their hearing loss was not understood by those nearest to them and therefore they felt very misunderstood and lonely.

Hearing loss is prevalent among older adults, and many people can anticipate developing some degree of hearing loss as they age. However, few are aware of what it means to acquire a hearing loss later in life. Those who lose their hearing in tandem with the aging process encounter difficulties unique to this population.

Sociological Effects of Hearing Loss

When hearing loss occurs, it begins to interfere with social efficiency. The more severe the loss, the more the person may be forced out of communication situations. Those seniors who experience a loss may begin to feel socially and/or psychologically disadvantaged as a result either of their hearing loss or because of the aging process. This occurs frequently in a society that has an obsession for youth and physical perfection. Many deafened older adults complain that when they attempt to interact in social situations, they are the victims of insensitivity, indifference, and cruelty due to the stigma of their hearing loss. They feel that the focus of attention is placed on their disability and that they are not recognized as anything other than a hearing impaired person. This presents a real dilemma for the older adult. They may question their involvement in social situations from several perspectives.

> Do I join other older adults?
> How will they react to my hearing loss?
> Do I join other adults who experience difficulty hearing?
> What do I share with them other than the loss of my hearing?
> Where do I fit in?
> Do I fit in at all? (Wax, 1987)

Society often views older people negatively. In addition, those with a disability are also viewed negatively. This frequently results in being treated differently by those around them. Older people are a kind of "minority group." People who have difficulty hearing fall into another category of a minority group. As a result, those individuals who fall into both groups are doubly disadvantaged when responding to society. It may be very difficult for deafened older adults to come to grips with themselves as they try to relate to the larger structure of society. In order for them to accomplish this task, they must have a healthy self-concept and be equipped to incorporate strategies that will further facilitate communication.

REHABILITATION FOR THE DEAFENED ADULT

It is estimated that six million Americans over the age of 65 experience a significant bilateral hearing loss, thus warranting consideration of hearing aids, yet only 17 percent of them use amplification (Alpiner, Kaufman, & Hanavan, 1993, p. 3). The majority of those with a progressive loss attribute it to the aging process and do not seek rehabilitation. Traditionally, aural rehabilitation has been known to consist of hearing aid evaluation and orientation, counseling for deafened individuals and their families, auditory training, and speech reading and speech conservation (Newby, 1972). In essence, it is broadly defined as an effort made to rehabilitate the hearing impaired through nonmedical procedures. Once a medical diagnosis from an otologist or an evaluation by an audiologist identifying the degree and type of loss is received, an overall rehabilitative program can be designed.

Determining the Feasibility of Hearing Aid Use

After a medical diagnosis has been assessed and it becomes apparent that surgical procedures will not benefit these individuals, they should be provided with information regarding alternative strategies. Usually the step that follows is to determine if they can benefit from amplification.

When one conducts hearing aid evaluations with elderly people, special considerations must be taken into account. One area of primary importance is the site of the lesion. As the site moves from a peripheral to a central location, the usefulness of a hearing aid diminishes. For those senior citizens exhibiting a middle ear disorder resulting in a conductive hearing loss, the success rate of utilizing a hearing aid is as high as 94 percent. However, for those experiencing a form of central auditory dysfunction, the success rate drops to only 6 percent (Otto & McCandless, 1982).

Audiometric measures testing both pure tones and speech reception thresholds (SRTs) need to be used when evaluating the senior citizen's hearing loss. The older adult will typically hear some of the vowel sounds but very few of the consonant sounds. Most of the loudness of speech is in the low frequencies where the vowel sounds occur. However, the clarity of speech is found in the upper frequencies where the consonants are heard. Therefore, when sounds occurring below 500 Hz are not heard, about 98 percent of the speech signal can still be understood. However, if the information heard around 1500 Hz is removed, only 65 percent of the signal will be understood (Fletcher, 1929). Because of this, most older individuals will do poorly on speech discrimination tests. Although they tend to hear sounds at a comfortable level, they are unable to decipher what is being said.

When audiologists administer a hearing battery, they attempt to assess the pure-tone average (average threshold of 500, 1,000, and 2,000 Hz), and obtain the speech reception threshold (SRT). These values may be compared with the 45 dB audiogram level, which is the average speech loudness when sitting three to four feet from someone speaking at a normal intensity. When the SRT level exceeds 45 dB, then conversation will be heard only when it is unusually loud (Schow et al., 1978).

Audiologists routinely recommend that individuals who experience a 40–60 dB loss wear a hearing aid on a continuous basis. They also recommend that they take advantage of other aural rehabilitation services. Hodgson (1977) suggested a cursory guide outlining those individuals who should be referred for a hearing aid evaluation. It is based on the pure-tone average or speech reception threshold (SRT) in the better ear. Specific recommendations are presented in Table 9-2.

Once it has been determined that an individual can benefit from a hearing aid and agrees to purchase one, training must be provided. Senior citizens may be in need of orientation on how to utilize their hearing aids. In addition, they may benefit from counseling sessions. These sessions enable them to become comfortable with their

TABLE 9-2 **Hearing Loss as It Relates to Amplification**

Hearing Loss in dB re: ANSI 1969	Need for Amplification
0–25	No Need
25–40	Part-time Need for Special Occasions
40–55	Frequent Need
55–80	Area of Greatest Satisfaction
80+	Great Need—Partial Help

hearing loss and develop strategies for enhancing their interpersonal communication skills.

The important components of hearing aid orientation and counseling sessions have been described by Sanders (1982) and Kasten and Warren (1977). In these sessions they suggest inclusion of the following hearing aid information:

1. Introducing the hearing aid, including its components and controls
2. Putting the aid on and listening to amplification
3. Caring for ear molds and batteries
4. Using the telephone, TV, alarm clocks, and other communication devices
5. Checking the aid and getting it repaired

In counseling they suggest:

1. Describing the levels of hearing such as primitive, warning, and symbolic (Ramsdell, 1970)
2. Explaining the audiological findings
3. Discussing the handicapping aspects of hearing loss
4. Describing the benefits and limitations of aids
5. Analyzing total communication needs
6. Finding solutions for communication problems (Schow et al., 1978)

It is imperative that senior citizens receive some orientation when they begin wearing hearing aids to insure that they will receive the maximum amount of benefit from them. In addition, in order for them to maintain a positive self-concept in light of their hearing loss, they may find counseling sessions beneficial.

Strategies for Coping with Hearing Loss in Later Life

When a diagnosis has been made and a hearing loss is confirmed, there are certain strategies that can be implemented to help individuals deal with their hearing loss. The first strategy involves assessing and understanding the physical extent of the loss. Once this has been determined, seniors can concentrate on their physical settings and communication strategies that will enhance their abilities to relate to others.

The Physical Setting: Coping Strategies

As hearing deteriorates, the use of the visual field becomes increasingly important. In order to receive information and comprehend what the speaker is saying, certain physical characteristics need to be taken into consideration.

1. Communication must be exchanged within the same room. If hearing people forget and attempt communicating from a distance, the deafened adult should tactfully remind them of his or her needs.

2. The speaker must face these listeners when addressing them. It is virtually impossible for individuals with a significant hearing loss to comprehend what is being said if the message is delivered behind them.
3. Light sources are extremely important. Speakers should avoid standing with their back to a light source; if this occurs it forces the deafened adult to look directly into a light source while attempting communication. This prohibits speech reading and enhances eyestrain.
4. In lecture situations, it is imperative for deafened and hard of hearing individuals to position themselves close to the speaker so that they can benefit from all visual cues.

Communication Tips: Coping with a Variety of Speakers

1. Whenever possible, those with a degree of hearing loss should "set up" the conversation in order to anticipate the response they will be getting.
2. When misunderstandings occur, repeat back the part of the conversation that was not clear so that the speaker will be advised of where the breakdown in communication occurred.
3. Ask the speaker to slow down and rephrase statements when misunderstandings occur. This may add clarity to the message.
4. If a specific number or word is misunderstood, request that the speaker spell or write it. In this way senior citizens can be sure they have received an accurate message.
5. When misunderstandings occur, ask for clarification of what the speaker said. Explain to the speaker what you thought you heard and proceed from there.

Additional strategies can be incorporated by hearing speakers that enable a smooth exchange of information between those who experience difficulty hearing and those who can hear. A few of the more critical strategies have been included below.

Communication Strategies: Tips for the Hearing Speaker

1. Use clear, distinct articulation, but avoid shouting.
2. Inform the individual of the topic you're discussing. When the topic changes it is imperative to inform the deafened listener.
3. Incorporate natural facial expressions when you are speaking, but avoid facial contortions and excessive exaggeration.
4. Avoid speaking with objects covering the mouth (pens, hands, paper, microphones, etc.), or speaking with objects in your mouth (food, gum, chewing tobacco, etc.).
5. Speak directly to the person with a hearing loss and not about him. Include him in conversations and listen to what he has to say.

Although speechreading is an art many deafened adults incorporate into their communication skills, it rarely provides total understanding by itself. Speechreading can be defined as that process through which listeners train themselves to be visually alert to all lip, facial, gestural, and environmental clues. In addition, ease of communication will occur more readily if the strategies listed above are incorporated by both parties.

SUPPORT GROUPS FOR THE DEAFENED ADULT

Throughout the past several years various organizations have been providing information for the deafened adult. Several of these provide inexpensive literature and periodicals that can be obtained by subscribing. A list of some of these agencies has been included below.

Alexander Graham Bell Association for the Deaf
3417 Volta Place, NW
Washington, DC 20007
(202) 337-5220 (Voice & TDD)

Provides information on speech reading, education, advocacy, aids and devices, and the psychological and social implications of deafness. The Oral Deaf Adults Section (ODAS), an active service group of adults encountering a deterioration in their hearing, offers special activities and programs for its members.

National Association of the Deaf
814 Thayer Avenue
Silver Spring, MD 20910
(301) 587-1788 (Voice & TDD)

Provides information for its members and other interested persons about deafness, programs and services for deaf people, communication skills, legislation, employment rights, and advocacy.

National Association for Hearing and Speech Action
10801 Rockville Pike
Rockville, MD 20852
(301) 897-8682 (Voice & TDD)

Provides consumer and public information about communication disorders. HELPLINE assists in finding professional assistance (call toll-free 1-800-638-8255).

Self Help for Hard of Hearing People, Inc.
7910 Woodmont Avenue, Suite 1200
Bethesda, MD 20814
(301) 657-2248
(301) 657-2249 (TDD)

Provides information about dealing with hearing loss, assistive devices, and adjustment to loss of hearing. Advocates on issues concerning hard-of-hearing people and encourages the establishment of state and local SHHH chapters.

American Speech-Language-Hearing Association
10801 Rockville Pike
Rockville, MD 20852
(301) 897-5700 (Voice & TDD)

ASHA provides public information about communication disorders, including deafness, and the role of speech and hearing professionals in rehabilitation. Information about local direct services is also available.

National Information Center on Deafness
Gallaudet University
800 Florida Avenue, NE
Washington, DC 20002
(202) 651-5051 (Voice)
(202) 651-5052 (TDD)

NICD provides information in all areas related to hearing loss and deafness, including education, communication with persons with hearing loss, and assistive devices. Makes referrals whenever possible to local and community services. (NICD, 1984, 1987)

SUMMARY

Approximately 80 percent of individuals with hearing problems are over 45 years of age, and nearly 55 percent of these are 65 years or older. It has been estimated that over 20 percent of the population of the United States between the ages of 45 and 54 have some hearing loss for high frequency pure tones. In individuals between the ages of 75 and 79 years, the frequency of hearing problems rises to about 75 percent of the population (Butler & Lewis, 1973).

However, within this population only 13 to 18 percent of the hearing impaired elderly population actually receive any form of amplification (Lichtenstein et al.,

1988). This can be attributed, in part, to their lack of awareness of resources available to them. In addition, several attribute their hearing loss to the aging process and see no reason to seek help for something they view as a natural phenomenon. As a result, many continue through the aging process experiencing communication difficulties that could be remediated through proper aural rehabilitation.

Older adults who experience difficulty hearing need to be aware of those materials and agencies that can help them learn how to improve their communication skills. They need to have the opportunity to engage in support groups, seminars, and educational activities that address the unique concerns of this population. By providing them with the opportunity to explore and understand the world of the deafened adult, they can become more comfortable with the disability and develop strategies for coping with the hearing public. As this occurs, one can anticipate a decline in communication problems, decreased feelings of isolation and fear, and an increased sense of a positive self-concept.

▶ 10

Myths and Misconceptions

Few hearing people know much about deafness. Because it is a low incidence handicap, the general public may not encounter many, if any, deaf individuals (those who are born with severe to profound losses). As a result, when they do come in contact with this population, they may have many preconceived ideas that are completely inaccurate. It is not uncommon for the hearing population to assume that deaf individuals can't read, can't drive, and that they rely on Braille for communication. Upon encountering a deaf individual for the first time, the hearing person, sensing a breakdown in the communication process, may first resort to shouting, hoping that the deaf person will hear. Upon realizing that this mode of communication will not work, the hearing person will attempt to discover if the deaf one can read.

Frequently, those outside the field of deafness assume that all deaf people can't talk, that they can all lip-read, and that hearing aids will cure their inability to hear. Further, they assume that deaf people are unable to deal with abstractions, cannot appreciate jokes, and produce all deaf offspring.

Not knowing people who are different from ourselves frequently leads to the invention of myths and misconceptions. To dispel these ideas, one needs to be provided with, and receptive to, accurate information and knowledge. By examining these misconceptions in light of current research and literature pertaining to this population, insights can be substituted for myths. In the ensuing pages, several of the more common myths and misconceptions surrounding deafness have been presented. Following each one, information has been included pertaining to deafness as a disability and the ramifications of it as a handicap.

DEAF PEOPLE CAN'T HEAR ANYTHING

It is not uncommon for members of the lay community, upon encountering a deaf individual for the first time, to assume that the person can't hear anything. As a result, phrases such as "stone deaf" and "deaf as a post" become incorporated into the hearing person's vernacular. The terms, which are of a derogatory nature, represent one of the fallacies associated with deafness.

The cause of one's loss, the type and severity of the impairment, and the age at onset all contribute to the extent to which the disability becomes a handicapping condition. Losses range from mild to profound and affect various frequencies. Although one individual may experience a loss in the high frequency range, others may hear those sounds satisfactorily but be unable to differentiate those sounds produced at lower frequencies.

In addition, two individuals may produce audiograms that appear identical; however, the effect of the loss on the individuals may be strikingly different. Although some may be able to compensate for their hearing deficits, utilize their residual hearing, and function as hard-of-hearing, others may find their loss to be significant and feel isolated from interactions within their social environment. The term "hard-of-hearing" refers to a score on an audiological evaluation and is not reflective of the individual's functioning ability. Therefore, those who have identical audiograms may function totally differently in various environmental situations.

The term "hearing loss" is broad, encompassing the hard-of-hearing at one end of the continuum, and the profoundly deaf on the other end. It is a heterogeneous group comprised of unique individuals. Their hearing losses differ, the sounds they are able to hear are diverse, and they vary in their abilities to capitalize on their residual hearing.

MYTHS SURROUNDING THE
CAUSES OF HEARING LOSS

Although the majority of those who are diagnosed as having a hearing loss can receive a medical explanation, there are some cases with unknown etiologies. As a result, parents, as well as concerned family members and friends, attempt to find reasons to justify the handicapping condition.

Misconceptions surrounding the causes of hearing loss include blows to the head, "brain fever," and high fevers that have "burned up the nerves" (Mindel & Vernon, 1987). These reasons may appear logical to parents when no other medical explanations are available. Nearly all parents can remember when their children have been sick and run a high fever or have taken a tumble. When searching for a cause for their child's deafness, they may feel that these events have contributed to their child's hearing loss.

However, fever alone does not cause hearing loss. In the event that the child contracts a disease, such as spinal meningitis, and runs a high fever, a loss may occur; but the fever by itself will not generate "burned up nerves" or create an auditory dysfunction. A blow to the head is not likely to create a loss either, unless it is severe enough to fracture the bones of the skull that protect the auditory mechanism. It is a rare occurrence when fractures occur simultaneously that damage both ears. At best, when people cite these reasons for causes of hearing loss, it is because the true medical diagnosis is unknown.

ALL DEAF PEOPLE CAN READ LIPS

The term "lipreading" has been used to denote the process that deaf individuals engage in while attempting to comprehend what the speaker is saying. However, upon closer examination, the term was changed to "speechreading," thus signifying the comprehensive scope of the process. Speechreading, unlike lipreading, not only includes lip movements, but also incorporates facial expressions, eye movements, and body gestures (Bevan, 1988). All of these factors assist hearing impaired individuals as they attempt to comprehend what the speaker or group of participants is saying. Speechreading, therefore, becomes a supplement to the communication process, assisting individuals in their receptive skills. It is not a substitute for one's hearing, but rather a technique that can be incorporated to enhance communication and promote understanding of the spoken message.

Members of the professional community have debated whether speechreading, itself, is an innate ability individuals possess or rather a skill that can be developed. Although there is no consensus on this point, certain issues within the domain of speechreading are generally agreed upon. Almost all professionals support the premise that speechreading has certain limitations. These limitations can be summarized as follows:

1. Between 40 to 50 percent of speech sounds encountered in the English language are not visible on the lips. Sounds such as i, e, g, h, a, and k remain hidden when they are vocalized, thus preventing the speech-reader from receiving words in their entirety.
2. There are only sixteen mouth movements that are distinguishable in the English language. These sixteen movements represent the thirty-eight English phonemes. Therefore, the mouth movements for differing speech sounds may look the same; the distinguishing features for these sounds are made by the tongue, or the larynx, both of which are invisible (Schein & Stewart, 1995). As a result, some of the sounds are homophonous (look alike on the lips) such as p, b, and m and add confusion as one tries to determine if the word is "mat, bat, or pat."

3. To benefit from speechreading, individuals must have a fairly extensive language background. Without this they are unable to fill in the gaps providing them with information that cannot be obtained through speechreading or hearing (Bevan, 1988, p. 106).

Hearing individuals outside of the field of deafness frequently assume that all deaf people can speech-read and fully comprehend what they are saying. This is a misconception, and deaf individuals are faced daily with frustrations as they attempt to understand what the speaker is saying. Although some deaf and hard of hearing individuals are excellent speech-readers, the majority are not, and they find themselves struggling in their efforts to understand what is being said.

When trying to surmount a breakdown in communication with a hearing impaired person, hearing people frequently resort to other methods in their attempt to convey their message. Oftentimes, the first question that arises pertains to whether or not the hearing impaired individual has the ability to read.

CAN DEAF PEOPLE READ?

Although the majority of deaf and hard of hearing individuals can read, their levels of comprehension vary dramatically. Some who are hard-of-hearing (possessing a mild to severe loss) achieve reading levels that are comparable to their hearing counterparts; however, others who experience a severe to profound loss rarely become really skilled readers.

National surveys, individual studies of reading achievement, and studies of specific aspects of the reading process all indicate that most deaf children (those who have a severe to profound loss) have difficulty reading the English language (Quigley & Paul, 1984). This can be attributed, in part, to their depressed general knowledge bank resulting from the isolation they experience on a daily basis. Hearing children have the benefit of gathering a substantial knowledge base as they interact with parents and significant others. These experiences are internalized through the spoken language process and become a part of the hearing child's practical knowledge. As a result, they enter the reading process with a language base to draw from. Children who are born deaf, or lose their hearing prior to the development of language patterns, encounter communication problems with those significant others and enter the domain of reading with a very impoverished knowledge base (Quigley & Paul, 1984, p. 137).

Studies conducted by the Office of Demographic Studies (ODS) at Gallaudet provide the most comprehensive information on reading achievement levels. Throughout the years, various studies have been undertaken and cited in the literature. They consistently reveal that those students with a severe to profound loss do not perform well at any age level on tests of general ability to read standard English text. The results of these studies are notable. A few of them have been cited below.

These studies represent the findings of the larger body of research and reflect the reading problems experienced by the deaf and hard of hearing populations.

- In the sixties, national norms for reading levels of deaf children were supplied by Wrightstone, Aronow, and Moskowitz (1963). They administered the elementary level battery of the Metropolitan Achievement Test to 5,307 deaf students between the ages of 10½ and 16½ years.
- Furth (1966) conducted an analysis on the data from that study and determined that only 8 percent of the national sampling of deaf and hard of hearing students read above the fourth grade level.

In addition, reading grade levels for the sample increased as follows:

> *a mean improvement to only 2.7 years between the ages of 10 and 11 increasing to only a 5.5 between 15 and 16 years of age, representing an increase of less than one grade level in five years (Quigley & Paul, 1984, p. 115).*

In the seventies, studies revealed that over a ten-year period, deaf and hard of hearing students between the ages of 8 to 18 increased their vocabulary, on the average, only as much as the average normal hearing child does between the beginning of kindergarten and the latter part of second grade.

Studies during this period also revealed that the reading ability of deaf students in special education increased very little between age 13 and 20 and that only one deaf young adult in ten could easily read a newspaper that is eighth-grade material (Benderly, 1980, p. 88).

- An additional study conducted by Trybus and Karchmer (1977) reported reading scores for a stratified random sample of 6,871 deaf students. They found that the median reading level at age 20 was a grade equivalent of only 4.5, a score that is reflective of the reading level they had obtained at age 14. Only 10 percent of the very best students enrolled in the reading group (consisting of 18-year-olds), could read at or above the eighth-grade level (Trybus & Karchmer, 1977).
- During the eighties, Allen (1986) analyzed data from the two norming projects (1974 and 1983) involving the Stanford Achievement Test scores normed on hearing impaired students. His analysis revealed that although deaf students as a group acquired reading comprehension skills more rapidly in 1983 than in 1974, they showed little or no gain in relation to their hearing cohorts (Allen, 1986).

The results of these studies reveal the difficulties experienced by deaf and hard of hearing individuals when presented with written material. Although they possess the intellectual abilities needed for comprehension to occur, they frequently lack the experiential, cognitive, and linguistic base required for fluency to develop.

DEAF PEOPLE CAN'T TALK

Hearing people typically assume that everyone can hear and speak. Upon encountering individuals who have hearing losses and observing them sign or write, they automatically assume that all deaf people are unable to speak. Speech is equated with language; the hearing individual may surmise that without speech, language does not develop and thought processes do not occur. Therefore, the deaf individual is perceived as lacking the resources to think, develop language, and use oral expression. Nothing could be further from the truth.

Unless there is an abnormality that occurs in the speech mechanism, such as the larynx, vocal chords, or the structures within the mouth involving the articulators, individuals have the capability to produce sound. However, the process involved in imitating speech sounds and producing intelligible words is highly complex. To produce accurate vocal utterances, air must pass through the mouth, and the individual must alter the flow of the air by changing the shape of the mouth or obstructing the airflow by utilizing the teeth or the tongue (Mindel & Vernon, 1987, p. 114).

Infants who have normal hearing listen to speech for an extended time before they are able to speak intelligibly. At the earliest stages, babies begin babbling, store the sounds they make in their memory, and retrieve them at will. By initiating these sounds and listening to them, they begin to monitor their own production of sound. As they develop, their babbling becomes incorporated into the elements of speech sounds that will later be used to form words. Their ability to hear themselves speak and to monitor sound production is critical to the development of the speech process. Through this form of feedback, children can determine how accurately they are producing any given sound. Throughout this process they rely on the acoustic images they hear, strive to imitate those speech sounds they perceive, and vocalize them as accurately as possible (Mindel & Vernon, 1987, p. 114).

Most prelingually deaf children do not develop comprehensible speech sounds. There are two reasons why this occurs: First, they cannot receive speech sounds auditorily; and, second, they have no way to monitor their production of sounds, thus interfering with the critical feedback process. Although amplification may be somewhat beneficial, it does not clarify speech sounds and deaf individuals are left wondering if they are saying things in the right manner.

Hearing individuals who have enrolled in a foreign language class understand the importance of speaking the language accurately. They spend hours mastering word order, accent, and vocabulary choice to ensure that their message will be understood and that no one will ridicule them. Those wishing to utilize their language in a foreign country want to ensure that they will be able to express themselves without the fear of embarrassment.

Deaf individuals experience the same challenge as they attempt to speak. However, their task becomes more difficult as they rely almost exclusively on their visual channel for cues. Hearing individuals have the benefit of hearing the foreign language spoken and can match their response accordingly. Deaf individuals, however, must master English, which to them is a foreign language, and must do so within the confines of a restricted sound environment.

Because they cannot hear how they sound or monitor how loud or soft they are speaking, many prefer not to use their voices. Others will attempt to speak and either realize that they are not being understood or feel ridiculed and, therefore, refrain from speaking.

ALL DEAF CHILDREN HAVE DEAF PARENTS

Deafness is a low incidence handicap, affecting only a small percentage of the total population. Recent information provided by the National Information Center on Deafness indicates that approximately 22 million Americans experience some form of hearing loss (one in every eleven persons). Of those who have difficulty hearing as many as 2 million have been diagnosed as having a severe to profound loss (NICD, 1990).

Frequently the assumption is made that deaf parents produce deaf children and that, therefore, all deaf children have parents with similar disabilities. However, this is generally not the case.

Research indicates that nine out of every ten children born to deaf parents hear normally (approximately 88 percent). Although hearing loss can be attributed to genetic causes, it does not occur frequently, affecting only a small percentage of the population.

Deaf children having two deaf parents comprise only about 3 to 4 percent of the general population, and fewer than 10 percent are known to have at least one deaf parent (Rawlings & Jensema, 1977).

DEAF CHILDREN CAN'T ATTEND SCHOOL

Prior to the seventies, it was not uncommon to hear deaf individuals or parents tell stories of how they or their children were denied access to the public school system. The majority of deaf students attended residential schools for the deaf, often traveling long distances and remaining at school throughout most of the school year. If the parents declined the services of the school for the deaf and elected to keep their child at home, it was often left to the discretion of the school board to determine if the child would be admitted to a regular public school. If the child had a secondary handicap or exhibited any characteristics denoting behavioral problems, he or she was often sent home, where he or she remained unless other educational facilities could be located.

However, in the mid-seventies this changed. On November 29, 1975, President Gerald Ford signed into law the "Education for All Handicapped Children Act of 1975" (Public Law 94-142), later renamed the Individuals with Disabilities Education Act

(IDEA) (Lane et al., 1996, p. 231). It was significant legislation for the handicapped because it charged the local, state, and federal governments with the responsibility of guaranteeing that each handicapped American child would receive a free, appropriate, public education. This law has not only opened doors for many deaf children but has had an impact on where they attend school.

In the early seventies, 48 percent of all school-aged deaf students attended classes away from home in residential schools, whereas in 1984, 74 percent attended day classes while living at home (Mindel & Vernon, 1987, p. 149). In addition, in 1984, 15 percent of the deaf student population attended regular classes with normally hearing students on a full-time basis (Mindel & Vernon, 1987, p. 150). Prior to the passing of P.L. 94-142, this practice was so rare that statistics are not available.

Today, deaf children have the option of attending public school or residential school facilities. Data from 1997–1998, compiled by the Gallaudet Research Institute, indicates that 29.9 percent of the deaf and hard of hearing school-aged population attend special schools. Thirty-two percent receive instruction in self-contained classrooms, 13 percent in resource rooms, 43 percent in mainstreamed settings, 2 percent at home, and 4.3 percent in other unspecified educational settings.

Furthermore, several postsecondary institutions, technical schools, and vocational training centers have designed specific programs with support services for this population.

HEARING AIDS ENABLE DEAF PEOPLE TO HEAR SPEECH

One of the common misconceptions surrounding deafness lies in the area of amplification. Hearing aids are frequently purchased with the preconceived idea that they will restore normal hearing to the hearing impaired person. Older adults, particularly, may become frustrated when they purchase an aid. They may find that the quality of sound they receive falls far short of their expectations. Although their level of hearing may be enhanced, they may find that what they are able to understand varies considerably.

Hearing aids serve the purpose of amplifying sounds. Speech sounds become loud enough that they are within the range of the individual's hearing. However, an aid cannot replace damaged nerve fibers and cannot clarify speech. The type of loss experienced will determine how beneficial the aid will be. If the loss is mild, the increased volume provided by the aid may permit excellent clarity. However, if the individual has severe damage to the nerve fibers located in the inner ear, amplification will not provide the same effect. Upon using an aid, these individuals will experience the ability to hear speech and environmental sounds, but they will not be able to clearly differentiate the speech sounds.

Those who have a sensorineural loss are unable to hear frequencies in the higher pitch range, where the greatest amount of speech sounds are located. Even with a hearing aid, amplified speech may still be distorted. When too many nerve fibers located in the inner ear are damaged, speech will never be completely clear. As a result, the individual may be able to hear the sound, but he will not be able to understand what is being said (Bevan, 1988, p. 58). Those with profound losses frequently benefit from an aid, as they are able to locate the source of environmental sounds. However, aids do not provide the individual with clear speech sounds.

With the advent of modern technology, cochlear implants have come to the forefront (see complete description in Chapter 12). These devices are used by 3.9 percent of the school-aged deaf population (1997–98 Annual Survey of Deaf and Hard of Hearing Children, Gallaudet Research Institute) and are designed to enhance spoken language acquisition.

The effectiveness of these devices is currently being investigated. Although the research thus far is limited, initial results, in the perception area, are promising. However, whether these improvements will result in improved spoken language production is highly controversial (Crouch, 1997; Lane & Grodin, 1997). It is too early to judge whether cochlear implants will grant individuals with profound losses total access into the larger hearing community where they can fully participate (Tomlin, Spencer, & Flock, 1999).

As with other hearing aids, one must not assume that this device can produce sounds that mirror the speech sounds that a hearing person receives. Rather, it is an aid designed to provide auditory stimulation for those who cannot hear. For even with a cochlear implant, the individual is still a person with a hearing loss who has the benefit of an aid.

ALL DEAF PEOPLE WISH THEY COULD HEAR

To the outsider, the world of the deaf often appears bleak, empty, and dismal. Hearing people tend to look on those who are deaf with pity, surmising that they are unhappy and helpless. They make the assumption that all deaf people want desperately to hear and are not content living in a silent world.

Although these are the feelings expressed by some prelingually deaf individuals, they are not reflective of the majority of the adult deaf population. Deaf people, for the most part, may struggle through childhood and adolescence but emerge as self-fulfilled, happy adults.

The Deaf community is comprised of dynamic, cheerful, and well-balanced people who live their lives and attend to business without much more visible distress than people who can hear. They attend deaf socials, engage in athletic events, and enjoy face-to-face communication providing them with the opportunity to exchange stories and anecdotes (Becker, 1980).

Deaf people are frequently asked if their deafness could be cured and their hearing restored, would they take advantage of the procedure. Answers to this question always vary. Younger members of this unique population periodically respond with an affirmative. However, those adults who have resided in the Deaf community for their entire life consider themselves members of a special subculture and have no desire to hear. They enjoy their friends, participate in social activities, and dislike being pitied.

Many feel there are advantages to being deaf and feel fortunate that they are not bothered with the cacophony of daily life bombarding hearing people. Others have become accustomed to their state of hearing and have no desire to experience the world from a hearing perspective.

DEAF PEOPLE ARE NOT AS INTELLIGENT AS HEARING PEOPLE

One's intelligence is often confused with one's ability to communicate. Upon encountering individuals who have weak expressive skills, there is a tendency to assume that the person has inferior intellectual functioning abilities. Hearing people place a high premium on communication skills, and the way individuals present themselves is often used as a baseline to determine how intelligent they are.

Word choice, sentence structure, grammar, and presentation are all used as measures by the hearing population to ascertain who is intelligent and who is not. Unfortunately, many individuals are stereotyped based on these criteria.

When deaf people express themselves vocally and the sounds they produce do not make sense to the hearing observer, the assumption is made that there is something wrong with them. In addition, if hearing impaired individuals repeatedly request the same information, the layperson frequently assumes that it is because they are "dumb" or "stupid," not realizing the difficulties they encounter with speechreading.

Research conducted with the deaf population indicates that their levels of intellectual functioning are comparable to that of hearing people. Studies conducted by Braden concluded that the average IQ score on the performance part of the WISC-R was 96.89, only slightly lower than the hearing children's norm of 100 (Braden, 1985, p. 499).

Because speech and language are often confused with thinking, deaf individuals are perceived as being intellectually inferior. However, one's ability to speak and the content of what one has to say are two entirely separate processes.

DEAF PEOPLE CAN'T DRIVE

Hearing people incorporate the use of both their eyes and ears when they are driving, thus alerting them to their surroundings. Sirens, the sound of screeching tires, and horns honking all provide warning signals for the hearing driver.

Because hearing individuals rely heavily on both senses to drive defensively, many assume that if your hearing is impaired, your ability to drive is also impaired. Members of the general public are oftentimes surprised to discover that deaf people do indeed drive and maintain very safe driving records.

A study conducted in 1968 by Sherman G. Finesilver (President's Advisory Committee on Traffic Safety) concluded that across the nation deaf individuals are only involved in one-fourth as many accidents as their hearing counterparts. In addition, when driver licensing officials were surveyed in all states, forty-one of the forty-nine responding ranked the deaf driver at least as good, and in many cases better, than the hearing driver (Finesilver, 1968).

Because 97 percent of the warning signals that reach the driver are gained through the visual channel (Greenmum, 1952), the deaf driver has the opportunity to survey his surroundings and respond accordingly. Their eyes become their primary information resource and they frequently wait at intersections when the light turns green to observe if any vehicles are not heeding the directive to stop. Although several states require that the hearing impaired driver purchase a side mirror for both sides of his car, generally no other restrictions are mandated.

DEAF INDIVIDUALS HAVE MORE SERIOUS EMOTIONAL PROBLEMS THAN HEARING PEOPLE

Although some deaf people suffer serious emotional disturbances, their rate of real maladjustment is not excessive, considering the rigors of their youth and the frustrations of their daily lives. Within the realm of psychiatric disorders, they suffer these disabilities with no greater frequency than the hearing population (Benderly, 1980, p. 65).

Hearing community dwellers periodically observe behaviors exhibited by deaf people as being abnormal or socially unacceptable. They, in turn, surmise that there is some psychological deficiency inherently characteristic of the deaf person. However, with accurate background information pertaining to this population, it becomes apparent that those behaviors, which may appear to be abnormal, are merely the result of deficiencies of social knowledge.

According to Yambert and Van Craeynest, much of what people with normal hearing learn is based on what they overhear. This is particularly true in the area of social knowledge. Much of what the child learns to be socially acceptable or unacceptable is gleaned through overhearing parental discussions. Being privy to information regarding someone else's behavior provides them with the opportunity to learn about cultural norms and expectations about behavior (Yambert & Van Craeynest, 1975).

Because deaf children cannot "eavesdrop" on parental conversations and because very few of their parents sign, this aspect of development may go untouched.

Hearing children automatically assimilate information and mimic behaviors by observing events that occur within their environment. However, this same information that emanates from an auditory environment must be taught to the deaf child. Those behaviors that, for all intents and purposes, appear to be everyday common knowledge escape the deaf person if they are not directly addressed.

This environmental deprivation results in the hearing public stereotyping them as immature, exhibiting unacceptable behaviors, or having severe emotional problems. However, when the deaf child is provided with ready access to this information and is challenged to grow, the potential for developing socially acceptable behaviors is present.

DEAF PEOPLE CAN'T WORK

Because deafness is a low incidence handicap, many employees may never encounter a deaf worker. As a result, their mind-set about deaf adults may revolve around the old stereotypes of the deaf adult peddling manual alphabet cards to earn a living. The general public may be unaware of the wide array of employment possibilities available to this population.

Historically, deaf individuals were employed in factories, as printers, dry cleaners, and in other forms of manual labor. However, with the advent of the Vocational Rehabilitation Act, a myriad of vocational opportunities were made available to disabled individuals.

Training programs were developed, support services provided, and deaf individuals began entering the competitive job market. Occupational surveys indicate that deaf individuals are employed in the managerial/professional sector; obtain jobs in the technical, sales, and administrative support areas; are employed as operators and precision production managers; and continue to work as fabricators (Welsh & Walter, 1988). Although unemployment and underemployment still plague this population today, hearing impaired individuals can be comparably trained and be equally capable of working in a comparative field.

These positions provide deaf individuals with a sense of accomplishment and also enable them to live independently within the community. They take great pride in being self-sufficient and self-supporting; they abhor those individuals who resort to peddling as a way of life.

Within the Deaf community, peddling is perceived as deviate behavior. Those members who have worked hard to gain their rightful place in employment see the peddlers as spoiling their image and jeopardizing their chances of being rightfully included in activities controlled by the hearing world (Higgins, 1980, p. 175). Historically, deaf individuals were perceived as being capable of earning a living only by peddling. As a result, the members, for the most part, have worked hard to dispel this image.

ALL DEAF PEOPLE KNOW SIGN LANGUAGE

Sign language has received considerable attention throughout the past several years. The general public has become more aware of interpreters and has observed them as they facilitate communication. Sign language classes are offered on a regular basis by community centers and college programs, as more people express an interest in learning the language.

As a result of this exposure, hearing individuals may assume that all deaf people can sign. Today, 95 percent of students with severe to profound impairments attend classes that incorporate some type of manual communication into their program (Mindel & Vernon, 1987, p. 149). However, not all of those who are deaf do sign. Hearing individuals periodically encounter a deaf person who does not know how to sign or who prefers to communicate orally.

DEAF PEOPLE ARE VERY QUIET

From a distance, or to the untrained eye, the first impression of a "deaf social event" is that deaf people are very quiet. However, upon closer examination one realizes that this is not the case. Deaf social events provide the participants with the opportunity to share stories with each other, tell jokes, and engage in lively entertainment. Peals of laughter, shrieks of excitement, and animated sounds are all characteristics of these events. It is not uncommon for one to pound on the table, shout out a name, or stomp the floor in order to get a bystander's attention.

When music accompanies these events, it is usually played at a level enabling the participants to feel the vibrations on the floor. The music, coupled with the typical sounds produced by deaf individuals, provide the hearing participant with an auditory, as well as visual, experience.

SUMMARY

Hearing individuals who have not encountered members of the Deaf community often "freeze" and withdraw when they meet a deaf person for the first time. Communication may be strained, misunderstandings may develop, and embarrassment may result. If the hearing person does not have the skills to permit a free exchange of ideas to occur, the deaf person remains on the outside trying to comprehend what is being conveyed. As a result, the exchange may end with both parties having formulated misconceptions about each other.

Throughout history, these types of interactions have led to the development of myths and misunderstandings that are still evident today. Only recently have deaf spokespersons come to the forefront, thus dispelling some of these preconceived ideas. However, the general public is frequently still in awe upon meeting a deaf person for the first time. Therefore, their uncertainty of what to expect and how to communicate interferes with their ability to relate effectively.

Deafness will probably remain a low incidence handicap. Consequently, the majority of hearing individuals residing outside the field of deafness may have little, if any, contact with the prelingually deaf population.

With the advent of modern technology, recent legislation, and support services, more people have become aware of the abilities of this unique population. Although myths and misconceptions still remain, some have been dispelled as deaf awareness spreads.

▶ 11

Deafness and the World of Work

"Employment" is a term that can be equated with a variety of meanings. For the economist, it provides a key to material welfare in our society. The psychologist views the world of work as critical to development of our self-concept as we mediate our values and structure our lives. It becomes the arena where we can balance our capabilities against career opportunities and experience feelings of self-worth. Through vocational experiences, individuals are provided with the option of responding in a responsible fashion, thus becoming contributing members of society.

Annually, thousands of deaf and hard of hearing students graduate from high school. Over 50 percent continue their education at vocational training centers and postsecondary institutions, while others attempt to enter the work force. Those possessing marginal academic and language skills can be directed into training. This training provides them with those skills necessary to enter the work force as semi-skilled or unskilled laborers. Those possessing above average academic and language skills are directed into areas of postsecondary study. However, those who exhibit average to above average language and cognitive skills but whose level of academic functioning reflects a poor or uneven pattern may find themselves entering employment in jobs below their abilities. This group may be considered the "occupational under-achievers" (Bolton, 1976).

Regardless of their backgrounds or their educational levels, the majority of deaf and hard of hearing individuals entering the work force are faced with the challenge of convincing hearing employers that they will make capable employees. Throughout the last decade there has been an onslaught of activities designed to heighten deaf awareness; however, barriers still exist, making it difficult for deaf individuals to secure employment.

BARRIERS TO EMPLOYMENT

When deaf and hard of hearing individuals apply for jobs, they frequently encounter employers who hold a variety of erroneous notions, myths, and stereotypes about deafness (Wang et al., 1989). Their misconceptions regarding the abilities and disabilities of this group contribute to unemployment as well as underemployment of the deaf population. Employers tend to perceive disabled persons as being more expensive to hire, train, and place than able-bodied workers, based on the support services that may be required throughout the initial training period (Bowe, 1978). As a result, disabled individuals who are hired may find themselves being placed in entry level positions that are "dead end" in nature, thus restricting their opportunities for job advancement.

When the issue of employing deaf workers is discussed, four attitudes generally prevail:

1. *Resistive*

"We don't want any deaf people working as employees here." They belong in a social welfare agency as they are more of a bother than they are worth.

2. *Permissive*

"If a deaf person applies, sure we'll consider him, but he better be able to function independently." We won't bend the organization to fit his needs, so he must be able to perform the tasks in standard ways.

3. *Accommodative*

"For a qualified deaf individual, we can restructure the job somewhat so he can perform the majority of the duties." Someone else can answer the phone and in meetings someone can sit next to him and take notes. Perhaps some of his coworkers will learn how to sign and fingerspell.

4. *Facilitative*

"Let's initiate some special programs to augment accommodative measures." Let's not wait for a qualified person; let's instigate the program (Jamison, 1983; Crammatte, 1987).

Those deaf individuals encountering the accommodative or the facilitative employer have the opportunity to utilize their skills. Those who are met with a resistive or permissive attitude may face discrimination and be denied access to positions for which they are qualified. However, employer attitude is only one dimension contributing to the barriers that prevent deaf individuals from securing employment. Lack of training, poor communication skills, and the inability of the deaf worker to engage in effective interpersonal relations all contribute to unemployment.

The term "lack of training" is used to refer to those deaf workers who are undereducated, as well as to those who possess limited work experience. These potential employees may not have competitive occupational skills that will render them marketable in today's work force. Their poor communication skills may result in training difficulties and they may be perceived by the employer as being inflexible workers. Furthermore, ineffective interpersonal relationships can be attributed to originating within the deaf individual. The deaf employee may experience feelings of low self-esteem, possess unrealistic career goals, exhibit poor work history, and/or may dress inappropriately. All of these components can contribute to barriers in employment.

Additional factors that may prevent the deaf person from securing employment include lack of job search skills, transportation problems, family attitudes, child care problems, and resistance to giving up government support. To eliminate barriers to employment, two components must be in place: First, deaf workers must receive those vocational educational skills that will render them competitive; and, second, discrimination expressed by employers must be eliminated. Provided with training and reduced discrimination, deaf individuals approach the world of work better equipped to deal with the hearing population and secure employment.

VOCATIONAL DEVELOPMENT, ASSESSMENT, AND CAREER EXPLORATION

From the time children enter elementary school, they begin to become aware of the various types of employment possibilities surrounding them. Through adult role models, bombardment by the media, and contact with their peers and their families, they begin to fantasize about possible career choices and their futures.

By the time children reach early adolescence, they begin to explore their own abilities and extrapolate those tasks that they perform well. They, in turn, view their talents and interests within the confines of what is deemed socially useful or desirable as a future career goal. Toward the end of the adolescent period and throughout their early adult years, young people continue to explore potential vocations. They do this with increasing concern for the amount of education required, potential job opportunities available, and amount of income the position will generate. Following this exploration period they begin working toward establishing themselves in a given occupation (Super & Overstreet, 1960, as cited in Bolton, 1976).

Vocational development can be viewed as a process involving two stages. Within the *prevocational stage,* individuals become aware of all the behaviors associated with the world of work. Although employability is not secured, vocational information is obtained, planning is initiated, and vocational aspirations are formed. As individuals enter the *vocational stage,* the concern becomes one of transferring these vocational behaviors to the actual world of work. The focus is placed on obtaining an appropriate job, performing it in a satisfactory manner, and achieving job satisfaction. The ability to arrive at this level is determined by several internal and external factors.

Internal factors include the individuals' vocationally related traits, including their abilities and interests, their knowledge base, and their predisposition to enter any given field. External factors that influence their vocational development can be attributed to general information they have received about jobs and work. This includes input from their parents, teachers, peers, and so forth, as well as several contingency factors pertaining to current economic conditions and the potential employee's geographic locale (Bolton, 1976).

It becomes apparent that true vocational behavior, including job-seeking skills, job placement, and job adjustment, can be attributed to a multitude of components. Figure 11-1 illustrates these factors.

During the vocational developmental process, the individual's behavior proceeds from a random and undifferentiated activity to a goal-directed specific activity.

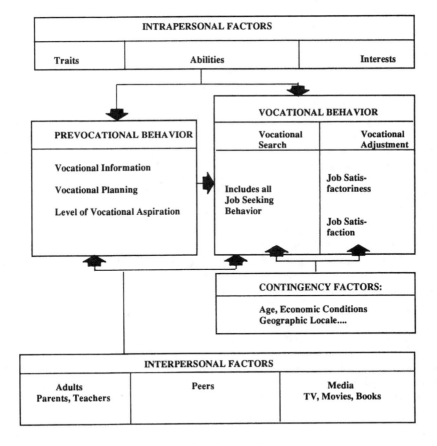

FIGURE 11-1 **Model of Vocational Development**

(From *Psychology of Deafness for Rehabilitation Counselors,* Brian Bolton. Copyright 1976 by University Park Press. Used by permission.)

Aspirations are transformed into the beginnings of their career development as individuals move from dependence to increasing independence.

Due to the ramifications of deafness, these individuals progressing through this developmental process may encounter different experiences when compared with their hearing peers. Their experiential base may be limited, their language and communication competence lowered, and the level of stimulation received in the home may be reduced. These factors may all adversely affect the vocational developmental process.

Effects of Deafness on Vocational Development

Hearing impaired high school graduates often lack an adequate understanding of their own proficiencies and limitations. They may not have a clear picture of the vocational options available to them or of the training that is required to enter the various occupations. This lack of information frequently results in unrealistic employment expectations (Wang et al., 1989).

White (1974) further supports this premise and states that there are at least three factors that contribute to the individual's understanding of him- or herself. These factors are instrumental in influencing his or her career development and include:

1. perceptual differences that can be attributed to altered self-perceptions of reality,
2. a restricted life space that decreases knowledge of and familiarity with areas outside the immediate social or geographic area, and
3. a limited sociocultural horizon (Farrugia, 1982).

Those students lacking exposure to the vast array of vocational opportunities available to them may cling to employment in the traditional unskilled or semiskilled areas, thus failing to aspire toward higher levels of ambition and skill development.

Career Exploration and Education

It can be assumed that the soundness of young deaf and hard of hearing adults' vocational decisions reflect the adequacy of their career education. One can further assume that those individuals who make appropriate job-related decisions will obtain employment commensurate with their skills and training (Wang et al., 1989). As a result, career exploration and education can play a significant role in preparing these students for positions that are consistent with their skills and training.

Career exploration can be viewed as a lifelong process that unfolds as individuals mature and grow. Experiences, both of a formal and informal nature, occurring within children's home and school environments are instrumental in influencing their fundamental awareness of the variety of occupational categories available to them. Throughout the elementary and middle school years, students enrolled in career exploration programs are exposed to a variety of occupations. Using this information, they begin to formulate their vocational interests and values. High school students who are enrolled in classes that incorporate career education as part of their curriculum are better prepared to define their vocational goals. Throughout their junior and senior years, they begin taking courses that will better prepare them for the transition into college or the world of work.

Career education programs can begin as early as kindergarten and extend through high school. Within the parameters of a vocational assessment curriculum originating at the elementary school level, the students' skills, aptitudes, values, interests, and temperament are continuously monitored. In addition, coursework is designed that injects career development concepts into subject matter classes. By being provided with a link between the subject matter and the world of work, students are able to begin formulating those career areas that are of interest to them. In addition, teachers and counselors are able to view the individual student's progress and direct them into those areas in which they can ultimately achieve success.

Although career education programs can provide students with positive vocational learning experiences, few school programs serving hearing impaired students incorporate this type of curriculum planning into their programming. In a recent study of sixteen residential and day high schools, Schroedel (1991), examined the types of career development activities that had been made available to high school seniors from the tenth through the twelfth grade. The target population examined were students who were graduating from high school with either an academic or a vocational diploma.

Of the students surveyed, 77 percent of the seniors at the residential school had prelingual onset of deafness compared to 57 percent of those enrolled in the day programs. The findings of his study merit discussion.

Within the residential school setting, approximately 58 percent completed a vocational interest test, 98 percent received vocational training, and 78 percent were provided with career counseling. However, only 4 percent had the opportunity to enroll in a career education class, and only 33 percent could participate in work study.

Of the day high school students surveyed, approximately 30 percent completed a vocational interest test, 64 percent received vocational training, and 91 percent were provided with career counseling. Eight percent of the students enrolled in a career education class, and 39 percent participated in work study (Schroedel, 1991, p. 332).

Further results of the study indicated that most high schools did not offer a formal career course and that some states had virtually no postsecondary training. Of the seniors surveyed, approximately 52 percent indicated that they wanted to attend college, 20 percent stated that they would pursue other kinds of training, and 25 percent sought jobs (Schroedel, 1991, p. 337).

Based on this study, it is apparent that very few schools provide career education courses. When these courses are available, careers are explored, vocational assessments are made, and work-related behaviors are examined. All of these topics are critical for inclusion in vocational programs when preparing deaf students for the world of work.

Vocational Assessment

Whether vocational assessment takes place in a curriculum-based program or in a vocational evaluation center, there are several key elements that should be included. First, real or simulated work experiences should be available. The more realistic the work experience is, the more beneficial it will be for the student and the more valid and useful the results will be.

Second, the assessment should be relevant for the types of employment being considered. The student's job skill strengths and weaknesses, specific to the job, need to be evaluated as well as his work behaviors and functional living skills (Peterson, 1989).

Peterson and Hill (1982) have outlined three components that should be considered in the design of vocational evaluation and curriculum development. They state that:

1. curriculum-based vocational assessment should start by the sixth grade. During this time prevocational skill development should be examined, and career orientation and exploration should be initiated,
2. vocational assessments should continue to be conducted at major vocational deciding points and prior to entry into any vocational education programs, and
3. vocational evaluations should be based on the needs of the individual student and designed accordingly (Peterson, 1989).

Although this is the ideal situation, recent investigators have cited that there is a lack of appropriate vocational assessment throughout the school years. In addition, career-related objectives and transitional planning appears to be weak (Cobb & Phelps, 1983). There may be a minimum of parental involvement. Counseling and career planning services may be lacking, and the students may not have the opportunity to engage in work experience programs while still in high school (Rusch & Phelps, 1987). As a result, students may leave high school unaware of training opportunities; out of touch with their abilities, skills, and limitations; and ill-equipped to enter this transitional period.

If educational experiences are broadened and strengthened and students are given the opportunity to explore their strengths and weaknesses, they will be better prepared to enter the job market or the postsecondary training sites. However, without better preparation, the likelihood of improving their employment prospects will be minimal at best (Rusch & Phelps, 1987). Deaf individuals must take an active role in their career planning. Together with educators, potential employers, and vocational rehabilitation counselors, they can improve employment possibilities.

VOCATIONAL REHABILITATION

One of the key agencies involved with disabled populations as they enter into the transitional phase from high school through job placement is the Federal Vocational Rehabilitation (VR) Program. The program is administered by the Commissioner of the Rehabilitation Services Administration (RSA) in the Department of Health, Education and Welfare. This agency operates in all of the fifty states and is primarily responsible for preparing disabled youth and adults for gainful employment.

The original Vocational Rehabilitation act was passed in 1954 and amended in 1966. The original Act, Public Law 88-565, provided a good deal of direct and indirect assistance to the deaf (Brill, 1974).

The rehabilitation process is threefold in nature. It involves making a diagnosis and evaluation to determine the extent and vocational implications of the disability(ies); it provides training that will enable the person to adjust to and overcome his or her limitations; and it prepares them for a specific vocation or cluster of vocations (Bowe, 1978).

In order to become a client of Vocational Rehabilitation, the individual must meet the eligibility requirements. These requirements are based on three criteria:

1. the client must demonstrate, usually through a medical exam, the existence of a disability
2. based on the disability, it must then be determined, usually by the individual vocational rehabilitation counselor, that the disability constitutes a "substantial handicap" to employment
3. there must be a certain level of expectation by the VR counselor, that there is a "reasonable" chance that through VR services the person may be enabled to engage in gainful employment (Bowe, 1978, p. 168).

Once a client is determined to be eligible for services, the client and the counselor work together to prepare a rehabilitation plan. The Work Plan (previously referred to as the Individual Written Rehabilitation Program [IWRP]), outlines the training, educational objectives, and career goals for the client. It is subject to review on a periodic basis and includes a listing of the types of services that will be purchased for the client. These services include training programs, medical treatment and restoration, hearing aids, interpreting services, and any other products and services that can reasonably be expected to enhance the client's ability to qualify for and obtain employment.

Within the Division of Rehabilitation, general counselors serve individuals with a myriad of disabilities. Visually impaired, orthopedically handicapped, deaf and hard of hearing, and mentally disabled persons are among the individuals for which Vocational Rehabilitation provides services. Frequently, counselors' caseloads are comprised of individuals who have different disabilities. Their caseloads are often heavy, and their clients' backgrounds may be as diverse as the individuals themselves. It is not uncommon to find counselors who are not prepared to deal with the varying disability groups.

Within the field of deafness this is particularly true. As many as 70 percent of the clients are seen by general counselors (Tully, 1970). Most counselors have a heavy caseload of hearing clients, a myriad of case management responsibilities, and not enough time or training to work extensively with deaf applicants (Casella, 1978;

Usdane, 1976; Zadny & James, 1979). The situation is compounded by the fact that often new counselors have minimal training in deafness, do not sign, have little understanding of the Deaf culture, and are not familiar with the attributes of this population. Although there are some exceptional VR counselors serving the deaf and hard of hearing, the turnover within the field is generally high and new counselors entering the field are not equipped to deal with the situation.

Those encountering deaf clients for the first time may become extremely frustrated. They are faced with individuals who have completed their formal education but who lack the necessary social, personal, and vocational skills needed to succeed in the world of work.

Rehabilitation counselors, upon attending meetings and workshops, frequently share the concerns and frustrations that stem from their deaf caseloads. Topics routinely discussed revolve around the fact that:

- deaf and severely hard-of-hearing students generally do not possess the personal and interpersonal skills needed for successful interaction with coworkers and supervisors
- they frequently display poor work behaviors and habits; they do not understand the value of work and they are unaware of most career fields and occupations
- many of them lack the language and reading skills required for job placement and in turn limit their opportunities for successful training and job placements
- additional problems discussed by the counselors include a concern for the clients' limited exposure to those experiences that contribute to the development of independent living skills, personal responsibility, and survival skills. These areas, together with a limited understanding of appropriate use of leisure time, may interfere with the client's ability to adjust to the postsecondary educational setting or to job training environments (Melton, 1987).

Additional factors impacting on the overall vocational development of deaf people have been cited in the literature. Areas that appear to function as barriers to gainful employment include:

- poor decision-making skills (DiFrancesca, 1978)
- lack of vocational information (Lerman, 1976)
- dependence on others (Roy, 1962)
- restricted experiential base (Mindel & Vernon, 1987; Sliger & Culpepper, 1979)
- poor development of interests (Hoemann, 1964; Lerman, 1976 as cited in Farrugia, 1982, p. 753).

Many of the concerns articulated by the VR counselors and cited in the literature pertain primarily to hearing impaired individuals. However, the majority of them are common problems that are experienced routinely by clients who are in the VR counselor's general caseload. These individuals have daily contact with Vocational

Rehabilitation and pose several of the same problems for them. As a result, Rehabilitation has established new programming. The aim of this programming is to provide client education directed toward those areas in which individuals are lacking in knowledge. This instruction is focused on topics pertaining to securing employment, as well as job retention strategies. This training often is placed under the umbrella of job-seeking skills, job clubs, or classes in self-directed job search strategies.

The clients are taught job-seeking skills in a classroom atmosphere and through these job clubs support is provided to them as they implement their job search (Dwyer, 1983). Topics discussed within the job club setting may include appropriate work behaviors, resume writing, interviewing techniques, the art of filling out applications, and strategies for getting along with coworkers on the job. Sessions may include role-playing exercises, visits from deaf role models (who are gainfully employed), and conversations with potential employers. Participants involved in job clubs are encouraged to explore their vocational interests, relate them realistically to their abilities, and view them in relation to the availability of employment possibilities. Watson and colleagues (1983) have cited benefits that have been realized by practitioners employing self-directed job search methods. Some of them include:

- a significantly higher number of job placements in less time (Keith, Engelke, & Winborn, 1977; Matthias, 1981; McClure, 1972; Salomone, 1971)
- an increase in client self-esteem, including one's internal locus of control, positive worker personality characteristics and attitudes, independent job-seeking behaviors and confidence in the ability to locate one's employment, resulting in a decrease in dependency on Vocational Rehabilitation (Fraser, 1978; Gardner & Beatty, 1980; Tesolowski, Jarecke, & Halpin, 1980)
- an increased ability on the part of the client to convey an image of self-sufficiency required by prospective employers (Baxter, 1979; Silver, 1974).
- a method to assist clients in obtaining lifelong learning when the need for supplemental training arises. In addition, they provide individuals with the opportunities to upgrade their careers and continue vocational development via planned job change (Maguran, 1974; Vandergoot & Swirsky, 1980; Veatch, 1980; Watson et al., 1983, pp. 20–21).

It has become apparent to those working within the field of Rehabilitation that deaf clients must be provided with the opportunity to master life skills and decision-making strategies. The youth of today must be trained in the art of "learning how to learn" rather than learning through rote memorization. It is imperative that they begin enhancing those skills that will assist them as they attempt to secure employment. Also, they must be provided with those strategies that focus on how they can transfer their skills into other job areas as additional vocational opportunities arise.

Vocational Rehabilitation serves as a vital link between the school years and the world of work. By including VR counselors as part of the multidisciplinary team while the students are still in high school, they can begin gaining insights into vocational opportunities. In addition, by providing them with early exposure to those experiences that are geared toward the enhancement of independent living skills, their career development opportunities will be broadened and the utilization of community resources will continue to be promoted. This, in turn, provides them with an edge on employment possibilities.

EMPLOYMENT

Employment can provide individuals with feelings of deep personal satisfaction and self-worth. It has the ability to offer daily stimulation and challenge, monetary compensation, and social interaction with a wide variety of people. In addition, those engaged in the work force have the opportunity to produce, create, and experience personal as well as professional growth.

In contrast, those individuals who experience forced idleness and are refused entry into the world of work may be denied the opportunity to develop feelings of self-worth. Remaining outside the work force results in reduced opportunities for personal growth and limited exposure to new experiences. As a result, the income generated may only produce a bare subsistence-level living, thus instigating intense feelings of self-hatred and disgust (Bowe, 1978, p. 166).

Those with disabilities may be prevented from earning a living, resulting in loss of self-confidence, deterioration of basic skills, and dependence on family members. To ensure that this cycle is not self-perpetuating, more Vocational Rehabilitation counselors are encouraging their clients to secure additional training and education after completing high school.

Education has been shown to have a significant effect on one's socioeconomic status (Bowen, 1977; Jencks et al., 1977). Typically, higher education results in graduates having less difficulty in securing employment, obtaining more satisfying and secure occupations, earning more income, and attaining a higher socioeconomic status (Welsh & Walter, 1988).

Throughout the past thirty-five years there has been a tremendous influx of deaf students attending college programs. In 1950 there were only 250 deaf students enrolled in colleges around the country. However, by 1985 the number had increased to more than 8,000 deaf students (Rawlings & King, 1986). Data collected in a 1986 survey reflects the importance of a postsecondary education with regard to employment and potential income that can be earned.

A study conducted by Welsh and Walter (1988) involving deaf students enrolled at NTID/RIT noted that college degrees opened several career options that were not available to many high school graduates. Persons with two-year degrees were found to be employed more than three times as often in managerial/professional occupations. Those holding bachelor's degrees were more than ten times as likely to be employed in professional occupations as compared to those who held no degree (see Table 11-1).

TABLE 11-1   **Occupations of Deaf High School Graduates and Deaf College Alumni**

	Percent of Graduates in Occupation		
Occupational Level	*No Degree*	*Sub-Bachelor's*	*Bachelor's*
Managerial/Professional	6.4	19.4	66.7
Technical Sales, & Administrative Support	35.5	58.4	27.8
Precision Production, Craft, & Repair	9.1	6.7	0.0
Operators, Fabricators, & Labor	30.9	13.2	1.9
Other	18.1	2.3	3.6

(From Welsh & Walter, JADARA, July 1988. Used with permission.)

The study further noted that when students earning a high school diploma were compared with those who had earned a sub-bachelor's degree, their likelihood of unemployment was reduced by more than 60 percent; the holding of a bachelor's degree reduced this figure by an astonishing 90 percent (Welsh & Walter, 1988, p. 16).

The study further surveyed incomes of deaf high school graduates and compared them with college graduates. They found that graduates with sub-bachelor degrees earned approximately 47 percent more than high school graduates. Salaries of bachelor degree recipients averaged more than twice as much as those persons with lower level earnings (Welsh & Walter, 1988, p. 16). Table 11-2 reflects the earnings of deaf high school graduates and deaf college alumni.

Although deaf and hard of hearing youth can benefit from continued education beyond high school and later secure employment within the professional sector, many set their sights too low and aspire toward low paying, semiskilled employment. Frequently, deaf individuals, particularly deaf women, do not see themselves as having leadership capabilities. Lacking self-pride and self-respect, they are not perceived as confident, active participants in the potential work force.

Farrugia (1982), utilizing the Wide Range Interest and Opinion Test (WRIOT) comparing deaf and hearing individuals ages 16–19, found significant differences between the two groups. As a group, the deaf students showed lower interests in educational and culturally related vocational areas when compared with their hearing peers. In addition, deaf students preferred manual activities (as determined by the WRIOT) over verbal activities. In attitudes, the deaf students tended to aspire toward lower levels of ambition and skill development than the hearing students (Farrugia, 1982, p. 758).

The aspirations toward lower-skilled jobs by deaf students have also been observed by Polansky (1979). While conducting vocational education classes, Polansky

TABLE 11-2   **1986 Weekly Earnings of Deaf High School Graduates and Deaf College Alumni**

	Weekly Earnings	
Group	*Mean*	*Std. Deviation*
No College Degree	$230	$168
Sub-Bachelor's Recipients	$339	$131
Bachelor's Recipients	$496	$218

(From Welsh & Walter, JADARA, July 1988. Used with permission.)

scheduled field trips for deaf and hard of hearing students. They frequented various job sites and returned to the classroom for discussions pertaining to the appropriateness of the various employment possibilities within each site. When employment opportunities with newspapers were discussed, students listed jobs that the deaf could handle as pressmen, dockworkers, or pasteup workers, but not as reporters, writers, or even typists.

In hospitals, the students felt the deaf could be food service workers, cleaners, or nurses' aides, but not doctors, nurses, or laboratory technicians (Polansky, 1979, p. 453). The students tended to see themselves in stereotypic positions and had a difficult time envisioning employment possibilities that were not limited to manual labor or semiskilled jobs.

Unfortunately, these studies are representative of how deaf students perceive their employment possibilities. Their opportunities for environmental exploration may be restricted, thus limiting their awareness of the full spectrum of vocational opportunities available to them. Because of this limited exposure, they may have lowered aspirations about what they believe they are capable of doing and therefore refrain from obtaining advanced training or education. This results in employment being secured in positions that require a minimal skill level and do not tap into potential abilities.

UNDEREMPLOYMENT

Underemployment can be defined as occurring any time individuals are employed in positions that are incompatible with their intelligence, skills, and education. It results in employees filling positions for the sake of "having a job" and usually results in "dead-end" employment. Characteristics of underemployment include failure to place employees in positions affording them the opportunity to draw upon their talents and abilities, reluctance to promote skilled employees into the upper managerial levels, and failure to compensate workers for the quality of the work they perform.

Historically, deaf people have lagged behind their hearing counterparts in most major measures of work achievement. Studies have shown that deaf persons are heavily underrepresented in less prestigious blue-collar occupations and typically earn substantially less than hearing workers (Schein & Delk, 1974; Walter, MacLeod-Gallinger, & Stuckless, 1987; Weinrich, 1972). Additionally, Schroedel (1976) noted that deaf workers experienced more restricted occupational mobility during a period of time (1920–1970) in which a great many Americans were upwardly mobile (Welsh & Walter, 1988, p. 14).

Due to severely limited achievements, many deaf and hard of hearing adults are often compelled to perform manual labor rather than technical work. Statistics show that nearly 90 percent of deaf as opposed to less than 50 percent of their hearing counterparts are employed in jobs requiring manual labor. Only 17 percent of deaf employees have white-collar jobs as compared with 46 percent of hearing people (Rosen, 1986).

In addition, those deaf individuals hired in entry level positions traditionally experience difficulties with upward mobility. Although employers hire deaf employees and make attempts to accommodate them, they frequently do not address the issues of career education and advancement. It is not uncommon to find deaf individuals in their same entry level positions after twenty years of working with the same company. Although they have the potential for advancement, the promotion is often given to the hearing individual who, from the employer's perspective, will be easier to train. Christiansen (1982) reports that although deaf and hard of hearing workers report a high degree of job satisfaction, they indicate that they have not had many opportunities for advancement and often remain in the same job for extremely long periods of time.

Johnson (1993) surveyed 490 workers who were deaf to determine longevity of employment and levels of promotion. Eighty-one percent of the workers who completed the questionnaire were between the ages of 31 and 60, and 44 percent had been employed for one to ten years. Forty-five percent had been employed for eleven to thirty years, and over half (52 percent) had been employed in their current job between eleven and twenty-nine years. Furthermore, 20 percent had held the same job for over thirty years. Of these workers, 55 percent had a high school or postsecondary vocational technical education, and 27 percent were college graduates. Thirty-six percent indicated that they were very satisfied with their jobs, 46 percent were somewhat satisfied, and 14 percent were not satisfied (Johnson, 1993, p. 347). While they remained in these entry level positions, their incomes remained relatively stagnant and their salary increases do not reflect gains made by the general population.

The discrepancies in salaries are not limited to those employed in the blue-collar work force. Income reported for Gallaudet-educated employees during 1983 was $23,500.00, far below the $28,110.00 figure reported for hearing individuals with similar college backgrounds (Chough, 1983). Figure 11-2 reflects the mean 1985 wages and salaries of deaf and hearing college graduates.

Thousands

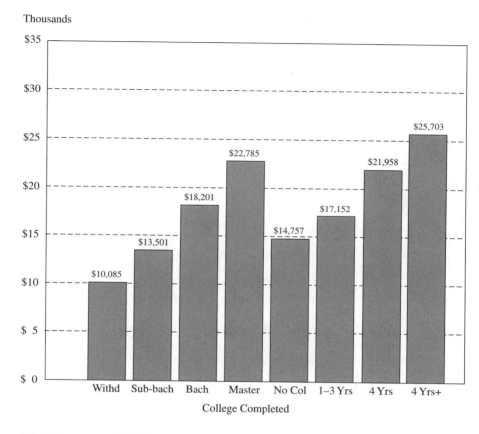

FIGURE 11-2 **1985 Wages and Salaries of Deaf and Hearing College Graduates**
(From Welsh & Walter, JADARA, September 1988. Used with permission.)

Additional data on salaries compiled from a survey of hearing impaired workers (from mild to profound hearing loss) in managerial, professional, and technical positions in 1982–83 indicated that the median salaries for these workers was $21,957—approximately $1,700 less than salaries earned by those workers employed in similar positions in the general population (Crammatte, 1987, p. 1). Although deaf individuals today are employed in a wider array of professional jobs (54 different professional occupations in 1982–1983 as compared with 28 types in 1960), their salaries are still substandard (Crammatte, 1987, p. 1). Figure 11-3 provides a salary comparison between deaf and hearing college graduates.

Thousands

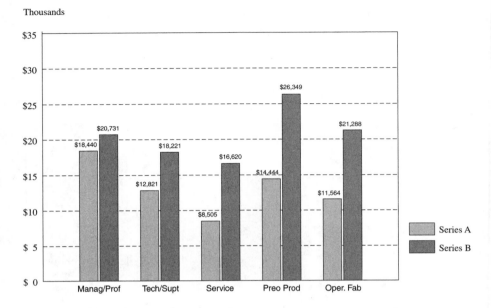

FIGURE 11-3 **Salary Comparison Between Deaf and Hearing College Graduates**
(From Welsh & Walter, JADARA, September 1988. Used with permission.)

There are several possible causes for underemployment within the Deaf subculture. Some of the chief reasons include:

- inadequate education
- inadequate social adjustment
- a poor public image
- isolation of deaf adults
- poor service by programs that should serve the adult deaf (Jacobs, 1980)

In addition, negative attitudes among employers influence the employment of disabled persons and their opportunities for advancement. They may perceive the disabled person as more expensive to hire, train, place, and provide support services to than other workers. Other factors involve a perceived lack of flexibility and ability to adapt to changed conditions and new responsibilities on the part of disabled individuals (Bowe, 1978).

Bolton (1976) has suggested that deaf workers with good social skills have greater opportunities to advance in their work. He further states that those deaf workers having acquired the highest level of skill but lacking good social and communication abilities are virtually locked into their positions and salaries (Bolton, 1976, p. 93). Bolton emphasizes that a person's ability to develop good relationships with coworkers and supervisors is critical to job advancement. He stresses that one must have the ability to engage in conversations pertaining to the formal and informal aspects of work in order to obtain salary increases and promotions.

Other reasons cited for reduced upward mobility include:

- entering the job market at the ceiling of their occupational potential, leaving little room for mobility without additional training
- difficulties in receiving incidental information that is pertinent to keep one current professionally at the higher occupational levels (Foster, 1988)
- securing employment in areas where the positions above theirs on the career ladder are managerial in nature, requiring excessive demands on communication skills (Welsh & Walter, 1988, p. 18)

Recent studies continue to support previous views on the barriers to job advancement. Level of English literacy, educational background, and career selection are all cited as potential barriers to career mobility. Due to their lack of postsecondary training and their depressed reading levels, the majority of deaf workers enter their careers at an average status, only slightly above that of service workers. There they remain for twenty years or more. In comparison, hearing people, on an average, begin their careers at a status level where deaf people are after twenty years, and throughout their tenure in the work force, they significantly increase their career status (Welsh, 1993).

Although the reasons for underemployment are many, the outcomes for the deaf employee are negative. He may remain in an entry level position for his entire career, only earning a salary of about 70 percent of the national average (Jamison, 1983).

There is considerable evidence to suggest that these individuals will not make any major gains in the world of work until there is a concentrated effort to identify and introduce interventions that will lead to their increased employment capabilities (Rusch & Phelps, 1987). While there has been considerable research conducted in the area of employment mobility for the general population, there exists very little evidence on the extent and pattern of mobility among hearing impaired workers (Lang & Stinson, 1982).

Continued research on the vocational development of deaf persons is needed. By obtaining a more global concept of the relationship between the vocational interests and attitudes of deaf workers as they interface with employment opportunities, discrepancies in job placement and upward mobility can be reduced.

VOCATIONAL OPPORTUNITIES FOR MINORITIES AND DEAF INDIVIDUALS WITH SPECIAL NEEDS

The deaf who have been served thus far are not the deaf who are most in need (Taft, 1983). Those who are poor, multihandicapped, and are hidden away in our inner cities and in our ghettos are particularly in need of services (Anderson, 1972). These individuals contribute to a hard-core unemployment group, comprised of approximately 20 to 25 percent of the deaf vocationally aged population (Vernon & Hyatt, 1981). Many are young and reside in urban areas. A disproportionate number are black or Hispanic. Many receive SSI, welfare, and other forms of government assistance.

Other characteristics of this group include individuals who are reading at a second or third grade level. Their domicile may be comprised of one-parent families. Frequently the father is not part of the family unit, and drug use and crime are model behaviors within their communities. This segment of the deaf population, at an early age, becomes part of the "permanent jobless underclass," and many of these youth will never enter the work force (Mindel & Vernon, 1987).

Bowe (1971) has postulated that although there is an absence of national studies pertaining to the nonwhite deaf population, enough information is available to provide a cursory overview. When examining this group, it becomes apparent that within the nonwhite deaf population, undereducation and underemployment are in excess of that found for white deaf persons (Bowe, 1971, p. 361).

Hairston and Smith (1973) have concluded that the effects of undereducation and underemployment contribute to other problems such as: deficiencies in communication skills, low socioeconomic status, and an unfavorable self-image (Taft, 1983, p. 453). This results in these individuals being placed in entry level positions that require very little educational preparation and/or skill. The opportunity for upward mobility within these positions is virtually nonexistent. The worker becomes trapped in a minimum wage earning category with only remote opportunities for advancement. Frequently, the amount of income generated in these positions is comparable to their government incomes. As a result the individual has no incentive to work. Compounding this problem is the fact that those jobs that produce income signal the end to health insurance benefits provided by the government. Often the cost of day-care facilities, coupled with transportation and health insurance costs, cannot be met by compensation paid to workers in entry level positions. As a result, they are forced to remain out of the work force and depend on government subsidies for their livelihoods.

The District of Columbia is unique in that the majority of the population is black. According to the 1982 Revised Census of the Office of Planning and Development, the black population in this area is comprised of 70.3 percent of the general population. According to figures compiled by Gallaudet University's Department of Demographic Studies, the estimated number of black deaf individuals is approximately 3,867. Based on percentages reported by Schein and Delk (1974), the number of black deaf individuals in this area who are unemployed is a staggering 1,547. This population represents an untapped segment of our society.

Further light can be shed on this situation by examining general unemployment trends among the deaf population. When Schein and Delk conducted the national census on deaf individuals they indicated that unemployment among nonwhite deaf males dramatically increased from 7.7 percent in 1972 to 40 percent in 1977, compared to an increase of 5.3 percent to 8.3 percent for white males during the same period of time (Taft, 1983, p. 456).

Jackson (1972) has referred to this group of individuals as the "culturally disadvantaged Black deaf" (p. 9). They are living in environments that are not conducive to the acquisition of those social, educational, and occupational skills that are procured by the hearing, working population. He further suggests that because they lack these opportunities, these deaf individuals develop low aspirations and values that are not always consistent with the goals of rehabilitation services. They see little opportunity to achieve in the world of work and, as a result, retreat to their communities and survive on subsistence incomes.

FUTURE EMPLOYMENT TRENDS

Deaf and hard of hearing youth entering the work force during the twenty-first century will be faced with challenges previously unknown to older generations of workers. The overall characteristics of the employee spectrum will be altered as individuals continue to immigrate into this country. Increased numbers of workers will be well-versed in foreign languages, and English will become their second language as they seek to communicate with their coworkers. Their cultures will be different, and they will add a unique dimension to the work force.

During the early part of this century, the workplace will continue to see an increase in the number of older individuals working outside of the home. As more Americans live longer and remain in good health, many are capable of working and will choose to do so. Although some will retire at the golden age of 65, many more will continue working and will be employed in some capacity, working either in full-time or in part-time capacities. The workplace will further be characterized by an increase in the employment of disabled workers. Modern medicine has enabled many more children to survive early childhood illnesses and congenital defects. As a result, they are attending special classes and are rapidly reaching the age in which they will be ready to seek employment.

This is particularly true for the deaf population. As they reach the secondary school level, the students, together with their parents, are looking forward to employment possibilities that will afford them the opportunity to enter the arena of business and industry. In order to compete with their hearing counterparts they will have to be qualified to apply for the jobs that await them.

The composition of the work force will change drastically in America during the next decade and will be mirrored in the transformation of new jobs as well. Many of the old jobs will disappear as America moves from an industrially based to a technically based society (Walter et al., 1987). According to employment projections published by the Bureau of Labor Statistics (February, 2000), the ten fastest growing occupations from 1998–2008 include computer engineers, up 108 percent; computer support specialists, up 102 percent; systems analysts, up 94 percent; database administrators, up 77 percent; and desktop publishers, up 73 percent.

In addition to these jobs, there will be an increase in paralegal and legal assistants, personal care and home health aides, medical assistants, social and human service assistants, and physicians' assistants.

Table 11.3 reflects the employment projections for the ten occupations that will incur the largest growth from 1998–2008.

Deaf and hard of hearing individuals must prepare for the future in the same way as others wanting to enter the work force. They will be required to have reading, writing, and mathematics skills comparable to those required of all persons wanting to gain access into the fields of business and industry. In addition, employers will expect that their employees have the capacity to communicate comfortably with supervisors, fellow employees, and with office staff.

Throughout this century, skills involving computer technology will be expected and required of many if not all of those employed in office settings. Most of those in the information industry will be required to have familiarity and, hopefully, a proficiency in computer operation (Fellendorf, 1985).

TABLE 11-3 **Occupations with the Largest Growth, 1998–2008**

Type of Employment	Approximate Number of Jobs 2008
Systems Analysts	1,194,000
Retail Salespersons	4,620,000
Cashiers	3,754,000
General Managers & Top Executives	3,913,000
Truck Drivers	3,463,000
Office Clerks, General	3,484,000
Registered Nurses	2,530,000
Computer Support Specialists	869,000
Personal Care & Home Health Aides	1,179,000
Teacher Assistants	1,567,000

(Based on Employment Projections Published by the Bureau of Labor Statistics, February, 2000)

SUMMARY

Employment opportunities for deaf workers hinge on two factors: the deaf individuals' abilities, skills, and educational attainments; and the attitudes of the employers engaged in the hiring process. Each factor impacts significantly on the employability and upward mobility of deaf individuals.

Research has indicated that annually many deaf students graduate from high school unprepared to enter either postsecondary settings or vocational training programs. They lack the necessary skills mandatory for entry level positions in high tech corporations. Far too many are resigned to the fact that they must accept those jobs involving manual labor or enter the ranks of the unemployed. Although some are fortunate and can continue their education, many more face the grim prospects of unemployment and underemployment.

Studies indicate that those entering the work force will be challenged with positions that change daily due to automation and advanced technology. This will force them to update their technical knowledge and personal skills in order to remain competitive. Those who are uncomfortable with career change and have no desire to move upward from their present situation will be left on the fringes of the labor market. To obtain higher levels of employment, appropriate intervention strategies must be incorporated. These strategies need to be designed with the education of this population in mind. It is imperative that they incorporate activities that will enhance feelings of self-confidence. Incentives need to be included that encourage the individual to strive toward upward levels of advancement. Teachers of the deaf, parents, and significant others must change their perceptions regarding the abilities of deaf individuals. These students should be challenged and encouraged to explore the wider range of vocational options available to them.

There are signs of a widening gap between the well-trained deaf worker and the unskilled worker. Unless there are dramatic changes in the training programs and rehabilitation efforts, the gap will continue to widen (Rosen, 1986). In addition, an influx of functionally illiterate deaf persons who are welfare dependent will continue. Students need to begin receiving career education classes in the elementary school years and continue receiving this type of instruction throughout high school. Course material containing information pertaining to the diverse world of work should be shared, and employment availability needs to be stressed. Stereotypic job placements need to be dissolved and replaced with positive attitudes. It is critical that emphasis be placed on job behaviors and socialization, as well as on technical skills.

In short, students must be taught how to learn if they are going to compete in the labor market. Fundamental changes must take place to insure that over 20 percent of the young deaf population will not remain in the unskilled work force (Bolton, 1976, p. 85). As the future economic growth of this country centers around higher levels of education, deaf individuals must receive training to meet this challenge, thus affording them the opportunity to compete equally with their hearing counterparts.

► 12

Deaf Individuals with Special Needs

Children with multiple disabilities comprise a unique segment of the deaf and hard of hearing population. Due to the nature of the disability, these conditions may accompany deafness and impact significantly on the child's development. These additional disabilities may impose physical limitations or result in cognitive/intellectual impairments. Because the extent and nature of particular disabling conditions vary enormously, each deaf and hard of hearing child with special needs must be viewed individually.

Although there have been articles written pertaining to this population since the mid-1800s, the most extensive data base on individuals with additional disabilities can be found in the Annual Survey of Hearing Impaired Children and Youth Residing in the United States (Wolff & Harkins, 1986). This survey is conducted by the Center for Assessment and Demographic Studies (formerly known as the Office of Demographic Studies, located at Gallaudet), which has been collecting information on hearing impaired children and youth since 1968 (Cherow, 1985).

To compile information for the Annual Survey, all educational programs known to be providing preschool, primary, or secondary school services to the deaf and hard of hearing populations are contacted, and data describing the characteristics of this population are gathered. Background information is compiled describing the cause and age at onset of hearing loss, as well as any disabilities the child may have in addition to his hearing loss.

The Annual Survey also provides data on all types of educational programs including schools for the deaf and public school programs. Although the survey is not comprehensive, it does provide information concerning approximately 70 percent of the deaf and hard of hearing school-age population (Karchmer, 1985).

PREVALENCE OF ADDITIONAL CONDITIONS

Of the 48,274 deaf and hard of hearing students included in the 1995–96 Annual Survey, 24.8 percent were reported as having one or more additional disabilities, and 8.5 percent of the total group had two or more additional handicapping conditions (Holt, Hotto, & Cole, 1994). Previous studies conducted throughout the past fifteen years indicate that these percentages have remained relatively stable (Karchmer, 1985, p. 39). Figure 12-1 illustrates the percentage of deaf and hard of hearing individuals exhibiting additional conditions.

These conditions can be classified under two general headings: those involving a physical condition and those affecting the cognitive/intellectual functioning of the individual. Physical conditions include blindness, brain damage, epilepsy, orthopedic problems, cerebral palsy, and heart disorders. Those that fall in the cognitive domain include mental retardation, emotional/behavioral problems, and specific learning disabilities.

Within the two general categories, conditions in the cognitive/intellectual area are far more prevalent than those of a physical nature. Table 12-1 includes information pertaining to the prevalence within each category.

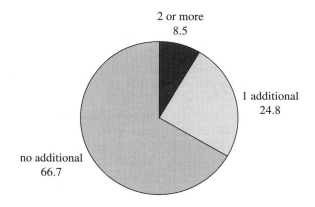

FIGURE 12-1 **Percentage of Deaf and Hard of Hearing Individuals Exhibiting Additional Handicapping Conditions**

(Additional handicapping condition(s) among deaf and hard of hearing students. This represents information on 48,274 students. Gallaudet Research Institute. Regional and National Summary Report of Data from the 1995–1996 Annual Survey of Deaf and Hard-of-Hearing Children and Youth. Washington, DC: GRI. Gallaudet University.)

TABLE 12-1 **Prevalence of Additional Conditions**

Cognitive Intellectual Disabilities	
Mental retardation	8.2%
Specific learning disabilities	9.0%
Serious Emotional/Disturbance	0.3%
Attention Deficit Disorder	4.3%

Physical Conditions	
Legally blind	1.5%
Cerebral palsy	2.9%
Other Conditions	2.6%

(Unpublished data from the Annual Survey of Hearing Impaired Children and Youth, 1997–98. Copyright 1998 by Gallaudet Research Institute.)

Deaf individuals with special needs may experience one or more disabling physical conditions in addition to deafness. It is also possible for an individual to have more than one cognitive/intellectual disability in conjunction with his hearing loss. Various combinations of both physical and cognitive/intellectual conditions can occur.

Closer examination of this information reveals that:

- special learning disorders and emotional/behavioral problems are the only conditions that are reported alone the majority of the time
- students exhibiting legal blindness, brain damage, epilepsy, and orthopedic disorders are reported as having other disabilities in over two-thirds of the cases
- students diagnosed as learning disabled are more likely to have emotional/behavioral problems than those where there is no evidence of learning disabilities
- those students with epilepsy, and brain damage also tend to have increased incidence of learning disabilities
- legal blindness, brain damage, epilepsy, and orthopedic disorders are found more frequently in tandem with mental retardation than in isolation by themselves (Karchmer, 1985, p. 53)

There are a multitude of factors that can contribute to additional disabling conditions. Diseases occurring during the prenatal period, genetic factors, conditions present at birth, early childhood diseases, and trauma can all impact significantly on the child's development.

When these situations occur, children may develop one or more disabling conditions that in turn will influence their physical, social, and psychological development. Frequently, the child will require a specialized educational placement with modifications being made within the curriculum, thus insuring that learning can occur.

The classification of deaf and hard of hearing individuals with special needs denotes a heterogeneous group. The characteristics of these additional conditions, concomitant with the degree of deafness, will influence the profile of the individual. By examining the characteristics of the additional disabling conditions as they relate to deafness, a greater understanding of this population can be gained.

DEAF AND HARD OF HEARING CHILDREN WITH SPECIAL NEEDS: COGNITIVE/ INTELLECTUAL CONDITIONS

Individuals Who Are Deaf or Hard of Hearing and Mentally Retarded

In 1961 the American Association on Mental Deficiency (AAMD) defined the term "mental retardation." Although the definition has been modified slightly over the past several years, it has remained relatively the same.

In essence, the AAMD defined retardation as a condition that exists when the individual possesses a significantly subaverage general intellectual functioning level existing before the age of 16 reflecting an impairment in adaptive behavior.

It can further be defined from a medical perspective and additionally clarified by examining the social psychological, educational, and adaptive behavior classifications as they relate to the definition. Within the confines of medicine, mental retardation can be discussed by examining the underlying disease process or defective biological condition that causes the disability to occur. Therefore, the focus of this classification is on the examination of the etiological (causal) factors of the disability (Kirk & Gallagher, 1979).

Grossman and colleagues compiled a list of the causal factors contributing to this disability. Included in this list are:

- infection
- trauma
- disorders of metabolism
- gross brain disease
- chromosomal abnormalities
- gestational abnormalities
- past psychiatric disorders
- environmental influences. (Grossman et al., 1973, pp. 135–150)

One of the most obvious manifestations of this dysfunction can be found in the response to intelligence testing. According to the AAMD, to classify individuals as mentally retarded their scores must fall within the following range:

	Intelligence Quotient Range
Mild mental retardation	50–55 to approx. 70
Moderate mental retardation	35–40 to 50–55
Severe mental retardation	20–25 to 35–40
Profound mental retardation	20–25 and below
Unspecified mental retardation	

In addition to low performance on intelligence measures, there must also be evidence of deficiencies in adaptive behavior. Adaptive behavior is not as easy to measure as intelligence. Test instruments designed to measure this function are not readily available. One measure that is frequently included in the test battery is the Vineland Social Maturity Scale. This instrument renders a single score and reflects a level of general social competence. The test is designed to sample various aspects of social ability, such as self-sufficiency, self-direction, communication, and social participation. This instrument also reflects the child's need for direction, assistance, and supervision by others. Although this scale tests a variety of behaviors and contains a section for young children as well as older children and adults, it does not yield the same type of levels found in intelligence testing.

Once there is evidence of significantly lower intelligence and maladaptive behavior, the child can be considered for placement in the special education setting. For educational purposes, classifications pertaining to mental disabilities are further defined.

	Measured Intelligence
Borderline or the slow learner	70–85
Educable mentally handicapped	Generally falls between two (2) and three (3) standard deviations below the mean*
Trainable mentally handicapped	Generally falls between three (3) and five (5) standard deviations below the mean*
Profoundly mentally handicapped	Generally falls below five (5) standard deviations below the mean*

* The assessed adaptive behavior also falls below that of other students of the same age and social cultural group. These scores are evaluated considering the child's capabilities and needs to assure proper placement occurs.

Borderline or the Slow Learner

Slow learners may attend public school classes and require special assistance to ensure that they can successfully complete their academic program. They are not considered mentally disabled because they are capable of achieving a moderate degree of academic success, even though they must go at a slower academic pace. They perform better in a classroom designed for the instruction of those students functioning slightly below the normal child. However, with support services they can complete their academic program, become gainfully employed, and be socially adjusted.

Educable Mentally Handicapped

This classification corresponds to the mildly retarded classification as defined by the AAMD. These students, because of their subnormal mental development, are unable to function in the regular classroom. However, they do have the potential to develop academically and progress through the advanced primary grade levels. They are generally socially adjusted to the point that they can interact independently in the community and ultimately become employed at the adult level. Although their employment possibilities may be restricted to the unskilled or semiskilled level, they can become totally or partially independent as they enter adulthood.

The Trainable Mentally Handicapped

This educational classification corresponds to the moderately and severely retarded children identified in the AAMD definition. Characteristics of this classification include minimal educational attainment occurring below a first grade level, development of self-help skills, the ability to adjust socially within the family and neighborhood, and economic usefulness within the sheltered workshop environment or an institutional setting. Unlike the educable mentally handicapped who can function independently within the community and become self-supporting, those who are trainable remain more dependent. Many live in a structured environment throughout adulthood.

The Profoundly Mentally Handicapped

Because of the severity of this disability, the individual is unable to be trained to a high level of self-care, socialization, or economic usefulness. This individual requires almost complete care and supervision throughout his lifetime and would be unable to survive without it.

Deafness and Mental Retardation

Within the field of deafness the task of identifying individuals with varying degrees of mental retardation can be challenging. The incidence figures on deafness and other disabling conditions reflect a wide variation in statistics. These discrepancies are influenced by the methods in which the data is collected, the definitions of educationally significant disabilities, and the accuracy of the data that is available on the students. Due to the difficulties teachers and other professionals encounter while developing adequate sign communication, students may be misdiagnosed when evaluations are conducted. Practitioners may misconstrue what is being said and therefore mislabel the child.

Those involved in the diagnostic process frequently encounter deaf individuals who have experienced familial and social isolation. As a result, communication skills are substandard, preventing the examiner from obtaining an accurate picture of their functioning abilities. In some instances, professionals must observe the child over an extended period of time in order to make an accurate diagnosis. Periodically, when a diagnosis of mental retardation is made, there is some discrepancy as to whether the deafness or the mental retardation is the primary disability. Since the late 1960s, a decline in the number of deaf individuals with mental retardation has been reported. This is due in part to professional awareness of the communication difficulties experienced by deaf individuals. However, 6 to 8 percent of students in programs for the deaf tend to be labeled mentally retarded, a label that is only used to identify approximately 3 percent of the hearing population (Kirk & Gallagher, 1979).

Deaf individuals who are mentally retarded differ from the hearing mentally retarded population in that they must rely almost exclusively on visual cues for instructional purposes. These visual cues differ from those utilized within the non-mentally disabled Deaf community in that "gross communication" becomes the communication link with deaf mentally disabled children.

Gross communication refers to isolated gestures with predetermined meanings. This form of communication runs parallel to the single-word verbal communication utilized with mentally disabled hearing children. Once these words are communicated, word combinations expressed in gesture form are conveyed until word clusters expressing thoughts or commands emerge (Johnson, 1972).

Due, in part, to the communication problems experienced by deaf mentally retarded children, they tend to exhibit a higher incidence of maladjustment than do hearing children who are also mentally disabled. In addition, because of their limited communication, they are inclined to become withdrawn and isolated. This withdrawal may affect their perception of the world around them and cause them to misinterpret other individuals' intentions and motivations, while interacting with them (Lapeer Project, cited in Johnson, 1972, p. 32).

Educational Personnel Serving the Deaf/Mentally Disabled Child

Since the mid-sixties, various studies have been conducted pertaining to educational programming for mentally disabled deaf children. The majority of this research indicates:

1. that there are few, if any, professional or paraprofessional workers who have had the benefit of training in the areas of both deafness and mental retardation (Stewart, 1971)

2. most educational programs serving deaf/mentally retarded children employ teachers of the deaf and through in-service training attempt to enhance their skills (D'Zamko & Hampton, 1985)

3. two-thirds of the instructors currently teaching deaf/mentally disabled children have revealed that they would prefer teaching deaf students without any additional disabling conditions (Anderson & Stevens, 1970)

Educating deaf children whose intelligence is intact can be a difficult task that becomes more complex when mental retardation is present. These children experience hearing loss, subaverage general intellectual functioning, and deficits in adaptive behavior (Healey & Karp-Nortman, 1975). The combination of these three factors working together require services that are different from those traditionally requested by the group of individuals exhibiting either mental retardation or deafness.

Specific Learning Disabilities

The label "learning disabilities" encompasses a wide array of disabilities. Those students, who in the past did not fit neatly into the traditional categories of disabled children, found themselves designated as learning disabled. Today the term has evolved to incorporate a heterogeneous group of children who share one thing in common: They all have discrepancies between their abilities and their achievements (Kirk & Gallagher, 1979).

From a medical perspective, specific learning disabilities can be identified based on the cause of the dysfunction and how the specific causes relate to abnormalities in the brain. Some of the medical terminology commonly used in describing this population includes brain injury, minimal brain damage, minimal cerebral dysfunction, and central nervous system disorders. However, not all learning disabilities can be verified medically, and not all students with medical evidence display learning disabilities.

Learning disabilities can be defined further by identifying the dysfunction according to the behavioral or psychological manifestations associated with it. Terminology utilized to describe these ramifications include conceptual disorders, reading disabilities, language disorders, arithmetic disabilities, and perceptual handicaps.

Thus, a child who is identified as having "minimal brain dysfunction syndrome" is referred to as one who has near average, average, or above average general intelligence with certain learning or behavioral disabilities ranging from mild to severe. These central nervous system deviations manifest themselves through various combinations of impairments that occur in perception, conceptualization, language, memory, control of attention, impulse, or motor functioning abilities (Clements, 1966, pp. 9–10). As a result, the child may have average intellectual functioning abilities but experience a disorder in one or more of the basic psychological processes. These processes may involve receptive or expressive language, convey either a spoken or a written format, reading, writing, or engaging in mathematical computations.

These discrepancies between abilities (potential) and achievement comprise only one of the three criteria needed to establish the fact that these children have a specific learning disability. In addition, they must meet the exclusion criterion and criterion that involves special education.

Exclusion Criterion

The exclusion criterion theoretically differentiates learning disabilities from other disabling conditions. When identifying this population, most definitions eliminate difficulties in learning that can be attributed to mental retardation, emotional disturbances, environmental deprivation, or visual or auditory disabilities. Individuals with these conditions can also be learning disabled. However, the intent here is to separate these contributing factors from the underlying cause of learning disabilities.

Special Education Criterion

Learning disabled children differ from children with environmentally deprived backgrounds. The latter group can be placed in the classroom, provided with educational enrichment programs, and develop into average academic students. In essence, they do not require a special education placement. In contrast, students with learning disabilities require special education programs that incorporate remedial programming in order for the child to learn.

Because learning disabilities may share similar characteristics of other disabling conditions, it is important that the professional identify the cause of the atypical behavior and differentiate it from other conditions. Through this process, referred to as making a differential diagnosis, remedial programs can be surveyed, and the most appropriate program can be selected. There are three general criteria taken into consideration when a differential diagnosis is determined.

1. Does the child have a specific learning disability? Is there a discrepancy between his abilities and level of achievement, or are there contributing factors that are primarily responsible for the disabling condition?
2. If it is determined that the child has a specific learning disability, it is important to ascertain what his abilities and disabilities are in relation to his own areas of development.
3. When the child's strengths and weaknesses have been determined, it is essential that the underlying causes of the discrepancy be examined. Determining the underlying cause of the deficit will aid the diagnostician in selecting the most appropriate program.

Deafness and Learning Disabilities

Ramifications of deafness tend to exacerbate difficulties experienced by the individual within the language arts area. As a result, significant delays in reading and writing may be evident. In addition, many of the behaviors typically exhibited in deaf and hard of hearing students are used as criteria to identify the learning disabled population. Therefore, the diagnostician must be cautious when attempting to identify the learning disabled deaf population. Although at first glance certain characteristics of these two groups may appear similar, the underlying causes contributing to each are decidedly different (see Table 12-2).

In recent years there has been extensive information published pertaining to the field of learning disabilities; however, only a scant amount of information is available in reference to the deaf and hard of hearing populations (Powers, Elliott, & Funderburg, 1987; Wolff & Harkins, 1986).

Because the criteria for identifying learning disabilities for hearing children are not appropriate for use within the confines of the deaf and hard of hearing population, it is difficult to identify and define characteristics specifically related to the learning disabled hearing impaired (LDHI) subgroup.

It has been estimated that between 6 and 7 percent of the deaf and hard of hearing students in the United States have a learning disability as an additional disability (Craig & Craig, 1987; Powers et al., 1987); however, these figures are not well-founded. Without a clear definition of LDHI students and with no specific criteria for identifying them, these figures present an estimate at best (Powers, Elliott, & Funderburg, 1988; Powers et al., 1987).

To determine how LDHI students are identified, Powers, Elliott, and Funderburg (1987) conducted a national survey of teachers of the deaf. They examined the methods that the teachers used for identifying and assessing deaf and hard of hearing students who have a learning disability as an additional handicap. They also examined program procedures that are used with these students. Results of their survey indicated that teacher observation and referral are the most frequently used methods for

TABLE 12-2 **Characteristics Shared by Two Populations with Different Underlying Causes**

Deaf and Hard of Hearing Without Learning Disabilities	Normal Hearing Learning Disabled
Average intelligence	
Depressed language scores due to an auditory deficiency	Discrepancy between estimated ability and academic performance
Social-emotional difficulties based on environmental problems/experiential deprivation	Social-emotional problems
Motor disorders related to etiology of deafness	Motor disorders
Lags in cognitive development based on language deficits	Metacognitive deficits

identifying LDHI students for assessment; however, due to the lack of clearly defined criteria for assessing this population, determination of specific cases can be difficult (Powers et al., 1987, p. 278).

In addition to teacher observation and referral, some instructors indicated that they rely on standardized tests such as the Wechsler Intelligence Scale for Children-Revised (WISC-R) and the Bender Visual Motor Gestalt Test for information. Others paid particular attention to unusual learning styles and language problems that are atypical of the deaf.

Instructors and administrators completing this survey indicated that the majority of the LDHI students (60 percent) receive services in self-contained classrooms for deaf and hard of hearing students. Additional itinerant services, or those services provided by a teacher trained to work with hearing students who have learning disabilities, were provided to over 50 percent of the students identified as LDHI (Powers et al., 1987, p. 283).

Teachers responding to this survey were asked to indicate the type of training they had received preparing them to work with this population. The vast majority of the teachers (83.9 percent) indicated that they had had little training and were not certified to teach LDHI students. Almost 78 percent indicated that they had received no training during their college program that would prepare them for this population. However, 88.3 percent responded with an affirmative when asked if they felt they could benefit from special training (Powers et al., 1988).

These data suggest that additional research is needed in the area of LDHI. Emphasis needs to be placed on establishing criteria that can be used for assessment purposes, developing curriculum materials that can be incorporated within the classrooms, and enhancing teacher training programs, thus providing school personnel with the information they need to better serve this population.

Emotional/Behavioral Problems

The term "seriously emotionally disturbed" as defined in P.L. 94-142 has been elaborated upon to serve as an advisory tool and to be utilized as a general guideline for those professionals responsible for identifying and providing services to this population. In essence, the definition states that the individual's educational performance is adversely affected over an extended period of time due to the following conditions:

1. An inability to learn that cannot be explained by intellectual, sensory, or health factors.
2. An inability to build or maintain satisfactory interpersonal relationships with peers and teachers.
3. Inappropriate types of behavior or feelings under normal circumstances.
4. A general, pervasive mood of unhappiness or depression.
5. A tendency to develop physical symptoms, pains or fears associated with personal or school problems.

This term also includes children who are schizophrenic. However, it does not encompass children who are socially maladjusted unless it is determined that they are seriously emotionally disturbed (Wang et al., 1988).

One of the problems facing educators is that the term itself covers the full gamut of behaviors, including aggression and hyperactivity at one end of the continuum, and withdrawal or the inability to make friends at the opposite end. Emotionally disturbed children frequently have additional disabling conditions, such as learning disabilities or mental retardation. As a result, it may become difficult to establish whether the academic difficulty the child is experiencing is the result of an emotional problem or if school failure is causing the emotional difficulty (Slavin, 1988).

Characteristics of Students with Emotional Disturbances

There is a multiplicity of characteristics that are associated with the area of emotional disturbance (Kneedler, 1984). However, the issue that merits particular attention is the degree of the behavior problem. Although any behavior exhibited over an extended period of time could be considered as an indication of an emotional disturbance, there are some general characteristics that are displayed by most students identified as emotionally disturbed. They include poor academic achievement, poor interpersonal relationships, and poor self-esteem (Kneedler, 1984).

Quay (1979) surveyed the literature pertaining to the characteristics of the emotionally disturbed population. He took the attributes that were displayed by the majority and grouped them into four categories. These categories reflect the various dysfunctions that occur under the umbrella of emotional/behavioral disorders: 1) conduct disorders, 2) anxiety/withdrawal behaviors, 3) factors pertaining to immaturity, and 4) socialized aggressive disorders.

Conduct Disorders

Emotionally disturbed children displaying conduct disorders frequently disrupt the academic setting and engage in fighting and other unacceptable school behaviors. Hyperactivity was also included in this category, due to the general disruptive nature of the dysfunction.

Anxiety/Withdrawal

Children within this category tend to be tense and fearful and may become overly anxious about their health. They have few, if any, friends and do not adjust well to the social/educational setting. They have difficulty constructing a positive self-image and experience feelings of depression. These perceptions can all interfere with their academic functioning.

Immature Behavior
Students lacking social skills experience difficulties focusing on academic studies. They may exhibit very short attention spans and be inattentive in class. They may have a difficult time focusing on tasks and struggle during extended periods of time in the classroom.

Socialized Aggressive Disorders
The behavior observed in these children is similar to that evidenced in the group reflecting conduct disorders. Although they may appear similar on the surface, this group's behaviors can generally be attributed to their home environments. Within these settings, aggressive behavior is reinforced and exhibited deviant behaviors are learned.

Specific characteristics of these categories, along with the outward manifestations of their corresponding behavior, have been included in Table 12-3. The characteristics alone do not constitute an emotional disturbance. Only when these conditions continue for an extended period of time and cause an adverse affect on the individual's academic achievement can they be viewed as attributed to emotional/behavioral problems.

The Deaf or Hard of Hearing Emotionally Disturbed Individual

Statistical data concerning the prevalence of emotional/behavioral problems in the school-age deaf population varies considerably. This is due to identification criteria incorporated by the school as well as formal reporting practices. A national survey conducted by Jensema and Trybus (1975) focuses on all forms of childhood illness and disability. They reported that 8 percent of the school-age deaf and hard of hearing population have emotional/behavioral problems. Among the multidisabled contingency, the number rose to 20.4 percent. However, these statistics varied considerably from those reported in an earlier study conducted by Pless and Roghmann (1971). Pless and Roghmann indicated that 30 percent to 50 percent of all chronically ill or disabled children had secondary social and emotional problems. Psychiatrists, such as Altshuler (1974), who has specialized in the treatment of emotionally disturbed deaf children, reviewed the literature and concluded that when low figures are reported pertaining to this population, it is reflective of the methodology used to record the incidents and should be viewed as a marked underrepresentation of the total population. Based on his professional experiences, he has estimated that between one and three out of every ten deaf students present significant emotional problems that warrant attention. These children display emotional problems ranging from mild to moderate and requiring special education services. Those with severe emotional problems frequently require institutionalization.

Causes of emotional disturbances in deaf children are varied. Some can be attributed to the impact of deafness on human development, the way those in the environ-

TABLE 12-3 **Emotional/Behavioral Problems, Characteristics, and Behavior Manifestations**

Characteristics	Manifestations of Behavior
Conduct Disorders	
Children who are frequently: disobedient distractible selfish jealous destructive impertinent disruptive	Children frequently engage in: fighting stealing destroying property refusing to obey teacher displaying other unacceptable school behaviors failing to respond to punishment
Anxiety/Withdrawal	

Children project images as being:
 fearful
 tense
 seclusive
 depressed
 hypersensitive
 timid
 bashful
	Children frequently:
	 have few friends
	 play with children much younger than
	   themselves or alone
	 have elaborate fantasies
	 have low self-image or grandiose
	   visions of themselves
	 are overly anxious about their health

Immaturity	
short attention span preoccupation inattention passivity poor coordination	Children often: appear odd or awkward at all times exhibit unusual or bizarre thinking lack social skills

Socialized Aggressive Disorder
   related to poor home conditions that
     model or reward aggressive behavior
	Socialized Aggressive Disorder
	   exhibit behaviors similar to those
	     involved in conduct disorders

(Based on literature provided by Quay, 1979)

ment respond to deafness, and the manner in which deaf individuals react to their environment. Other cases can be attributed to immaturity and poor home environments.

Theoretically, there is another significant component that may be responsible for this disabling condition. It involves an interactional effect of both the loss of hearing and of other central nervous system lesions associated with the condition causing the deafness. Impulse disorders, psychosis, general behavioral disorders, and aphasoid disorders can also be accounted for, in part, due to pathology located within the central nervous system (Vernon & Rothstein, 1967). Additional research conducted by Rainer and Altshuler (1966) has suggested that some deaf mentally ill individuals exhibit symptoms that are similar to characteristics found in brain injured people. In addition, research conducted by Chess and Fernandez (1980) has also documented physiological findings. In studies of children with rubella-related deafness, a high incidence of emotional and behavioral difficulties was noted. This further supports studies cited in the Annual Survey whereby conditions such as rubella, birth trauma, and complications during pregnancy were cited in conjunction with emotional/behavioral problems (Schildroth & Karchmer, 1986, p. 76).

Physiological causes, strained familial and peer relationships, social difficulties, educational environment, and communication factors can all contribute to emotional and behavioral difficulties. Once a dysfunction of this nature has been identified, professional treatment must be secured. However, as with other areas of deafness, there is a scarcity of mental health professionals trained to work with this population (Cantor & Spragins, 1977), and the special needs of this group are not always met (Edelstein, 1977).

PHYSICAL CONDITIONS

Legal Blindness and Uncorrected Visual Problems

Individuals with visual problems can be classified into two categories: 1) the blind; and 2) the partially seeing, or individuals with low vision (Kirk & Gallagher, 1979, p. 237). A legal-medical definition of blindness can be found in the Fact Book prepared by the National Society for the Prevention of Blindness (1966). The definition for blindness is as follows:

- visual acuity for distance vision of 20/200 or less in the better eye
- with acuity of more than 20/200 if the widest diameter of field of vision subtends an angle no greater than 20 degrees

The partially seeing are defined as:

- persons with a visual acuity greater than 20/200
- but not greater than 20/70 in the better eye with correction

When testing for visual acuity, the most widely used assessment tool is the Snellen Chart. Individuals read letters on the chart to measure what they can distinguish at various distances. Based on the Snellen Chart, ratings can be interpreted in the following way:

- 20/20—the individual can distinguish at 20 feet what a normal eye can see at 20 feet
- 20/200—the individual sees at 20 feet what the normal eye can distinguish at 200 feet
- 5/200—the individual can distinguish at 5 feet what a normal eye can distinguish at 200 feet

Historically, children were placed into classes based on this legal-medical definition. However, during the sixties educators began to realize that the functional visual efficiency, the way in which children use their vision, is more appropriate for placement purposes. As a result, functional definitions of visual impairments were devised.

Barraga (1976) has developed a classification system in which one's visual disability can be relegated into three functional categories. *Blindness* is used to describe those people who experience only light perception; they have no vision and must learn through Braille and other related media. Those identified as having *low vision* are capable of seeing objects or materials within a few inches of them but experience limitations in their ability to see things at a distance. The third group is referred to as those who experience *limited vision.* These individuals can be considered sighted if their vision can be corrected (Barraga, 1976, p. 14).

According to Kirk & Gallagher (1979), the major causes of blindness are categorized as follows: infectious diseases, accidents and injuries, general diseases, and prenatal influences, including heredity (p. 242).

The Deaf-Blind Individual

The deaf-blind child has a combination of both visual and hearing impairments. This combination causes severe communication and developmental problems requiring that education programs be specifically designed for them. These children cannot be served in programs solely for children with hearing impairments, visual impairments, or severe disabilities without supplemental assistance (Miles, 1998). This is one of the most challenging of the multihandicapping conditions to work with because both of the primary sensory avenues are dysfunctional. The individual is cut off from the surrounding sights and sounds of daily living experiences.

Each deaf-blind person sustains both a visual impairment and an auditory impairment. However, the degree of severity with which they occur can vary. Certain individuals can rely on some residual hearing, while others experience a profound loss with partial sightedness. Some are in a transitional stage, adjusting to a second disability acquired long after the first. The severity of each impairment and the specific combination in which they are found will influence the types of instructional and rehabilitative techniques that are incorporated. Deaf-blind individuals may be categorized according to primary disability, severity of each, and time of onset. Table 12-4 illustrates these categories.

TABLE 12-4 **Variables Associated with Deaf-Blindness**

First Disability	Second Disability	Communication Modes
Congenital sensorineural loss resulting in profound hearing loss	Progressive loss in vision	Function as a deaf person, may utilize a sign system or other modes of communication
Congenital visual impairment rendering the person legally blind	Progressive hearing loss	Function as a blind person, may be skilled in Braille
Profound impairments in both disabilities		Utilize alternative modes of communication
Simultaneous progressive blindness and deafness		Communication strategies are learned in respect to the severity of the primary disability

Usher's Syndrome
Within the field of deafness, a particular hereditary genetic disorder deserves special attention because it is responsible for more than half of the deaf-blindness in the United States (Davenport & Omen, 1977; Vernon, 1969). Usher's syndrome is an autosomal, recessively inherited condition characterized by a moderate-to-severe sensorineural hearing impairment combined with retinitis pigmentosa (RP). The hearing loss is believed to be present at birth, while the initial overt symptoms of RP do not usually occur until the second or third decade of life. The RP association with Usher's syndrome is slowly progressive: The symptoms include night blindness, tunnel vision, decreased activity, and cataracts (Fillman et al., 1987).

Usher's syndrome is rare in the general population (3 per 100,000). However, 2 percent to 5 percent of the genetic deaf population have the disease (Vernon, 1973). This inherited condition is also the cause of more than half of all deaf-blindness in adults.

Because RP is progressive in nature, early identification is important. Students with this syndrome need to be informed that they have it and also of the disabling conditions. Frequently, their visual field and dark adaptation abilities deteriorate so that they may need additional assistance during the evening hours.

In previous years, education of the deaf-blind has primarily been conducted in private residential schools. Affluent parents were the only ones who could afford to send their children for training. Because so few children could benefit from this type of education, the federal government passed legislation in 1968 to establish ten model centers for deaf-blind children. The purpose of these centers was to provide family counseling services, medical and educational diagnoses, itinerant home services, as well as teacher training opportunities. As a result more deaf-blind children have been able to receive specialized services.

The majority of children who are diagnosed as having Usher's syndrome or classified as being deaf-blind have not lost the complete use of both senses. Students with this classification have some degree of residual hearing or residual vision. Instruction occurring in this area relies almost exclusively on other senses, such as touch, for conveying information.

Cerebral Palsy and Deafness

Within the general population, the prevalence of cerebral palsy affects between 0.1 percent to 0.6 percent (Nelson, 1959, p. 1138). Within the general population of deaf children, the rate is 15.8 percent or about 100 times greater. Further data indicate that over half of the children deafened by the Rh factor have cerebral palsy (Vernon, 1982, p. 18).

The term "cerebral palsy" was coined by Winthrop Phelps, an orthopedic surgeon and a pioneer in this field. Cerebral (referring to the brain) palsy (a motor disability) is not a disease but can be defined as a disorder of posture and movement due to a nonprogressive lesion in the brain that occurs in the developing central nervous system (Harryman & Warren, 1985, p. 202). Capute and others (1978) have stated that cerebral palsy is no longer considered a condition with a pure motor component. Rather, it is viewed as a multidimensional disorder in which the type and distribution of the motor disability has become a neurodevelopmental marker for underlying associated disabilities of a neurologic, cognitive, or perceptual nature. It is not uncommon to find visual problems, hearing disorders, intellectual disabilities, and speech and learning difficulties among individuals diagnosed with cerebral palsy.

Deaf and hard of hearing students who also have cerebral palsy function in a variety of ways. The severity of the palsy, the degree of the neuromuscular involvement, and the site of the lesion will all influence their ability to progress educationally and independently. Educational placements are based on the multidimensional characteristics of the disorder and the individual's motivation to explore his or her potential.

Other Disabling Conditions

Other disabling conditions noted in the Annual Survey include orthopedic handicaps, epilepsy, and heart disorders. In relation to deafness, statistics reveal that these are low incidence disabilities. The severity and the way in which they interface with deafness will determine the types of support services necessary for the individual to enter the mainstream of society.

SUMMARY

Approximately one-third of the deaf and hard of hearing population have secondary disabilities. These disabilities are varied and are the result of both physical and cognitive/intellectual dysfunctions. Some attend special education facilities while others become institutionalized. Within certain specialized areas, the support services are adequate, while in others there has been very little progress made.

Throughout the past decade research has been conducted that sheds new insights into the domain of the deaf population with special needs. Additional research needs to be done within this field. Educators' interests must be sparked, and programs must be developed to ensure that the potential that lies within this unique group of individuals is tapped.

▶ 13

Hearing Aids and Modern Technology

Statistics indicate that there are 22 million hearing impaired people in the United States. Within this population, only 1 million wear hearing aids (Mahon, 1983). This can be attributed to limited economic resources, perceptions of self-image, and a lack of accurate information.

The majority of individuals exhibiting some type of hearing loss can benefit from some form of amplification such as hearing aids, assistive listening devices and systems, and/or medical/surgical treatment. If amplification is the chosen habilitative or rehabilitative mode, individual assessments must be scheduled in order to determine which type of amplification will be the most advantageous for the hearing impaired consumer.

THE HEARING EVALUATION

The purpose of an audiological evaluation is to identify the cause and type of hearing loss the individual has and to determine what form of amplification, if any, will be beneficial. Frequently, a medical doctor (an otolaryngologist or an otologist) will do the initial evaluation to determine if the loss results from a medical problem. A hearing evaluation, performed by an audiologist or medical doctor, assists in determining the location of a hearing impairment along the auditory peripheral or central pathway. If there is no obvious problem, the person may be scheduled for a hearing evaluation with an audiologist.

A hearing evaluation is conducted in a controlled environment, usually a sound room. Each ear is tested individually to determine if there is a loss in either or both ears, the degree of loss in each ear, as well as the location of the impairment.

Incorporated in the evaluation is a series of tests designed to determine how clearly the individual understands words and the level at which they can best be comprehended. After the test, the results are evaluated and options for treatment are discussed.

In the event that amplification through the use of hearing aids is deemed necessary, a hearing aid evaluation will be scheduled. The purpose of this evaluation is to assist individuals in selecting the most appropriate aid, orient them to the hearing aid components, explain how they work, and what can be realistically expected when using it.

THE FUNCTION AND COMPONENTS OF HEARING AIDS

The basic function of a hearing aid is to amplify sounds, making them more intense or loud for the individual with a hearing loss. It operates like many other amplifying devices incorporating a microphone, amplifier, and receiver into its system (see Figure 13-1).

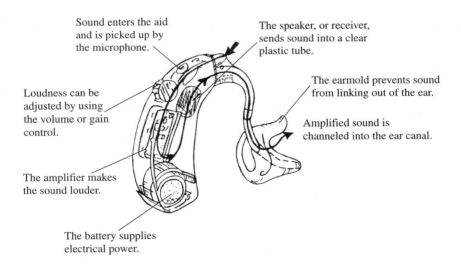

Sound enters the aid and is picked up by the microphone.

The speaker, or receiver, sends sound into a clear plastic tube.

Loudness can be adjusted by using the volume or gain control.

The earmold prevents sound from linking out of the ear.

Amplified sound is channeled into the ear canal.

The amplifier makes the sound louder.

The battery supplies electrical power.

FIGURE 13-1   **The Basic Design of a Hearing Aid**

Sound enters the aid through the **microphone.** Once received, the **volume control** can be used to adjust the intensity. Sounds are made louder by the **amplifier.** The battery supplies electrical power to the aid. Sound is transmitted to the **speaker** or **receiver** and enters a clear plastic tube. The tube enters the earmold. The earmold fits snugly within the ear, thereby preventing sound from "leaking" out of the ear. The amplified sound is directed into the ear canal. (Courtesy of Carnell Roberts)

Microphones

The purpose of the microphone is to pick up sounds in the environment. The electret microphone, which utilizes an electric field as opposed to a magnetic field (Killion & Carlson, 1974), is almost universally used for hearing aids. This is due to its size, sensitivity to sound, frequency response, low internal noise, and insensitivity to mechanical vibration.

Within the microphone the electret is made from a fluorocarbon plastic that holds a permanent electric charge. A very thin plastic diaphragm with a metallic coating is placed adjacent to the electret layer. As sound waves enter the microphone, the diaphragm vibrates, sending a small electrical voltage to the amplifier (Katz, 1985).

Amplifier

The amplifier serves two basic purposes. First, it amplifies the original environmental sound, which is received as a pulsating electrical signal from the microphone. This amplification is an optimal volume for assistance with hearing. Second, it limits the amount of sound pressure that the aid can deliver in order to avoid exceeding the user's level of comfort.

The amplifier consists of a series of integrated circuits (ICs). These circuits are comprised of transistors, diodes, and resistors on a silicon chip to provide the individual with the desired electronic output (Katz, 1985).

Receiver

The function of the receiver is to convert the electrical signal back to an acoustical signal that is louder than the original environmental one that was received by the microphone. The amplified acoustical sound signal is channeled through a receiver sending sound impulses into a plastic tube that directs the sound into the ear canal. When behind-the-ear hearing aids are utilized, the tube is guided into the ear canal by a supporting structure called an earmold.

Earmolds

The earmold is a plastic plug designed to fit the ear so that sound can be transmitted into the ear canal and on to the eardrum. It prevents sound from leaking out of the ear and has a strong effect on the overall performance of the aid. It is essential that the earmold is acoustically designed to enhance the sound as it courses down the ear canal, that it fits comfortably, appears cosmetically attractive, and can be easily cleaned.

There are three main types of earmolds:

1. The regular or receiver

In this type the earmold fills a considerable part of the concha and extends into the ear canal.

2. The skeleton or one of a similar type

With this mold, only the amount of material necessary for sealing, retention, and comfort is utilized. It is designed with a tip that extends into the ear canal and seals against its walls.

3. Open or nonoccluding

This type of mold is designed to keep the ear canal as unoccluded as possible. An open or unoccluded type of mold is used with tubing or a small diameter tip that projects into the ear canal (Katz, 1985).

If an earmold does not fit properly, the overall functioning of the aid will be affected. In addition, a loose-fitting mold may permit leakage of sound transmitted by the aid, thus producing a whistling sound commonly referred to as feedback.

Additional Components

Hearing aids have additional highly sophisticated circuitry to enhance their performance. Although not all of the controls are available on all aids, most share the more common ones.

Volume Control

Volume controls (sometimes referred to as gain controls) enable the hearing aid wearer to adjust the level of sound to a comfortable listening level as it is delivered to the ear. If the control is set too loud, headaches and dizziness may occur. See Figure 13-2.

Pitch or Tone Control

A pitch or tone control is used to alter the frequency response or the pitch emphasis of the amplified sound. Unlike the volume control, this control is set by the audiologist or hearing aid dispenser and should not be altered. This circuitry is especially beneficial for those individuals experiencing a loss in one primary frequency range. Those individuals experiencing normal hearing in only the low frequency range can benefit from an aid whose tone control is set to emphasize the high frequency sounds.

Telecoil Circuitry

Many hearing aids have circuitry built into the aid to make it easier to hear what is being said over the telephone. In 1988 the Hearing Aid Compatibilities Act was passed by the House (House Bill H-22213) and the Senate (S-314) mandating that

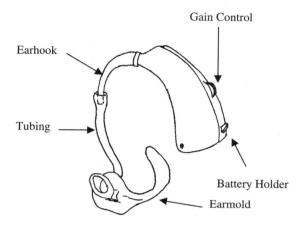

FIGURE 13-2   **External View of an Over the Ear (OTE) Hearing Aid**
(Courtesy Marie A. Scheetz)

all public telephones be compatible for use with telecoils. Hearing aids incorporating this circuitry utilize a telephone switch, usually labeled "T" on the hearing aid case. When turned on, the "T" switch activates the telecoil.

Telecoils function by responding to a magnetic field generated by the receiver within the telephone handset. Due to the variety of handset construction, in some units an adequate magnetic field is not generated. Adaptors can be purchased and attached to the earphone portion of the handset to correct this problem. They will change the acoustic energy of the earphone into a useful magnetic field. Other modifications installed directly within the handset can also produce the desired magnetic field. In addition to providing the wearer with increased telephone use, telecoils increase one's options for accessing various assistive listening devices such as closed-circuit "loop" systems found in large meeting rooms, theaters, churches, and synagogues. The telecoil receives the magnetic energy produced by these other devices. Subsequently, the hearing aid amplifies, then converts the energy into an audible sound.

Batteries

Batteries supply the electrical power to the aid and are currently of two main types. Currently, zinc air batteries are the most widely used. They have a significantly longer shelf life than mercury batteries and will last approximately twice as long while in use in the hearing aid (Shelfer, 1990).

TYPES OF HEARING AIDS

The earliest form of amplification utilized was probably man's hand cupped behind his ear. Acoustic amplifiers such as horns and speaking tubes followed the concept of cupping one's hand. These were followed by carbon hearing aids which were based on the principle of the telephone. Around 1938, vacuum tube hearing aids appeared which offered much greater amplification possibilities, wider frequency response, and lower harmonic distortion (Katz, 1985).

Today's hearing aids come in a variety of types and styles (see Figure 13-3) and are based on the invention of the transistor by Bell Telephone Laboratories. This discovery enabled manufacturers to design aids that are much smaller and more powerful. Individuals experiencing a hearing loss have a variety of aids to select from.

Over the Ear (OTE) or Behind the Ear (BTE)

This was the principal type of aid used for several years. The aid fits behind the pinna with the tubing going over the ear and carrying sound to the earmold. Within this type of aid there is enough room for several fitting adjustments. They are durable and are easily serviceable. Because they are able to produce a significant amount of power, OTEs/BTEs are frequently used by individuals with severe to profound losses. The basic design of this aid provides enough distance between the microphone and the earmold tip to facilitate increased power usage without encountering problems with feedback. In addition, many assistive devices are designed for use with OTE/BTE aids either through the use of the T-coil or a boot that can plug into the aid. The boot is a connection that is attached at the bottom of the hearing aid and allows a cord to be plugged into it. The cord is then connected to the signal receiving device of the assistive listening device enabling the hearing aid user to hear the sound being generated by the assistive listening device through their own personal hearing aid (see section regarding Assistive Listening Devices).

Eyeglass Hearing Aids

In 1959, nearly half of the hearing aids sold in the United States were of the eyeglass type (Berger, 1984). Sales decreased to approximately 2.7 percent in 1983 (Hearing Industries Association, 1984). In the eyeglass aid, all of the hearing aid parts (microphone, amplifier, and receiver) are enclosed in the earpieces (bows of the glasses). Historically, eyeglass aids were once popular but now they are rapidly disappearing. A common problem with eyeglass hearing aids is the fact that two sensory corrective (prosthetic) devices are linked together. If the hearing aid requires repair, one may need a spare pair of glasses and a spare hearing aid that can be used without an eyeglass frame. In addition, with the current size variations of in-the-ear hearing aids, often hearing losses can be accommodated successfully

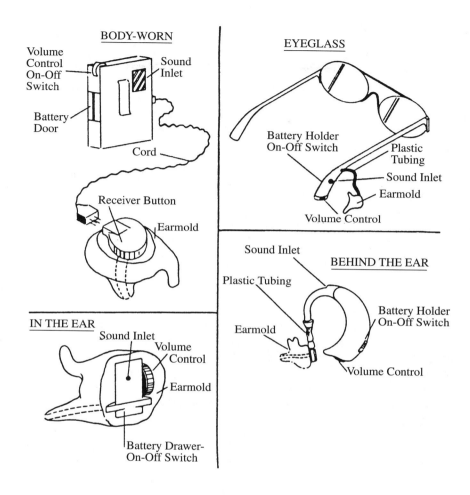

FIGURE 13-3 **Styles of Hearing Aids**
(From *Communication Disorders of the Aged,* Schow et al., 1978. Reprinted with permission.)

with a hearing aid style that will not interfere with a person's use of eyeglasses. This eliminates the need for eyeglasses and hearing aid. Before the development of smaller in-the-ear hearing aids, people often utilized OTE/BTE aids in conjunction with eyeglasses. This caused difficulties in keeping eyeglasses adjusted, as well as the discomfort of added weight due to the eyeglass temple piece, hardware, and the hearing aid resting on the pinna.

Body Hearing Aids

Prior to the development of eyeglass aids in the middle fifties, body aids were essentially the only available wearable type. Today, less than 2 percent of the aids sold in the United States are body type (Berger, 1984).

Today, body aids are primarily used with severely hearing impaired children in the school setting. They can provide more amplification without feedback than an ear level aid. In addition, they are designed with larger controls, benefitting both young children and the older adult population. Utilization of this type of aid requires a separate air or bone receiver connected to the aid by a cord.

The disadvantage of body aids lies in their size and visibility and their ability to absorb noise as clothing comes in contact with the aid. In addition, because body aids receive sound at the torso and not at the head or ear level, localization of sound is virtually impossible. Due to technological advances, OTE/BTE aids are, for the most part, as effective for the severely to profoundly hearing impaired population as the body aids. For these reasons, the majority of hearing impaired individuals select the behind-the-ear style.

All In the Ear (AIE) or In the Ear (ITE)

Hearing aids that fit entirely in the ear have become increasingly popular in the United States. In 1983 they accounted for 49.4 percent of the hearing aid sales (Hearing Industries Association, 1984). Recent technology has facilitated the miniaturization of electret microphones, correspondingly small receivers, and batteries. These advances have allowed the aid to be designed to fit within the concha and the ear canal.

In-the-ear aids are primarily of a custom design; however, modular units are also available. Custom aids are built into a shell made from an impression of the user's ear. Modular ITE aids are built into a case of fixed shape that fits into a matching depression in a custom earmold.

There are three main styles of custom in-the-ear aids.

1. *Standard Custom ITE*
   This aid is the most common of this type utilized. It occupies the entire concha area of the ear and extends into the canal. It permits the greatest flexibility in circuit design and fitting flexibility.
2. *Lower Concha Custom ITE*
   This aid occupies the concha, cavum and canal. Because it is smaller, there is less room available for the circuits and components, limiting its potential for gain and output.
3. *Custom Canal ITE*
   This style of aid is the least visible of all. It fits in a small space at the beginning of the ear canal. The sound quality of these aids can be quite good as the bowl of the ear is open and can help collect sounds. In addition, the tip of the aid is closer to the eardrum for better high frequency hearing.

Low Profile Aids

This type of aid utilizes the same full size cases as the regular all-in-the-ear aids. However, it has an additional feature. Low profile aids have an inset faceplate so that the microphone, battery cover, and volume control are recessed. They are less apparent, wind and noise are reduced, and the ear bowl helps gather sounds.

CROS Hearing Aids

CROS (Contralateral Routing of Signals) hearing aids are designed for individuals who have an essentially nonfunctional or unaidable ear and a good ear. Encased in a hearing aid body worn on the nonfunctioning ear, a microphone picks up sound from the nonfunctioning ear and routes it to the good ear. A hearing aid device is also utilized on the good ear that receives the sound from the poor ear and directs it into the good ear. Both hearing aid devices are connected by a cord that extends around the back of the head, or by a small, wireless FM radio transmitter, allowing the signal to be transferred from one ear to the other. A detailed diagram of the CROS aid is shown in Figure 13-4.

This type of aid is particularly beneficial for the individual experiencing deafness in one ear and a high frequency loss in the other. By utilizing a nonoccluding, open earmold design on the good ear, the tubing permits good amplification in the high frequency range while reducing the low frequency response. Sound from the

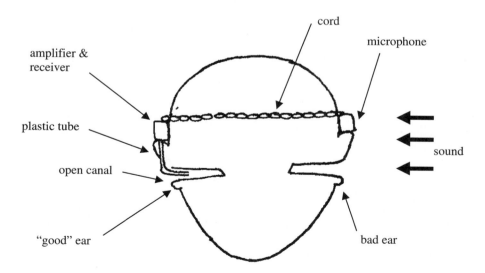

FIGURE 13-4 **Drawing Depicting the CROS Hearing Aid Principle**
(Courtesy of Marie A. Scheetz)

poor ear's side of the head is transmitted to the good ear, which also receives added amplification needed by the good ear to assist in hearing sounds in the high frequency range where the hearing loss exists (Shelfer, 1990).

The transcranial CROS differs from the conventional CROS in the way that sound is transferred from the impaired ear into the good ear. When employing this technique, a high gain–high output ITE or BTE aid is placed in the impaired ear. The sound is then transmitted through the cranial structures of the temporal bone into the cochlea of the better ear. Thus, sound travels by way of bone conduction (Valente et al.,). Recipients of the transcranial cross have reported "that amplified sound presented through their transcranial CROS was more 'natural' than the sound processed through their conventional CROS" (Freyman, Nerbonne, & Cole, 1991, p. 420).

IROS Hearing Aids

The term IROS (ipsilateral routing of signals) implies a standard hearing aid with an open earmold on the same side. It came into use after the open tubing effect of the CROS aid proved beneficial for sharply falling sensorineural hearing losses. This design can be utilized with BTE/OTE aids. When incorporated, the tubing itself projects into the ear canal with a nonoccluding "free-field" earmold. Those individuals exhibiting mild to moderate sensorineural losses are able to benefit from this type of configuration and enjoy the comfort of not having an earmold that is occluding the ear. This allows the ear's natural resonance to be utilized, enhancing the amplification of the high frequencies where the hearing loss is being experienced.

Bone Conduction Hearing Aids

Bone conduction aids operate by applying sound vibrations to the bones behind the ears. Although some sounds can be heard this way, the performance of this aid is poor when compared to aids which utilize earmolds (such as air conduction hearing aids). Very frequently bone conduction aids are only used where there is no ear canal or where there is chronic ear canal drainage.

Traditionally, bone conduction aids were used in individuals who experienced a large discrepancy in their ability to hear sounds as they were received through the auditory canal and temporal bone vibrations. When the air-bone gap exceeded 35 dB, conductive aids were employed. However, because of the success of stapes surgery in reducing the air-bone gap, the need for bone conduction aids has diminished.

Currently, there are two major types of conventional bone conduction aids being used. One incorporates a body aid while the other utilizes the eyeglass aid. When a bone conduction aid is used in conjunction with a body aid, a bone receiver is substituted for the air receiver and is held against the mastoid processes of the user by a headband. When eyeglasses or an over-the-ear (OTE) aid is used, the bone receiver is incorporated into one end of the eyeglasses or a headband is utilized.

Implantable Bone Conduction Hearing Aid Device

For individuals who cannot utilize either the conventional bone or the air conduction hearing aid, but would benefit from a bone conduction type hearing aid, an implantable temporal Bone Stimulator has been developed. People who have chronically draining ears or an ear deformity such as atresia of the ear canal, or absence of the pinna, may be candidates for this type of device. This is a medically implanted device that requires medical and audiological management. Basically, this unit is an electromagnetic device that directly stimulates the cochlea via a magnet implanted in the temporal bone. Individuals whose bone conduction thresholds are no worse than 40 dB HL in the speech frequencies appear to benefit most. The audiologist adjusts the device to provide maximum use of the auditory response of the cochlea.

Implantable Middle Ear Hearing Aids

Individuals who experience a conductive or mixed loss, due to middle ear transmission problems, may benefit from an implantable aid. Still in an experimental stage, these aids are designed to directly drive the ossicles, thus providing more "comfortable" speech reception for the listener.

Two designs are currently being explored: the partially implantable hearing devices (PIHD) and the totally implantable hearing device (TIHD). Although they differ in which components are housed externally, both provide direct magnetic stimulation to the tympanic membrane or the ossicular chain (Goode, 1995, p.143, Maniglia, 1989, p. 186–190).

Digital Technology

The term "digital hearing aid" can be used to encompass anything from an aid that incorporates touch volume controls to those instruments that have been computer programmed to meet the individual needs of the consumer. Digital systems can be programmed for eight different listening situations. As wearers move from one sound environment into another, they can adjust the performance program by pressing the hearing aid's up or down digital control buttons. In certain situations the program can tell the system to reject "noise" and amplify only "speech." In a noisy environment, the hearing aid analyzes incoming sound, both noise and speech, compares both to coded data in its memory, and then processes the speech differently—all within five to ten microseconds (Engebretson et al., 1986; Glattke, 1977). This technology can be especially beneficial for individuals who have poor speech discrimination/understanding, even under ideal listening conditions (see Figure 13-5).

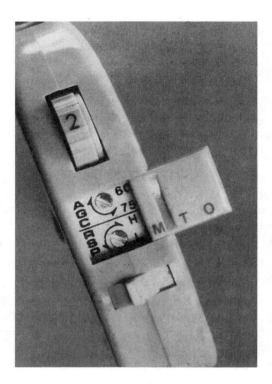

FIGURE 13-5 **View of Adjustment Controls on an OTE Hearing Aid**
(Courtesy of Starkey Labs)

Cochlear Implants

Cochlear implants involve a surgical procedure in which electrodes are implanted into the ear within the cochlea. Small electric currents delivered by the implanted electrodes stimulate the auditory nerve. Information from an external microphone, shaped by a speech processor, is used to generate the signal to the electrodes.

Viable candidates for cochlear implants are those who have profound losses that occurred after speech was acquired. These individuals have found traditional hearing aids to be of no significant benefit. These implants provide rudimentary hearing to profoundly deaf persons and improve their speech-reading ability. Additional factors that contribute to the success of the implant include the person's motivation to hear as well as possible and the determination to undergo the expense and discomfort of the surgical procedure (see Figure 13-6).

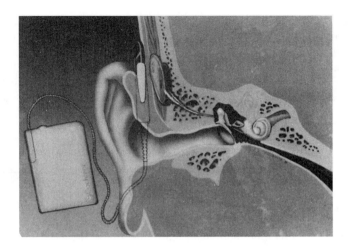

FIGURE 13-6 **Illustration and Explanation of How a Cochlear Implant System Works**

Sound enters the system through a tiny microphone behind the individual's ear. The sound is transmitted from the microphone to the speech processor through the thin cord that connects them. The speech processor selects and codes the elements of sound that are most useful for understanding speech. These electronic codes are sent back up through the thin cable to the transmitter. The transmitting coil, a plastic covered ring about 1 inch in diameter, sends the codes across the skin to the receiver/stimulator. The receiver/stimulator contains an integrated circuit that converts the codes into special electrical signals and sends them along the electrode array. The electrode array is a set of 22 tiny electrode bands arranged in a row around a piece of tapered flexible tubing. Each electrode has a wire connecting it to the receiver/stimulator. The coded electrical signals are sent to specific electrodes. Each electrode is programmed separately to deliver signals that can vary in loudness and pitch. These electrodes then stimulate different hearing nerve fibers, which send the messages on to the brain. Your brain receives the signals and interprets them. You experience a sensation of sound.

(Illustration and information provided courtesy of Cochlear Corporation)

Binaural and Monaural Hearing Aid Fittings

Research has been conducted over the past several years to determine if binaural aids (two aids) are more beneficial for the consumer than monaural aids (one aid). Studies show that those wearing binaural over monaural aids can hear signals in noise better. They also provide the individual with greater versatility in social situations (Ross, 1980).

People hear better with two ears than with one. Sounds are clearer and stronger with binaural aids, and they provide the listener with a stereo effect similar to that of normal hearing. In addition, two aids assist the individual as he attempts to determine the directionality of sound and locate the individual who is speaking.

HEARING AID ORIENTATION

Following the hearing evaluation an appropriate aid is selected and an earmold is designed. Instruction is then necessary to familiarize the user with the device. The purpose of hearing aid orientation is to help the hearing impaired people adjust to the use of their aid. At this time individuals learn how to use the aid and what benefits to expect. In addition to acquiring information regarding the physical characteristics of the aid, individuals need to receive counseling addressing the psychological and emotional ramifications of hearing loss.

Physical Aspects of Hearing Aid Use

During this orientation period the hearing impaired individual will need to be provided information pertaining to the following topics:

1. How to insert, remove, and clean the earmold
2. How to utilize the various switches:
   on-off switch
   gain control
   telephone switch
   tone control
3. What type of batteries the aid uses, where to purchase them, and how to change them
4. What the device can and cannot do to improve communication
5. What the user's communication abilities and limitations may be with the hearing aid

Psychological and Emotional Ramifications of Hearing Loss

Throughout the orientation session, it is imperative that the audiologist foster acceptance and objectivity regarding the hearing loss in a way that helps the consumer feel comfortable in utilizing an aid. The following topics may need to be discussed with the hearing impaired individual:

1. understanding of the hearing problem
2. understanding the nature, advantages, and limitations of hearing aids
3. learning acceptance of the loss and making a commitment to use amplification
4. learning how to inform other people of the loss and providing them with communication tips that will benefit the hearing impaired individual (see Table 13-1)

TABLE 13-1　**The Estimated Usefulness of Hearing Aids According to the Degree of Hearing Loss Experienced by Individuals and Their Degree of Motivation**

High Frequency Average in dbHL	Motivation	
	Positive	*Negative*
Mild loss		
25 dB	Aid is rarely used; may be used in special situations.	Aid is not needed; usually it is not accepted.
35 dB	Aid can be beneficial; might be accepted by the individual but expectations need to be explained realistically.	Aid could be beneficial; might be tolerated.
Moderate loss		
45 dB	Aid is accepted and is helpful.	Needs aid, but may refuse it.
55 dB	Aid is essential; used willingly.	Aid is needed, but may need support and encouragement to try it.
Severe loss		
65 dB	Successful use of aid. Aware of limitations. Makes adjustments.	Needs aid to function. May still refuse it. Encourages friends to talk louder.
75 dB	Uses aid constantly.	Uses aid sparingly. Not satisfied with it.
Profound loss		
85 dB 95 dB	Is very skilled in use of aid; does well except under adverse listening conditions. Uses visual means for information; uses acoustic clues for understanding.	Attempts to control conversations; avoids listening and bluffs way through conversations. Usually does not use aid; depends on visual contact; converses through written or manual language.

(Based on information found in *Handbook of Clinical Audiology* (1986) by Jack Katz)

In addition, the person who is going to wear an aid needs to know when to wear it. This will be determined by the magnitude of the loss, the demands on the individual's hearing, and the environment in which listening occurs. Individuals with slight or mild hearing losses may benefit from wearing aids on a part-time basis, utilizing them in quiet surroundings where people speak softly. Individuals experiencing a moderate loss may find wearing an aid the majority of the time beneficial with removal in "cocktail party" listening situations helpful. Listeners with severe or profound losses who use amplification generally wear their aids on a full-time basis. Although aids do not afford them the opportunity to understand speech, they do keep them in contact with the environment.

When individuals begin wearing an aid, they may become aware of environmental sounds that they had forgotten existed. They may hear the internal hum of the aid or the sound of clothing rubbing against a body aid. Some new hearing aid users make an easy adjustment and wear their aid from the time they purchase it. Other individuals, especially those with very mild or quite severe losses, may require a long time to adjust (Schow et al., 1978). Throughout the orientation period, the hearing impaired person is provided with suggestions, thus providing the necessary tools to enter into the arena of amplification.

GROUP LISTENING SYSTEMS

In addition to individual aids, group listening systems are available for people with severe losses. They can also prove helpful for those people experiencing a mild loss, provided the individual accepts the loss and is willing to seek help. There are four major types of group systems: audio loops, FM systems, AM systems, and those incorporating infrared light waves.

Audio Loops

Audio loops consist of a microphone, an amplifier, and a length of wire that loops the seating area. Within an audio loop sounds are converted to magnetic forces that emanate from wires under floors and around the walls. Hearing aids with telephone switches (T-coils) pick up these forces and change them back into sounds.

FM (Frequency Modulation) Systems

This system is very easy to install. Within this unit, transmitters broadcast sound using the same methods as radio stations. The listener uses a personal receiver for making sounds available to the ear. Not only is this system easy to install, but the signals can be transmitted over a three hundred foot range.

AM Systems

This works on the same principle as the FM system; however, it is more prone to static.

Infrared Systems

Infrared systems are one of the newer types of group listening devices. These systems are designed to convert sounds into infrared light waves that are converted back to sounds again by the listener's infrared receivers. This system is easy to install and is virtually static-free. However, the range is limited to line-of-sight propagation and the infrared light waves will not pass through obstructions such as walls or around corners.

INDIVIDUAL AMPLIFICATION SYSTEMS

Assistive Listening Devices

Assistive Listening Devices (ALDs) are designed to be used alone or in conjunction with a hearing aid. They send the desired signal directly from the sound force into the listener's ear. The signal is not affected by room noise or room acoustics. This allows listeners the opportunity to perceive the sound as if they are listening under ideal conditions. They require both the speaker and the listener to wear a unit about the size of a cigarette pack. The signal is usually transmitted by an infrared or FM signal. They are equipped with a microphone (for the speaker), amplifier, and receiver (for the hearing impaired person), and can be utilized one-on-one by those individuals attempting to participate in lecture or one-on-one communication situations. For individuals whose hearing impairment involves central auditory processing problems, conventional hearing aids often provide little benefit. Personal Assistive Listening Devices tend to be much more effective due to the superior signal-to-noise ratio achieved by ALDs, which significantly reduces if not entirely eliminates unwanted background.

Telephone Amplifiers

Some hard-of-hearing individuals can better communicate on the phone if their telephone can be equipped with an amplified handset. The amplifier, which is built into the phone handle, can be adjusted to an appropriate sound level.

Portable amplifiers are also available and are small enough to be carried in one's pocket or purse. These slip over most telephone receivers and virtually serve the same purpose. All phones are not designed to work with portable amplifiers. However, telephone adaptors can be purchased to facilitate usage.

ADDITIONAL DEVICES FOR INDIVIDUALS WHO EXPERIENCE DIFFICULTY HEARING

Hearing aids, cochlear implants, assistive listening devices, and portable amplifiers are only some of the aids available to assist individuals with hearing losses. Other products have been devised to alert the hearing impaired person to sounds within his environment.

Visual signals have been developed to alert the hearing impaired person to the doorbell, telephone, alarm clock, smoke alarm, and security systems. Additional devices have been designed to alert parents when their infants are crying. Light sources, increased amplification, and vibrotactile methods are employed when designing assistive devices.

In the event individuals' hearing loss prevents them from communicating over the telephone with amplification, they may invest in a telecommunication device (TDD). Instead of engaging in conversation through voice, TDDs permit conversation in print. TDDs are designed with typewriter keyboards, and the conversation appears either in a readout panel or on paper. In order for conversation to occur, each individual must have a compatible machine.

SUMMARY

There are a variety of aids and assistive listening devices available today. Modern technology has made great strides in providing the hearing impaired individual with stronger and more powerful forms of amplification. These new devices, coupled with orientation and consumer usage training programs, provide the wearer with opportunities not previously available.

In the next decade one can expect to see additional research into the development of implantable hearing aids, designed for the middle ear as well as the auditory brain stem. Continued attention will be paid to cosmetics as aids that fit entirely in the ear canal are modified and perfected. Furthermore, research will continue in the area of digital technology to enhance these aids.

Although hearing frequently cannot be restored to within the normal functioning range, these devices can enhance their ability to become aware of sounds within the environment, assisting them in communication.

▶ 14

Support Services

Support services frequently provide the vital link between deaf individuals and their hearing counterparts. They may be employed to facilitate communication, relay messages, or promote deaf awareness. Support services take many different forms. Some services can be found within the professional sector. Interpreters, notetakers, tutors, speech therapists, advocates, and social service employees are only a few of the professionals who provide a valuable service. Agencies and organizations functioning at both the national and the state levels provide another critical resource. These organizations, coupled with trained professionals and advanced technology, furnish the deaf and hard of hearing communities with numerous avenues, thus fostering independence.

SUPPORT PERSONNEL

Interpreting Services

Interpreters play an important role in relationships between hearing and deaf individuals. They serve as communication facilitators, ensuring that both parties have the opportunity to have their messages conveyed accurately and with the intent for which they are intended.

    Interpreters working in the educational, medical, legal, social, and rehabilitative settings generally require professional training and certification. Certification may be obtained through the national certifying body, The Registry of Interpreters for the Deaf (RID), or through quality screening programs that have been established by individual states.

    Interpreters, like other professionals, operate under a set of guidelines or a code of ethics. Due to the nature of their work, it is critical that they are proficient in their skill area, remain impartial, and serve only as a facilitator of information. RID has developed a Code of Ethics with the aim of protecting the rights of deaf consumers, those hearing individuals who are involved in the communication process, and the interpreter.

Code of Ethics
A code of ethics, such as the one established by RID, protects interpreters and lessens the arbitrariness of their decisions by providing guidelines and standards that can be followed. Some of the general guidelines of the RID Code can be stated as follows: (Note: The use of the term "transliterator" can be substituted for the word "interpreter."

- Interpreters shall keep all assignment-related information strictly confidential.
- Interpreters shall render the message faithfully, always conveying the content of the message and the spirit of the speaker, using language most readily understood by the person(s) whom they serve.
- Interpreters shall not counsel or advise those whom they serve, or interject personal opinions.
- Interpreters shall accept assignments using discretion with regard to skill, setting, and the consumers involved.
- Interpreters shall request compensation for services in a professional and judicious manner.
- Interpreters shall function in a manner appropriate to the situation (Frishberg, 1990).

Registry of Interpreters for the Deaf
The Registry of Interpreters for the Deaf (RID) was founded in the United States in 1964 and incorporated in 1972. The primary mission of this organization has been threefold. First, to provide training for those individuals wishing to pursue a career in this area. Second, to serve as a certifying body for those achieving certain skill levels and, third, to provide a registry for those seeking to contact the services of a professional interpreter.

Additional information regarding this organization including the availability of interpreting services within various geographic areas, levels of certification, fee schedules, and location of training programs can be obtained by contacting:

Registry of Interpreters for the Deaf
8630 Fenton Street, Suite 324
Silver Spring, MD 20910

The term "interpreting" has been used by the general public to describe the process that occurs whenever an individual is "signing" for the benefit of both hearing and deaf individuals. However, upon closer examination, this global term can be further defined to describe the communication process.

Interpreting.   Interpreting more accurately refers to the process of changing messages produced in one language immediately into another language. Within the field of deafness, this refers to communicating from English into American Sign Language (ASL) or from ASL into English.

Transliterating. Transliterating, on the other hand, refers to the process of utilizing manual communication to convey, in English word order, the message as it originates from the speaker. In transliterating, the language base remains the same; the difference is within the manual mode in which it is expressed.

Oral Interpreting. Oral interpreting involves the art of clearly, but inaudibly, mouthing the words as they are presented by the speaker. Words, which are difficult to understand through speechreading, may be altered in order to insure that the maximum amount of comprehension will be achieved.

Real-Time Captioning

Recent technological advances have made real-time captioning a viable option for many deaf and hard of hearing consumers. When provided, individuals are afforded the opportunity to participate in the monologue or dialogue by reading what is being said. As speakers address the audience, their commentaries are simultaneously projected on a screen, thus alerting the consumer to topics being discussed.

Notetaking

Because deafness is not a visible disability, hearing people frequently forget how difficult it is for the deaf consumer to lip-read or focus on an interpreter and take notes at the same time. In the classroom setting, as well as in the job setting, deaf individuals may find themselves in situations where it is critical to receive the information at the moment it is being given, but it is imperative to have the same information later in order to refer back to it. Unlike their hearing colleagues who can listen and write simultaneously, hearing impaired individuals must sacrifice one of the two levels of communication. Either they must listen, keeping their eyes focused on the interpreter or the speaker, or they must shift their gaze to write on the paper, thus losing the full intent of the message as it is delivered. To compensate for the visual demands of this disability, notetakers are frequently employed. By securing the services of a notetaker, the individual has the benefit of listening to the material as it is presented orally, as well as receiving a copy of the speaker's notes for later reference.

Current research suggests that what people *see* is not remembered or learned as well as what is *heard* (Fritz & Smith, 1985). Therefore, it is critical that notes be made available for the hearing impaired individual wishing to recall important information. Notes provided for the hearing impaired should contain the following characteristics:

1. They should be written in clear, legible handwriting
2. Everything should be included in complete sentences whenever possible; partial sentences and sentence fragments can be confusing when recalled

3. Information pertaining to specific times, dates, responsibilities, deadlines, and so forth, should be emphasized clearly
4. Wide margins and spaces between lines should be included enabling individuals to add their own notations
5. When abbreviations are included, the words should be written out the first few times to insure that these will be understood
6. Notes should be taken as if the deaf or hard of hearing person did not attend the event
7. Points that received special emphasis during the lecture or presentation need to be highlighted within the notes, either by incorporating a highlighter or some other form of indication (capitalization, underlining, etc.)
8. Notes should be dated, and each page should be numbered accordingly
9. Notes should be given to the consumer in a timely fashion in order to reinforce lecture material

With the advent of laptop computers, some individuals now have the opportunity to receive notes via disk or computer printout. When produced in this manner, points receiving special emphasis can be indicated by bold print or otherwise illustrated in a distinctive fashion.

Individuals requiring notetaking services are frequently enrolled in training programs, educational settings, or are part of the work force. As these services are needed, the individuals can usually access them through appropriate agency personnel.

Tutoring

Within the classroom, the work environment, or when training becomes necessary, it may be beneficial to provide tutoring services for the deaf and hard of hearing participants. Due to the large amount of verbal information that may be presented, the written material that may accompany it, and the comprehension level required of those involved, tutoring may prove to be essential. Oftentimes lecture material includes terminology that may be foreign to those encountering it for the first time. The concepts may be complex and require additional explanations in order for them to be assimilated by the individual. For the hearing impaired community, this is particularly true. Due to the environmental isolation experienced by this population, they may realize their language deficiencies and thus benefit from additional tutorial services.

Individuals assuming the role of tutor function in the following ways:

1. They are there to answer questions as posed by the deaf and hard of hearing individuals
2. They serve to clarify new information including vocabulary words, procedures, textbook information, and lecture notes
3. They can supply missing information or clarify misperceptions of content areas

4. They serve in the capacity of reviewing information the students have received either in notes or from their textbooks
5. They can provide a resource, placing the student or employee in contact with individuals or sources who can further clarify questions they may have

Tutoring may take place prior to formal instruction or after it occurs. Depending on the content of the material to be discussed, it may be beneficial for the individual to have exposure to the terminology and the concepts before the actual training takes place. When extremely complex materials are being covered, tutoring that occurs both prior to and at the end of the training session can be valuable to the program participants.

Speech Therapy

Speech therapists are trained to assist children who are experiencing difficulties with speech production. Their function is to provide corrective and remedial services for children and adults whose existing speech lacks clarity. They work with individuals who have an interest in improving their speech quality in order to verbally communicate with other persons.

Deaf children with profound hearing losses can receive speech training from teachers of the deaf. Once speech becomes part of their communication patterns, a speech therapist becomes an important reinforcer of this effort, offering individualized assistance in such areas as pronunciation and enunciation, phraseology, sentence production and pitch inflection and intonation, and articulation (Katz, Mathis, & Merrill, 1974).

Through the efforts of the speech therapist, individuals who are deaf and hard of hearing have the opportunity to work on their speech, correct those articulation errors that they may possess, and enhance their oral communication skills.

Those seeking information pertaining to speech therapists can contact either:

Alexander Graham Bell Association for the Deaf
3417 Volta Place NW
Washington, DC 20007

or

American Speech-Language-Hearing-Association
10801 Rockville Pike
Rockville, MD 20852

Counseling Services

Counseling services are administered by a wide array of professionals. In the school setting, guidance counselors frequently meet with students, addressing questions concerning academic planning, career development, and test scores. When problems arise requiring in-depth psychological testing, psychological counselors are often contacted to provide this service. Based on results obtained from assessment instruments, the psychologist is able to make recommendations and referrals to the appropriate sources.

As deaf individuals reach young adulthood and are preparing to leave the secondary school setting, vocational rehabilitation counselors become instrumental in the area of career planning. Through their efforts the students receive advice and counsel about college or vocational opportunities. Those students wanting to forgo training and secure immediate employment also receive services from vocational rehabilitation counselors. They are very instrumental in accessing job readiness programs, meeting with employers, and providing those necessary support services for the transition into the work force.

Individuals interested in obtaining information pertaining to counseling services can contact:

American Deafness and Rehabilitation Association
P.O. Box 727
Lusby, MD 20657

Social Workers

Social workers provide a major link between the school and the home. If problems arise in the home due to the ramifications of deafness, social workers can oftentimes intervene and assist in resolving the parents' dilemmas. When problems occur in the school setting, social workers may be called on to make a personal visit to the home to gather background information on the child's home environment. When the school is provided with background information pertaining to the parents' life-style, discipline patterns, and overall acceptance of deafness, school personnel can more adequately meet the needs of individual students.

The personnel listed above serve in a support capacity promoting independence within the Deaf community. The primary function of these professionals is to provide those support services that will allow deaf individuals access into their communities. This group of professionals, together with national organizations and agencies, provide the hearing impaired community with the necessary tools required to achieve and maintain independence.

ORGANIZATIONS AND AGENCIES

There are several organizations and agencies that have been established to provide services for the deaf and hard of hearing. Some are National Professional Organizations while others have been designed to operate at the state and local levels. Included below is an annotated list of resources of those agencies providing services for this population.

Alexander Graham Bell Association for the Deaf
3417 Volta Place,
NW Washington, DC 20007

Oral Hearing Impaired Section (OHIAS)
International Parents' Organization (IPO)
American Academy of Otolaryngology/Head and Neck Surgery
1101 Vermont Avenue NW, Suite 302
Washington, DC 20005

Promotes the art and science of medicine related to otolaryngology/head and neck surgery, including providing continuing medical education courses and publications. Distributes patient leaflets relating to ear problems and makes referrals to physicians.

American Association of the Deaf-Blind
814 Thayer Avenue, Room 302
Silver Spring, MD 20910-4500

American Association of the Deaf-Blind is a national organization for individuals who have both hearing and vision loss. AADB is available to deaf-blind individuals as well as those who are closely linked to them such as family or friends. They promote independent living for individuals who are deaf-blind and provide technical support for them and their family/friends.

American Athletic Association of the Deaf
3607 Washington Blvd., #4
Ogden, VT 84403-1737

Fosters and regulates athletic competition among member clubs. Provides special activities of interest to deaf members and their friends. Promotes state, regional, national, and world games for the deaf, and gives an award for The Outstanding Deaf Athlete of the Year.

American Hearing Research Foundation
55 E. Washington Street, Suite 2022
Chicago, IL 60602

Keeps physicians and laypersons informed of latest developments in hearing research and education.

American Society for Deaf Children
1820 Tribune Road, Suite A
Sacramento, CA 95815

Membership organization providing information and support to parents and families with children who are deaf or hard-of-hearing. ASDC promotes Total Communication as a way of life for deaf children and their families and encourages strong ties with deaf adults who enable families to better understand the deaf adults their children will become.

American Tinnitus Association
P.O. Box 5
Portland, OR 97207

Provides education and information about tinnitus to patients and professionals. Provides telephone counseling and self-help support and raises money for research.

Association of Late Deafened Adults
1145 Westgate St., Suite 206
Oak Park, IL 60301

The Association of Late Deafened Adults (ALDA) is an international organization for individuals who lose their hearing later in life.

Better Hearing Institute
5021-B Backlick Road
Annandale, VA 22003

Dedicated to informing persons who are hard of hearing, their friends and relatives, and the general public about hearing loss and available medical, surgical, and amplification assistance.

Captioned Media Program
1447 E. Main Street
Spartanburg, SC 29307

This company distributes captioned films, both educational (requires at least one individual who is deaf or hard of hearing) and general interest (requires at least six individuals who are deaf or hard of hearing). Contact Captioned Media Program for an application.

Cochlear Implant Club International
5335 Wisconsin Avenue NY, Suite 440
Washington, D.C. 20015

The Cochlear Implant Club International is an organization for people who have received implants and their families.

Convention of American Instructors of the Deaf (CAID)
P.O. Box 377
Bedford, TX 76095-0377

An association of teachers, administrators, and other professionals in North America banded together to promote educational services to deaf children; directly concerned with school-aged children who are deaf or hard of hearing and the educational facilities provided for them. In conjunction with the Conference of Executives of American Schools for the Deaf, publishes the American Annals of the Deaf.

Conference of Educational Administrators of Schools and Programs for the Deaf, Inc.
P.O. Box 1778
St. Augustine, FL 32085-1778

Promotes the management and operation of schools for the deaf along the broadest and most efficient lines. Also, promotes professional growth of all those who work closely with deaf people.

Council for Exceptional Children (CEC)
1920 Association Drive
Reston, VA 20191-1589

A national organization representing public, professional, and parent interests in regard to children who need special services. An advocate for the rights of exceptional children. Has an extensive stock of materials and publications for distribution.

Council on Education of the Deaf (CED)
P.O. Box 77090
Washington, D.C. 20013-7090

A confederation of the Alexander Graham Bell Association for the Deaf, the Conference of Executives of American Instructors of the Deaf, and Conference of Educational Administrators Serving the Deaf. Engaged in setting professional standards for educational programs and for persons engaged in providing educational services to hearing impaired children and youth.

Gallaudet University Alumni Association
Gallaudet University
800 Florida Avenue, NE
Washington, DC 20002

Seeks to preserve and increase the influence and prestige of Gallaudet College and to extend the sphere of its influence and benefits to those for whom it was established. Most chapters undertake projects of service to the Deaf community.

Hearing Dog Center—Red Acre Farm
P.O. Box 278
Stow, MA 01775

Provides information on hearing dogs, their ability, accessibility, and how to obtain them.

Helen Keller National Center for Deaf-Blind Youths and Adults
111 Middle Neck Road
Sands Point, NY 11050

The single national facility that provides comprehensive evaluation and vocational rehabilitation training; conducts an extensive network of field services through regional offices, affiliated programs, and a national training team; and maintains National Register of Deaf-Blind Persons.

House Ear Institute
2100 West Third Street
Los Angeles, CA 90057

Nonprofit organization that conducts research and provides information on hearing and balance disorders. Their Center for Deaf Children does evaluation and therapy.

John Tracy Clinic
806 West Adams Boulevard
Los Angeles, CA 90007

Provides a correspondence course for parents of young children throughout the world. Maintains a comprehensive diagnostic and research center on deafness, a day preschool program, guidance and education programs for parents, and a training center for teachers of the deaf that is affiliated with the University of Southern California.

Junior National Association of the Deaf Youth Program
814 Thayer Avenue
Silver Spring, MD 20910-4500

Develops leadership skills among deaf high school students by creating opportunities where students can get hands-on experience.

National Association of the Deaf (NAD)
814 Thayer Avenue
Silver Spring, MD 20910

The NAD is the oldest national organization of deaf people in America. Halex
House on Thayer Avenue serves as headquarters for several agencies serving the deaf
and is owned by the NAD. Official publication: *The Deaf American.*

National Captioning Institute (NCI)
1900 Gallows Road, Suite 3000
Vienna, VA 22182

NCI is a nonprofit corporation whose goal is to expand closed-captioned television. The staff writes captions for television programs, and they design, manufacture,
and distribute the decoder device that is attached to the user's television set.

National Center for Law and the Deaf
800 Florida Ave., NE
Washington, DC 20002

Provides legal representation, services, information, and education for the benefit of the deaf and hard of hearing individuals throughout the United States. Assists
with preparing legislation, filing petitions for rule making, and commenting before
government agencies. Provides legal counseling for Washington, D.C., area deaf persons and helps deaf students seeking entrance to law school.

National Center on Employment of the Deaf
National Technical Institute for the Deaf
Rochester Institute of Technology
1 Lomb Memorial Dr.
Rochester, NY 14623

Primary focus is on providing job-search assistance to NTID students and graduates. In addition, services are also available to deaf people seeking job-search assistance or to employers needing help in working with their deaf employees.

National Cued Speech Association
23970 Hermitage Road
Cleveland, OH 44122-4008

Provides information pertaining to cued speech: where to receive training, how to contact cued speech transliterators, and programs that include cued speech in their delivery system.

National Information Center on Deafness
Gallaudet University
800 Florida Ave., NE
Washington, DC 20002-3625

NICD works to educate the public about deafness and deaf people. Individuals having questions about hearing loss, deafness, or Gallaudet University can obtain information by contacting NICD.

National Fraternal Society of the Deaf
118 South Sixth Street
Springfield, IL 62703

A fraternal life insurance organization with more than 120 chapters in the United States and Canada, incorporated in 1907 for the primary purpose of insuring deaf persons. Also promotes gainful employment and the welfare of adult deaf persons.

National Theatre of the Deaf
5 West Main Street
P.O. Box 659
Chester, CT 06412

A theater group comprised of deaf and hard-of-hearing artists. This group tours nationally providing deaf individuals the opportunity to view theater productions through American Sign Language.

Quota International, Inc.
1420 21st Street, NW
Washington, DC 20036

Major service project, Shatter Silence, serves individuals with hearing and speech handicaps. Offers fellowships and annual outstanding Deaf Woman of the Year Program.

Registry of Interpreters for the Deaf, Inc. (RID)
8630 Fenton Street, Suite 324
Silver Spring, MD 20910
(Description included earlier in chapter)

Self Help for Hard of Hearing People, Inc.
7910 Woodmont Avenue, Suite 1200
Bethesda, MD 20814
(Description included in chapter on Deafened Adults)

Telecommunications for the Deaf Inc. (TDI)
8630 Fenton Street, Suite 604
Silver Spring, MD 20910-3803

TDI addresses issues related to telecommunications for the deaf. In addition to publishing an annual directory of TDD numbers, it is a consulting agency that provides information and assistance on telecommunication issues. TDI also publishes a quarterly newsletter, *GASK,* which includes information about telecommunications.

DEAF SERVICE CENTERS

Before leaving the section on professional organizations and agencies serving deaf individuals, particular mention needs to be made regarding Deaf Service Centers.

Although these agencies are not located in every state and every city, there are enough of them within the United States to merit discussion. Deaf Service Centers (also referred to as Deaf Action Centers) have been established as social service agencies and provide a host of support services to deaf and hard of hearing individuals. Frequently their goal is to provide services that will enable deaf and hard of hearing consumers access into other community services.

These agencies frequently provide the following types of services: interpreting, message relay via TDD, counseling, referral services, community education classes, and social activities. In addition, they promote deaf awareness and oftentimes serve as advocates for the population comprised of deaf and hard of hearing individuals.

TECHNICAL AIDS: SPECIAL EQUIPMENT AND PRODUCTS

In recent years new technology has been developed providing deaf individuals with additional avenues enabling them to pursue their independence. Telephone communication devices, visual signaling equipment, and telecaptioning devices have all been designed to help this population enter the mainstream of their communities. The following information from *Signaling and Assistive Listening Devices for Hearing-Impaired People* has been included courtesy of Alexander Graham Bell Association of the Deaf.

Telecommunication Devices (TDDs)

Telecommunication Devices for the Deaf, originally known as teletypewriters or TTYs, are machines that have the appearance of a small typewriter. They can be utilized with regular telephone handsets and allow deaf people to communicate with each other via typed words rather than speech. TDDs are made up of a typewriter-like keyboard, a telephone coupler, and some form of visual display.

The TDD user places a telephone handset on the coupler and types in the message he wishes to send. When a character on the keyboard is pressed to type in the message, a series of tones is generated. There is a different set of tones for each character. These tones that form the typed message are sent over telephone lines to the telephone on the other end of the line. This telephone also must be linked to a TDD so that the message can be decoded and displayed. A TDD allows a deaf or hard of hearing person to send and receive telephone calls just as a hearing individual can.

Signaling Devices

Signaling Devices have been designed to assist deaf and hard of hearing individuals in a variety of ways. Using the equipment is a substitute for hearing the sound. There are two ways for equipment to signal: with *light,* or with *vibration.*

One device sometimes can be used as a signaler for different sounds. Devices with microphones will be sensitive to sounds such as the doorbell, voices, a baby crying, a dog barking, the telephone, TV or radio, and smoke or burglar alarms. When using this kind of device, it is important to place the microphone near the chosen sound and adjust the microphone sensitivity to reduce the influence of other sounds in the room. Some sounds will have a distinctive rhythmic pattern, like the telephone ringing, and can be identified easily.

Sophisticated light systems have been incorporated and are used to alert deaf individuals to sounds within their environment. Some of the more common ones are discussed below.

Wake-up Alarms

Wake-up alarms include *digital* and *standard clocks, bed vibrators,* and *timers.* Clocks that use a flashing light as the alarm are useful for people easily awakened by light. Some clocks have a very bright strobe light. For heavy sleepers or deaf-blind persons, there are several kinds of bed-vibrating units. Some can be placed under a pillow or mattress, while others are small enough for travel.

Timers or clocks with built-in electrical outlets permit a choice of using a lamp, a strobe, a bed vibrator, or a fan, depending on the best method for awakening the person. When a lamp is used, an inexpensive *flasher button* will make an ordinary lamp flash 65 to 85 times per minute.

Telephone/Doorbell Signalers

This type of device incorporates the use of a *transmitter* and a *remote receiver.* The transmitter is placed next to or attaches to the telephone base or doorbell. The remote receiver plugs into a wall outlet. A lamp, strobe, or vibrator plugs into the remote receiver. The light or vibrator turns on or off when a signal is sent from the transmitter. Remote receivers can be moved from room to room as needed.

Some transmitters plug into a modular telephone. There are portable doorbell signalers with batteries that can be used for travel. These devices can be used for both the telephone and the doorbell.

Emergency Warning Devices

Some *multipurpose systems* can be used for alerting people to as many as six different sounds, including the telephone ring, baby cry, doorbell, alarm clock, smoke detector, and burglar alarm.

These systems consist of a receiver and a chosen number of transmitters. The receiver plugs into an electrical outlet. Separate battery-operated transmitters pick up different sounds. The transmitters are placed near the possible sound sources or connected to the sound source. The transmitter may or may not be plugged into a wall outlet. The lamp, strobe, or vibrator is plugged into the receiver. The receiver is set up to identify the different sounds. When the sound occurs, the light or vibrator turns on.

If a person needs to know when only one or two of these sounds occur, a multipurpose system may be unnecessary.

Many deaf or hard of hearing persons worry about being able to hear the alarm from their smoke detector. Some smoke detectors combine a built-in horn and a strobe light. Others have a separate horn that plugs into an electric outlet in the bedroom or elsewhere in the house. A lamp, strobe, or vibrator can plug into a portable receiver.

Emergency Alarm Devices

These can automatically call the fire department and give the person's address when a *smoke detector* goes off. Other emergency alarm devices call an emergency service (police, fire, or ambulance) and play a recorded message at the press of a button.

For automobile drivers, a *signaling device* for the car turns on a light when police or ambulance sirens or car horns are nearby.

TV, Radio, and Stereo Assistive Listening Devices

TV, radio, and stereo listening devices allow people to increase the loudness of sound without disturbing other people. Some devices can be connected to the TV, radio, or stereo:

- when using an audio input hearing aid
- by using earphones instead of a hearing aid
- by using an induction loop

A *TV caption decoder* is especially helpful for watching captioned programs. The decoder attaches to the TV and captions are seen only by people using the decoder.

Other assistive listening devices do not connect to the TV, radio, or stereo. These include the *infrared transmitter* and *receiver,* the *FM transmitter* and *receiver,* and the *TV band radio* or similar device. A TV band radio can be tuned in to the TV channel, with the volume adjusted, and placed close to the ear of the deaf or hard of hearing person.

Telephone Amplifiers

Telephone listening devices increase the loudness of sound coming through the telephone. They can be used with or without a hearing aid. Styles of telephone amplifiers are available in three categories with different models available in each category: (1) *built-in amplifier* is a part of the telephone handset; (2) *a portable amplifier* fits onto the telephone handset and uses a small battery for power; (3) *a modular amplifier* connects directly to a modular telephone.

Some amplifiers will work with audio input hearing aids. The amplifier connects directly to the hearing aid.

Hearing Ear Dogs

In addition to the mechanical devices, hearing ear dogs are being trained to assist deaf individuals. These dogs are trained to tell people when different sounds occur in the environment. In the event the phone rings or someone is at the door, the dog will lead the deaf individual in the direction of the sound.

SUMMARY

Support services enable deaf individuals to enter the mainstream of society. Through personnel, agencies, and mechanical devices they are able to interface with their surroundings and function as totally independent individuals.

Although the list of support services included in this chapter is not comprehensive, it provides the reader with resources to contact in order to acquire additional information. The purpose here has been to acquaint the reader with those professionals, agencies, and devices that are available to deaf and hard of hearing consumers, thus promoting their independence.

References

Allen, T. E. (1986). Patterns of academic achievement among hearing impaired students: 1974 and 1983. In A. Schildroth & M. Karchmer (Eds.), *Deaf children in America* (pp. 161–206). San Diego: College-Hill Press.

Allen, T. E. & Woodward, J. C. (1986, May). *How teachers communicate with deaf students today.* Paper presented at a seminar on sign language for Deaf culture, Gallaudet Research Institute, Washington, DC.

Alpiner, J., Kaufman, K., & Hanavan, P. (1993). Overview of rehabilitative audiology. In J. Alpiner & P. McCarthy (Eds.), *Rehabilitative audiology: Children and adults.* Baltimore, MD: Williams & Wilkins.

Altshuler, K. Z. (1963). Personality traits and depressive symptoms in the deaf. In T. Wortis (Ed.), *Recent advances in biological psychiatry,* Vol. 6 (pp. 63–73). New York: Plenum Press.

Altshuler, K. Z. (1974). Social and psychological development of the deaf child. *American Annals of the Deaf, 119,* 365–366.

Altshuler, K. Z., Deming, W. E., Vollenweider, J., Rainer, J. D., & Tendler, R. (1976). Impulsivity and profound early deafness: A crosscultural inquiry. *American Annals of the Deaf, 121,* 331–345.

Anderson, G. B. (1972). Vocational rehabilitation services and the black deaf. *Journal of Rehabilitation of the Deaf, 6,* 126–129.

Anderson, K. (1985). College characteristics and change in students' occupational values. *Work and Occupations, 12,* 307–328.

Anderson, R. M., & Stevens, G. D. (1970). Policies and procedures for admission of mentally retarded deaf children to residential schools for the deaf. *American Annals of the Deaf, 115,* 30–36.

Andrews, J., & Mason, J. (1986). How do deaf children learn about pre-reading. *American Annals of the Deaf.* July, 1986, pp. 210–216. In W. Teale & E. Sulzby (Eds), *Emergent literacy.* Norwood, NJ: Ablex.

Andrews, J., & Akamatsu, C. (1993). Building blocks for literacy: Getting the signs right. *Perspectives, 11*(3), 1–5.

Andrews, J., Winograd, P., & DeVille, G. (1996, Spring). Using sign language summaries during prereading lessons. *The Council for Exceptional Children.*

Andrews, J., & Zmijewski, G. (1997). How parents support home literacy with deaf children. *Early Child Development and Communication, 127–128,* 131–139.

Andrews, J., & Mason, J. (1991). Strategy use among deaf and hearing readers. *Exceptional Children, 57* (6).

Atelsek, F., & Mackin, E. (Eds.). (1971). *Diversifying job opportunities for the adult deaf.* Washington, DC: Department of Health, Education, and Welfare.

Athey, I. (1985). Theories and models of human development: Their implications for the education of deaf adolescents. In

D. Martin (Ed.), *Cognition, education, and deafness.* Washington, DC: Gallaudet College Press.

Baker, C., & Battison, R. (Eds.). (1980). *Sign language and the Deaf community.* Silver Spring, MD: National Association of the Deaf.

Baker, C., & Cokely, D. (1980). *American sign language: A teachers' resource text on grammar and culture.* Silver Spring, MD: T. J. Publishers.

Baker-Shenk, C. (1985). The facial behavior of deaf signers: Evidence of a complex language. *American Annals of the Deaf, 130,* 297–304.

Baron, N. (1992). *Growing up with language.* Reading, MA: Addison-Wesley.

Barraga, N. (1976). *Visual handicaps and learning.* Belmont, CA: Wadsworth Publishing Co.

Baumrind, D. (1967). Child care practices anteceding three patterns of preschool behavior. *Genetic Psychology Monographs, 75,* 43–88.

Baumrind, D. (1980). New directions in socialization research. *American Psychologist, 35,* 639–652.

Baxter, N. (1979). Disabled workers and the career counselor. *Occupational Outlook Quarterly, 23*(3), 2–14.

Becker, G. (1980). *Growing old in silence.* Los Angeles: University of California Press.

Belenky, M. F. (1984, June). The role of deafness and education in the moral development of hearing impaired children and adolescents. In A. Areson & J. DeCaro (Eds.), *Teaching, learning and development* (Volume 1, pp. 3–23).

Bender, R. E. (1970). *The conquest of deafness.* Cleveland: The Press of Case Western Reserve University.

Benderly, B. L. (1980). *Dancing without music.* Garden City, NY: Doubleday.

Benninga, J. S. (1988, February). An emerging synthesis in moral education. *Phi Delta Kappan,* 415–418.

Berger, K. W. (1984). *The hearing aid, its operation and development* (3rd ed.). Livonia, MI: National Hearing Aid Society.

Bergman, M. (1980). *Aging and the perception of speech.* Baltimore, MD: University Park Press.

Berk, L. (1998). *Development through the lifespan.* Boston: Allyn & Bacon.

Berlin, C. I. (Ed.). (1984). *Hearing science.* San Diego, CA: College-Hill Press.

Bernstein, E. (Ed.). (1989). *1989 Medical and health annual.* Chicago, IL: Encyclopedia Brittannica.

Best, B. (1970). *Development of classification skills in deaf children with and without early manual communication.* Unpublished doctoral dissertation, University of California, Berkeley.

Bevan, R. C. (1988). *Hearing-impaired children: A guide for concerned parents and professionals.* Springfield, IL: Charles C. Thomas Publishers.

Beyer, M. (1986, September-October). Overcoming emotional obstacles to independence. *Children Today,* 8–12.

Biehler, R. F., & Snowman, J. (1986). *Psychology applied to teaching.* Boston: Houghton Mifflin Co.

Binder, P. J. (1971). The relationship between verbal language and impulsivity in the deaf (doctoral dissertation, Wayne State University, MI, 1970). *Dissertation Abstracts International, 32,* 5614B–5615B.

Birk-Nielsen, H. (1974). Effect of monaural versus binaural hearing aid treatment. *Scandinavian Audiology, 3,* 183–187.

Birren, J. E., & Schaie, K. W. (Eds.). (1985). *Handbook of the psychology of aging.* New York: Van Nostrand Reinhold Company.

Bloom, L., & Lahey, M. (1978). *Language development and language disorders.* New York: John Wiley & Sons.

Bolton, B. (Ed.). (1976). *Psychology of deafness for rehabilitation counselors.* Baltimore: University Park Press.

Bonvillian, J. D., Charrow, V. R., & Nelson, K. E. (1973). Psycholinguistic and educational implications of deafness. *Human Development, 16,* 321–345.

Bornstein, H. (1973). A description of some current sign systems designed to represent English. *American Annals of the Deaf, 118,* 457–463.

Bornstein, H., Saulnier, K., & Hamilton, L. (Eds.). (1983). *The comprehensive signed English dictionary.* Washington, DC: Gallaudet University Press.

Bouvet, L. (1990). *The path to language: bilingual education for deaf children.* Cleveland, Avon, England: Metalingual Matters.

Bowe, F. (1971). Non-white deaf persons: Educational, psychological, and occupational considerations: Review of the literature. *American Annals of the Deaf, 116,* 357–361.

Bowe, F. (1973). Crises of the deaf child and his family. In D. Watson, *Readings on deafness.* New York University School of Education.

Bowe, F. (1978). *Handicapping America.* New York: Harper & Row.

Bowen, H. R. (1977). *Investment in learning.* San Francisco: Jossey-Bass.

Braden, J. P. (1985). LPAD applications to deaf populations. In D. Martin (Ed.), *Cognition, education, and deafness.* Washington, DC: Gallaudet College Press.

Braden, J. P. (1985). The structure of nonverbal intelligence in deaf & hearing subjects. *American Annals of the Deaf, 130,* 496–501.

Bragg, B. (1973). Ameslish—Our American heritage: A testimony. *American Annals of the Deaf, 118,* 672–674.

Brannon, J. (1968). Linguistic word classes in the spoken language of normal, hard-of-hearing and deaf children. *Journal of Speech and Hearing Research, 11,* 279–287.

Bredberg, G. (1977). Innervation of the organ of Corti as revealed in the scanning electron microscope. In E. F. Evan & J. P. Wilson (Eds.), *Psychophysics & physiology of hearing.* London: Academic Press.

Brice, P. J. (1985). A comparison of levels of tolerance for ambiguity in deaf and hearing school children. *American Annals of the Deaf, 130,* 226–230.

Brill, R. (1969). *The superior IQs of deaf children of deaf parents.* Riverside: California School for the Deaf.

Brill, R. G. (1974). *The education of the deaf.* Washington, DC: Gallaudet College Press.

Burton, C. A., & Nugent, M. P (1974). *A social learning curriculum—An alternative for the noncollege bound student.* Report of the Proceedings of the Forty-sixth Meeting of the Convention of American Instructors of the Deaf. Washington, DC: U.S. Government Printing Office.

Butler, R., & Lewis, M. (1973). *Aging and mental health: Positive psychosocial approaches.* St. Louis: C. V. Mosby.

Calderon, R., & Greenberg, M. T. (1983). *Social support and stress in hearing parents with deaf vs. hearing children.* Paper presented at the Western Psychological Association, San Francisco, CA.

Canney, J. F. et al. (1985). *Working on words.* Washington, DC: Gallaudet College Press.

Cantor, D., & Spragins, A. (1977). Delivery of psychological services to the hearing-impaired child in the elementary school. *American Annals of the Deaf, 122,* 330–336.

Capute, A., Accardo, P., Vining, E., Rubenstein, J., & Harryman, S. (1978). *Primitive reflex profile.* Baltimore: University Park Press.

Carter, P. D. (1982). Sensory changes with age—implications for learning research. *Lifelong Learning: The Adult Years,* June.

Casella, L. C. (1978). The deaf job seeker and employment agencies. *Journal of Rehabilitation of the Deaf, 11,* 23–25.

Catlin, F. I. (1978). Etiology and pathology of hearing loss in children. In F. N. Martin (Ed.), *Pediatric audiology* (pp. 3–34). Englewood Cliffs, NJ: Prentice-Hall.

Cetron, M. J. (1983, June). Getting ready for the jobs of the future. *The Futurist,* 15–22.

Chall, J. (1983). *Stages of reading development.* New York: McGraw Hill.

Champie, J. (1984). Is total communication enough? The hidden curriculum. *American Annals of the Deaf, 129,* 317–318.

Cherow, E. (Ed.). (1985). *Hearing-impaired children and youth with developmental disabilities.* Washington, DC: Gallaudet College Press.

Cheskin, A. (1982). The use of language by hearing mothers of deaf children. *Journal of Communication Disorders, 15,* 145–153.

Chess, S., (1975). Behavior problems of children with congenital rubella. In D. Naiman (Ed.), *Needs of emotionally disturbed hearing impaired children.* New York: New York University School of Education.

Chess, S., & Fernandez, P. B. (1980). Neurologic damage and behavior in rubella children. *American Annals of the Deaf, 125,* 998–1001.

Chess, S., Korn, S. J., & Fernandez, P. B. (1971). *Psychiatric disorders of children with congenital rubella.* New York: Brunner/Mazel.

Chough, S. K. (1983). Mental health planning for deaf citizens in Michigan. In G. D. Tyler (Ed.), *Critical issues in rehabilitation and human services.* Silver Spring, MD: American Deafness and Rehabilitation Association.

Christiansen, J. B. (1982). The socioeconomic status of the deaf population: A review of the literature. In J. B. Christiansen & J. Egelston-Dodd (Eds.), *Socioeconomic status of the deaf population.* Washington, DC: Gallaudet College.

Clarke, B. R., & Kendall, D.C. (1980). Learning disabled or hearing impaired:

A folly of forced categories. *British Columbia Journal of Special Education, 4(1),* 13–27.

Clements, S. D. (1966). Minimal brain dysfunction in children. (Public Health Services Publication No. 14.15). Washington, DC: Department of Health, Education, and Welfare.

Cobb, R. B., & Phelps, L. A. (1983, September). Analyzing individualized education programs for vocational components: An exploratory study. *Exceptional Children,* 62–64.

Cohen, O. P. (1978). The Deaf adolescent: Who am I? *Volta Review, 80,* 265–274.

Cohen, O., & Lerman, A. (1971). Residential care: A new concept. *American Annals of the Deaf, 116,* 369–371.

Cokely, D. (1983). When is a pidgin not a pidgin? An alternative analysis of the ASL-English contact situation. *Sign Language Studies, 38,* 1–24.

Colby, A., & Kohlberg, L. (1981). *Invariant sequence and internal consistency in moral judgement stages.* Cambridge, MA: Harvard University Graduate School of Education. (ERIC Document Reproduction Service No. ED 223514).

Collins, J. L. (1969). *Communication between deaf children of pre-school age and their mothers.* Unpublished doctoral dissertation, University of Pittsburgh.

Combs, A. (1988). *Hearing loss help.* Santa Maria, CA: Alpenglow Press.

Conrad, R. (1979). *The deaf school child.* New York: Harper & Row.

Conrad R., & Weiskrantz, B. C. (1981). On the cognitive ability of deaf children with deaf parents. *American Annals of the Deaf, 126,* 995–1003.

Conway, L. (1990). Issues relating to classroom management. In M. Ross (Ed.), *Hearing impaired children in the mainstream* (pp. 131–157). Parkton, MD: York Press.

Corbett, E., & Jensema, C. (1981). *Teachers of the hearing impaired: Descriptive profiles.* Washington, DC: Gallaudet College Press.

Corso, J. F. (1971). Sensory processes and age effects in normal adults. *Journal of Gerontology, 26,* 90–105.

Craig, W., & Collins, J. (1970). Analysis of communicative interaction in classes of deaf children. *American Annals of the Deaf, 115,* 79–85.

Craig, W. N., & Craig, H. B. (1984). Schools and classes for the Deaf in the U.S. *American Annals of the Deaf, 129,* 117–186.

Craig, W. N., & Craig, H. B. (1985). Educational programs and services. *American Annals of the Deaf, 130,* 132–133.

Craig, W. N., & Craig, H. B. (1987). Educational programs and services. *American Annals of the Deaf, 132,* 1–125.

Crammatte, A. B. (1987). *Meeting the challenge.* Washington, DC: Gallaudet University Press.

Crammatte, A. B. (1988). Questions and answers about employment of Deaf people (pp. 1–4). (Available from National Information Center on Deafness, Gallaudet University.)

Crouch, R. (1997). Letting the deaf be deaf: Reconsidering the use of cochlear implants in prelingually deaf children. *Hastings Center Report, 27*(4), 14–21.

Cruickshank, W. M. (1963). *The psychology of exceptional children and youth* (2nd ed.). Englewood Cliffs, NJ: Prentice-Hall.

Davenport, S., & Omen, G. (1977). The heterogeneity of Usher's Syndrome. In J. W. Littlefield, F. J. Ebling, & I. W. Henderson (Eds.), *Fifth International Conference on Birth Defects* (pp. 87–88). Amsterdam, The Netherlands: Excerpta Medica.

David, M., & Trehub, S. E. (1989). Perspectives on deafened adults. *American Annals of the Deaf, 134,* 200–204.

Davis, A. N. (1974). *Me, myself and who? Or how the deaf child looks at himself.* Proceedings of the Forty-Sixth Meeting of the Convention of American Instructors of the Deaf. Washington, DC: U.S. Government Printing Office.

Davis, H., & Silverman, R. (Eds.). (1960). *Hearing and deafness.* New York: Holt, Rinehart and Winston.

Day, C. W. (1982). Current screening procedures for the usher syndrome at residential schools for the deaf. *American Annals of the Deaf, 127,* 45–48.

Deafness: A fact sheet. (1990). National Information Center on Deafness. Washington, DC: Gallaudet Press.

DeCaro, J. J., Evans, L., & Dowaliby, F. J. (1982). Advising deaf youth to train for various occupations: Attitudes of significant others. *British Journal of Educational Psychology, 52,* 220–227.

DeCaro, J. J., Stuckless, E. R., et al. (1985). A framework for considering educational and non-educational influences on the attainments of deaf persons. *American Annals of the Deaf, 130,* 206–211.

DeCaro, P. A., & Emerton, R. G. (1978). *A cognitive developmental investigation of moral reasoning in a deaf population.* Paper presented at American Educational Research Association Meeting, Toronto. (ERIC #154–572).

Denton, D. (1971). Educational crisis. In P. Culton (Ed.), *Proceedings from Operation Tripod (Toward rehabilitation involvement by parents of the deaf).* (pp. 32–38). Washington, DC: U.S. Department of Health, Education, and Welfare Social and Rehabilitation Service.

Dicker, L. (Ed.). (1982). *Facilitating manual communication for interpreters, students, and teachers.* Washington, DC: RID.

Dickinson, D., Wolf, M., & Stotsky, S. (1993). Words move: The interwoven development of oral and written language. In J. B. Gleason (Ed.), *The development of language.* Boston: Allyn & Bacon.

DiFrancesca, S. (1978). Developing thinking skills in career education. *Volta Review, 80,* 351–354.

DiPietro, L. J. (Ed.). 1978. *Guidelines on interpreting for deaf-blind persons.* Washington, DC: Gallaudet College.

Dirks, D. D. (1964). Factors related to bone conduction reliability. *Archives of Otolaryngology, 79,* 551–558.

Dworetzky, J. P. (1987). *Introduction to child development.* St. Paul, MN: West Publishing Co.

Dwyer, C. (1983). Job seeking and job retention skill training with hearing-impaired clients. In D. Watson et al. (Eds.), *Job placement of hearing persons: Research and practice.*

D'Zamko, M., & Hampton, I. (1985). Personal preparation for multihandicapped hearing impaired students. *American Annals of the Deaf, 130,* 9–14.

Edelstein, T. (1977). *Development of a milieu intervention program for treatment of emotionally disturbed deaf children.* Paper presented at the Annual International Convention, The Council on Exceptional Children (55th), Atlanta, GA.

Edwards, J. R. (1979). *Language and disadvantage.* U.K.: Edward Arnold.

Egelston-Dodd, J. (1977). Overcoming occupational stereotypes related to sex and deafness. *American Annals of the Deaf, 122,* 5, 489–491.

Elkind, D. (1970, April 5). Erik Erikson's eight ages of man. *New York Times Magazine.*

Engebretson, A. M., Popelka, G. R., Morley, R. E., Niemoeller, A. F., & Heidbreder, A. F. (1986). A digital hearing aid and computer-based fitting procedure. *Hearing Instruments, 37*(2), 8–14.

Erikson, E. (1968). *Identity, youth and crisis.* Toronto: W. W. Norton & Company.

Erting, C. (1978). Language policy and deaf ethnicity in the United States. *Sign Language Studies, 19,* 139–152.

Etholm, B., & Belal, A. (1974). Senile changes in the middle ear joints. *Annals of Otolaryngology, 23,* 49–54.

Evans, A. (1975). Experiential deprivation: Unresolved factor in the impoverished socialization of deaf school children in residence. *American Annals of the Deaf, 120,* 545–552.

Farrugia, D. (1982). Deaf high school students' vocational interests and attitudes. *American Annals of the Deaf, 127,* 753–762.

Fellendorf, G. W. (1985). *New opportunities for employment in the 1990s.* Paper presented at the International Congress on Education of the Deaf, Manchester, England.

Ferris, C. (1980). *A hug just isn't enough.* Washington, DC: Gallaudet College Press.

Feuerstein, R. (1979). *The dynamic assessment of retarded performers: The learning potential assessment, device, theory, instruments, techniques.* Baltimore: University Park Press.

Feuerstein, R. (1980). *Instrumental enrichment: An intervention program for cognitive modifiability.* Baltimore: University Park Press.

Fillman, R. D. et al. (1987). Screening for vision problems, including Usher's Syndrome, among hearing impaired students. *American Annals of the Deaf, 132,* 194–198.

Finesilver, S. G. (1968). *The driving records of deaf drivers.* Statement by Sherman G. Finesilver, Denver District Judge, Denver, CO.

Finton, L. (1996). Living in a bilingual-bicultural family. In Paranis, I. (ed.) (1996). *Culture, language, diversity, and the deaf experience.* New York: Cambridge University Press.

Fischler, I. (1985). Word recognition, use of context, and reading skill among deaf college students. *Reading Research Quarterly, 120,* 203–218.

Fischler, R. S. (1985). The pediatrician's role in early identification. In E. Cherow (Ed.),

Hearing impaired children and youth with developmental disabilities. Washington, DC: Gallaudet College Press.

Fletcher, H. (1929). *Speech and hearing.* New York: Van Nostrand.

Foster, S. (1988). Life in the mainstream: Deaf college freshmen and their experiences in the mainstreamed high school. *Journal of the American Deafness and Rehabilitation Association, 22*(2), 27–35.

Fox, N., & Ysseldyke, J. (1997). Implementing inclusion at the middle school level: Lessons from a negative example. *Exceptional Children,* (1): 81–98.

Fraser, R. T. (1978). Rehabilitation job placement research, a trend perspective. *Rehabilitation Literature, 39*(9), 258–264.

Freeman, R. D. et al. (1981). *Can't your child hear? A guide for those who care about deaf children.* Baltimore, MD: University Park Press.

Freyman, R., Nerbonne, G., Cole, H. (1991). Effect of consonant-vowel-ratio modification on amplitude envelope cues for consonant recognition. *Journal of Speech Hearing Research, 34,* 415–426.

Fried, C. (1970). *An anatomy of values.* Cambridge, MA: Harvard University Press.

Frishberg, N. (1990). *Interpreting: An introduction* (rev. ed.). Silver Spring, MD: Registry of Interpreters for the Deaf.

Frishberg, N., & Gough, B. (1973). *Time on our hands.* Paper presented at the Third Annual California Linguistics Conference, Stanford, CA.

Fritz, G., & Smith, N. (1985). *The hearing impaired employee: An untapped resource.* San Diego: College-Hill Press.

Frumkin, B., & Anisfeld, M. (1977). Semantic and surface codes in the memory of deaf children. *Cognitive Psychology, 9,* 475–493.

Furth, H. G. (1966). *Thinking without language: Psychological implications of deafness.* New York: The Free Press.

Furth, H. G. (1974). The role of language in the child's development. *Proceedings of the 1973 Convention of American Instructors of the Deaf.* Washington, DC: U.S. Government Printing Office.

Furth, H. G. & Youniss, J. (1965). The influence of language and experience on discovery and use of logical symbols. *British Journal of Psychology, 56,* 381–390.

Gage, N. L., & Berliner, D.C. (1988). *Educational psychology.* Boston: Houghton Mifflin Co.

Gallagher, J. J., Beckman, P., & Cross, A. (1983). Families of handicapped children: Sources of stress and its amelioration. *Exceptional Children, 50,* 10–19.

Gallaudet Research Institute. (1997–1998). *Annual survey of hearing-impaired children and youth.* Center for Assessment and Demographic Studies. Washington, DC: Author.

Galloway, V. H. (1973). Les miserables. In D. Watson, *Readings on Deafness.* New York University School of Education.

Gannon, J. R. (1981). *Deaf heritage: A narrative history of deaf America.* Silver Spring, MD: National Association of the Deaf.

Gardner, D. C., & Beatty, G. J. (1980). Locus of control change techniques: Important variables in work training. *Education, 100,* 237–242.

Gardner, H. (1982). *Art, mind & brain.* New York: Basic Books, Inc.

Gardner, H. (1983). *Frames of mind.* New York: Basic Books, Inc.

Gardner, J. N., & Jewler, A. J. (Eds.). (1985). *College is only the beginning.* Belmont, CA: Wadsworth Publishing Company.

Garrett, J. F., & Levine, E. S. (Eds.). (1962). *Psychological practices with the physically disabled.* New York: Columbia University Press.

Gerber, S. E., & Mencher, G. T. (1980). *Auditory dysfunction.* Houston: San Diego: College-Hill Press.

Gilbert, J. G. (1952). *Understanding old age.* New York: Ronald Press.

Gilbert, J. G., & Levee, R. F. (1971). Patterns of declining memory. *Journal of Gerontology, 26,* 70–75.

Gilligan, C. (1982). *In a different voice.* Cambridge, MA: Harvard University Press.

Giolas, T. G. (1982). *Hearing-handicapped adults.* Englewood Cliffs, NJ: Prentice-Hall.

Glass, L. E. (1985). Psychosocial aspects of hearing loss in adulthood. In H. Orlans (Ed.), *Adjustment of adult hearing loss.* San Diego: College-Hill Press.

Glattke, T. J. (1977). Some implications for research. In W. R. Hodgson & P. H. Skinner (Eds.), *Hearing aid assessment and use in audiologic habilitation.* Baltimore, MD: Williams & Wilkins Co.

Goff, R. N. (1970). Language used by mothers of deaf children and mothers of hearing children. *American Annals of the Deaf, 115,* 93–96.

Goffman, E. (1963). *Stigma: Notes on the management of spoiled identity.* Englewood Cliffs, NJ: Prentice-Hall.

Goldin-Meadow, S., & Mylander, C. (1983). Gestural communication in deaf children: Noneffect of parental input on language development. *Science, 221,* 372–374.

Goode, R. (1995). Currency status and future of implantable electromagnetic hearing aids. Middle and inner ear electronic implatable devices for partial hearing loss, *Otolyarngologic Clinics of North America, 28* (1 11), 1–15.

Goodman, M. (1973). The deaf student in the hearing class. *Proceedings: National Conference on Program Development For and With Deaf People.* Washington, DC: Gallaudet College.

Goodman, Y. (1986). Children coming to know literacy. In W. Teale & E. Sulzby (Eds.), *Emergent literacy.* Norwood, NJ: Ablek.

Goslin, D. A. (1969). *Handbook of socialization theory and research.* Chicago: Rand McNally & Co.

Goss, R. N. (1970). Language used by mothers of deaf children and mothers of hearing children. *American Annals of the Deaf, 115,* 93–96.

Gough, P. (1972). One second of reading. *Visible Language, 6:* 291–320.

Graybill, P. (1996). Another new birth: Reflections of a deaf native signer. In I. Paranis (Ed.), *Culture, language, diversity, and the deaf experience.* New York: Cambridge University Press.

Greenberg, M. T. (1980). Hearing families with deaf children; Stress and functioning as related to communication method. *American Annals of the Deaf, 125,* 1063–1071.

Greenberg, M. T. (1980). Social interaction between deaf preschoolers and their mothers: The effects of communication method and communication competence. *Developmental Psychology, 16,* 465–474.

Greenberg, M. T., & Marvin, R. S. (1979) Attachment patterns in profoundly deaf pre-school children. *Merrill-Palmer Quarterly, 25,* 265–279.

Greenmum, Robert M. (1952, September). Stop! That driver's deaf! *Safety Education.*

Griffith, J. (Ed.). (1969). *Persons with hearing loss.* Springfield, IL: Charles C Thomas.

Groce, N. (1981). *Heredity deafness on the island of Martha's Vineyard.* Ph.D. dissertation, Brown University, Providence, RI.

Groce, N. (1985). *Everyone here spoke sign language.* Cambridge, MA: Harvard University Press.

Grossman, H. J. et al. (1983). *Classification in mental retardation.* Washington, DC: American Association on Mental Defiency.

Grushkin, D. (1998). Why shouldn't Sam read? Toward a new paradigm for literacy and the deaf. *Journal of deaf studies and deaf education.* Chapel Hill, NC: Oxford University Press.

Haas, W. H. & Crowley, D. J. (1982). Professional information dissemination to parents of preschool hearing-impaired children. *Volta Review, 84,* 17–23.

Hairston, E. E. & Smith, L. D. (1973). Ethnic minorities amongst the deaf population. *Journal of Rehabilitation of the Deaf: Deafness Annual III, 3,* 195–202.

Hannley, M. (1986). *Basic principles of auditory assessment.* San Diego, CA: College-Hill Press.

Hansen, C., & Riske-Nielsen, E. (1965). Pathological studies in presbycusis. *Archives of Otolaryngology, 82,* 115–132.

Hanson, V. (1982). Short-term recall by deaf signers of American Sign Language: Implications of encoding strategy for order recall. *Journal of Experimental Psychology: Learning, Memory, and Cognition, 8,* 572–583.

Hanson, V. (1991). Phonological processing without sound. In S. Brady & Shankweiler (Eds.), *Phonological processes in literacy: A tribute to Isabelle Y. Liberman.* (pp. 153–161). Hillsdale, NJ: Erlbaum.

Hanson, V. L., & Fowler, C. A. (1987). Phonological coding in word reading: Evidence from deaf and hearing readers. *Memory and Cognition, 15,* 199–207.

Hare, R. M. (1972). *Essays on the moral concepts.* London: Macmillan.

Harford, E. R. & Dodds, E. (1982). Hearing status of ambulatory senior citizens. *Ear and Hearing, 3,* 105–109.

Harris, R. I. (1978). The relationship of impulse control to parent hearing status, manual communication, and academic achievement in deaf children. *American Annals of the Deaf, 123,* 52–67.

Harryman, S., & Warren, L. (1985). Physical and occupational therapy models for motor evaluation. In E. Cherow (Ed.), *Hearing Impaired Children and Youth with Developmental Disabilities.* Washington, D.C.: Gallaudet College Press.

Hart, B., & Risley, T. (1995). *Meaningful differences.* Baltimore: Paul H. Brookes.

Healey, W. C., & Karp-Nortman, K. (1975). The hearing impaired mentally retarded: Recommendations for action. Rockville, MD: American Speech-Language Association. Hearing Industries Association (1984). Special Report.

Hefferman, A. (1955). A psychiatric study of fifty preschool children referred to hospital for suspected deafness. In G. Caplan (Ed.), *Emotional problems of early childhood.* New York: Basic Books.

Heider, G. (1948). Adjustment problems in the deaf child. *Nervous Child, 7,* 38–44.

Henggeler, S. W., & Cooper, P. F. (1983). Deaf child-hearing mother interaction: Extensiveness and reciprocity. *Journal of Pediatric Psychology, 8(1),* 83–95.

Hess, R., & Shipman, V. (1965). Early experience and the socialization of cognitive modes in children. *Child Development, 36,* 869–886.

Higgins, P. C. (1980). *Outsiders in a hearing world.* Beverly Hills, CA: Sage Publications.

Himes, J. (1973). Tell it like it is. *National Conference on Program Development for and with Deaf People.* Washington, DC: Gallaudet College.

Hinchcliffe, R. (1962). The anatomical locus of presbycusis. *Journal of Speech and Hearing Disorders, 27,* 301–310.

Hodgson, W. R. (1977). Special case hearing aid assessment: CROS aids. In W. R. Hodgson & P. H. Skinner (Eds.), *Hearing aid assessment and use in audiologic habilitation.* Baltimore: Williams & Wilkins.

Hodgson, W. R. (1986). *Hearing aid assessment and use in audiologic habilitation* (3rd ed.). Baltimore: Williams & Wilkins.

Hoemann, H. (1964). The deaf and vocational choice. *Rehabilitation Record,* pp. 17–21.

Hoemann, H. W. (1972). The development of communication skills in deaf and hearing children. *Child Development, 43,* 990–1002.

Hoffman, M. (1977). Moral internalization: Current theory and research. In L. Berkowitz (Ed.), *Advances in experimental social psychology* (Vol. 10). New York: Academic Press.

Hoffman, M. L. (1977). Personality and social development. In M. R. Rosenweig & L. W. Porter (Eds.), *Annual review of psychology* (Vol. 28). Palo Alto, CA: Annual Reviews, Inc.

Hogan, R., & Emler, N. P. (1978). Moral development. In M. E. Lamb (Ed.), *Social and personality development,* (pp. 200–233). New York: Holt, Rinehart and Winston.

Hollos, M., & Cowan, P. A. (1973). Social isolation and cognitive development: Logical operations and role taking abilities in three Norwegian social settings. *Child Development, 44,* 630–641.

Holstein, C. B. (1968). *Parental determinants of the development of moral judgement.* Unpublished doctoral dissertation, University of California, Berkeley.

Holt, J., & Holt, S., Cole, K. (1994). *Demographic aspects of hearing impairment: Questions and answers* (3rd ed.; pp. 1–13). Center for Assessment and Demographic Studies, Gallaudet University. Retrieved October 28, 1999 from the World Wide Web: http://gri.gallaudet. edu/Demography/factsheet.html.

Humphries, T., Padden, C., & O'Rourke, T. (1980). *A basic course in American Sign Language.* Silver Spring, MD: T. J. Publishers.

Jackson, C. (1972). The black deaf & rehabilitation services: Some socio-cultural and psychodynamic considerations. *Proceedings of the Working Conference on Minority Deaf,* pp. 8–48.

Jackson, L., & Schimke, R. (1979). *Clinical genetics: A source book for physicians.* New York: Wiley.

Jacobs, L. (1974). The community of the adult deaf. *American Annals of the Deaf, 119,* 41–46.

Jacobs, L. (1980). *A deaf adult speaks out.* Washington, DC: Gallaudet College Press.

Jacobsen, D., Eggen, P., & Kauchak, D. (1999). *Methods for teaching.* Saddle River, NJ.: Merrill.

Jaffe, B. (1972). Heredity and congenital factors affecting newborn conductive hearing. *Conference on Newborn Hearing Screening,* pp. 87–101. Washington, DC: Alexander Graham Bell Association for the Deaf.

Jamison, S. L. (1983). Professional employment of deaf persons through the turn of the century. In G. D. Tyler (Ed.), *Critical issues in rehabilitation and human services.* Silver Spring, MD: American Deafness and Rehabilition Association.

Jencks, C. et al. (1977). Who gets ahead? The determinants of economic status in America. New York: Basic Books.

Jensema, C. J. (1975). The relationship between academic achievement and the demographic characteristics of hearing impaired children and youth. Series R, Number 2. Washington, DC: Gallaudet College, Office of Demographic Studies.

Jensema, C., & Trybus, R. J. (1975). *Reported emotional/behavioral problems among hearing-impaired children in special educational programs:* United States 1972–73. Washington, DC: Office of Demographic Studies, Gallaudet College.

Jerger, J. (1960). Observations on auditory behavior in lesions of the central auditory pathways. *Archives of Otolaryngology, 71,* 797–806.

Jerger, J. (Ed.). (1984). *Hearing disorders in adults.* San Diego: College-Hill Press.

Jerger, J., & Hayes, D. (1977). Diagnostic speech audiometry. *Archives of Otolaryngology, 102,* 216–222.

Jerger, J., & Jerger, S. (1971). Diagnostic significance of PB word functions. *Archives of Otolaryngology, 93,* 573–580.

Johnson, D. D. *The adult deaf client and rehabilitation.* Unpublished manuscript.

Johnson, R. K. (1972). Educational programming with retarded deaf children. In L. Stewart (Ed.), *Proceedings of the Special Study Institute on Deafness and Mental Retardation* (pp. 29–34). Rome, NY: New York University School of Education.

Johnson, V. (1993). Factors impacting the job retention and advancement of workers who are deaf. *The Volta Review. 95:* 341–356.

Jones, N., & Mohr, K. (1975). *A working paper on plurals in ASL.* Unpublished manuscript, University of California, Berkeley.

Jordan, I., Gustason, G., & Rosen, R. (1976). Current communication trends at programs for the deaf. *American Annals of the Deaf, 121* (5), 527–531.

Jordan, I., Gustason, G., & Rosen, R. (1979). An update on communication trends in programs for the deaf. *American Annals of the Deaf, 124,* (3), 350–357.

Karchmer, M. (1985). A demographic perspective. In E. Cherow (Ed.), *Hearing impaired children and youth with developmental disabilities.* Washington DC: Gallaudet College Press.

Karchmer, M., & Belmont, J. (1976). *Assessing and improving performance in the cognitive laboratory.* Paper presented at the American Speech and Hearing Association Annual Convention, Houston, TX.

Karchmer, M., & Petersen, L. (1980). *Commuter students at residential schools for the deaf.* Washington, DC: Office of Demographic Studies, Gallaudet College.

Karp, A. (1985). Hearing loss associated with retinitis pigmentosa. *Journal of Visual Impairment & Blindness, 79,* 404–405.

Kasten, R. N., & Warren, M. P. (1977). Learning to use the hearing aid. In W. R. Hodgson & P. H. Skinner (Eds.), *Hearing aid assessment and use in audiologic habilitation.* Baltimore: Williams & Wilkins.

Katz, J. (Ed.). (1972). *Handbook of clinical audiology.* Baltimore: Williams & Wilkins.

Katz, J. (Ed.). (1985). *Handbook of clinical audiology* (3rd ed.). Baltimore: Williams and Wilkins.

Katz, L., Mathis, S. L., & Merrill, E. C. (1974). *The deaf child in the public schools.* Danville, IL: Interstate Printers and Publishers.

Keith, R. D., Engelke, J. R., & Winborn, B. B. (1977). Employment-seeking preparation and activity: An experimental job-placement training model for rehabilitation clients. *Rehabilitation Counseling Bulletin, 21(2),* 159–165.

Kelly, L. (1990). Congnitive theory guiding research in literacy and deafness. In D. Moores, & K. Meadow-Orlands (Eds.), *Educational and developmental aspects of deafness.* Washington, DC: Gallaudet University Press.

Kelly, L. P. (1993). Recall of English function words and inflections by skilled and average deaf readers. *American Annals of the Deaf, 138*(3); 288–296.

Kelly, L. (1995). Encouraging faculty to use writing as a tool to foster learning through writing across the curriculum. *American Annals of the Deaf, 140*(1), 16–22.

Kennedy, A. E. C. *The effects of deafness on personality.* Unpublished manuscript.

Killion, M. C., & Carlson, E. V. (1974). A subminiature electret-condenser microphone of new design. *Journal of the Audiological English Society, 22,* 237–243.

Kimmel, D. C. (1980). *Adulthood and aging.* New York: John Wiley & Sons.

King, C. A., & Quigley, S. P. (1985). *Reading and deafness.* San Diego: College-Hill Press.

Kirk, S., & Gallagher, J. J. (1979). *Educating exceptional children.* Boston: Houghton Mifflin.

Klein, G. (1962). Blindness and isolation. *Psychoanalytic Study of the Child, 17,* 82–93.

Kneedler, R. (1984). *Special education for today.* Englewood Cliffs, NJ: Prentice-Hall.

Kohlberg, L. (1969). Stage and sequence: The cognitive development approach to socialization. In D. A. Goslin (Ed.), *Handbook of socialization theory and research.* Chicago: Rand McNally.

Kohlberg, L. (1976). Moralization. In T. Lickona (Ed.), *Moral development and behavior.* New York: Holt, Rinehart and Winston.

Kohlberg, L. (1981). *The philosophy of moral development.* New York: Harper & Row.

Konigsmark, B. W., & Gorlin, R. J. (1976). *Genetic and metabolic deafness.* Philadelphia: W. B. Saunders.

Kretschmer, R. & Kretschmer, L. (1978). *Language development and intervention with the hearing impaired.* Baltimore: University Park Press.

Kuntze, M. (1998). Literacy and deaf children: The language question. *Topics in Language Disorders, 18* (4), 1–15.

Kurtines, W., & Greif, E. B. (1974). The development of moral thought: Review & evaluation of Kohlberg's approach. *Psychological Bulletin, 81,* 453–470.

Kusche, C. A., Greenberg, M. T., & Garfield, T. S. (1983). Nonverbal intelligence and verbal achievement in deaf adolescents: An examination of heredity and environment. *American Annals of the Deaf, 128,* 458–466.

LaBerge, D., & Samuels, S. J. (1974). Toward a theory of automatic information processing in reading. *Cognitive Psychology, 6,* 293–323.

LaBue, M. (1995). Language and learning in a deaf education classroom. Practice and a paradox. In C. Lucas (Ed.), *Sociolinguistics in deaf communities* (Vol. 1, pp. 164–220). Washington, DC: Gallaudet University Press.

Lane, H., & Gordon, M. (1997). Ethical issues in cochlear implant surgery. An exploration into disease, disability, and the best interests of the child. *Kennedy Institute of Ethics Journal, 7* (3): 231–251.

Lane, H., & Grosjean, F. (Eds.). (1980). *Recent perspectives on American Sign Language.* Hillsdale, NJ: Lawrence Erlbaum Assoc.

Lane, H., Hoffmeister, R., & Bahan, B. (1996). *A journey into the DEAF-WORLD.* San Diego, CA: Dawn Sign Press.

Lang, H., & Propp, G. (1982). Science education for hearing- impaired students: State-of-the-art. *American Annals of the Deaf, 27,* 860–869.

Lang, H., & Stinson, M. (1982). *Career education and socioeconomic status of deaf persons: Concepts, research and implications.* Unpublished manuscript, National Technical Institute for the Deaf at the Rochester Institute of Technology.

Lartz, M. N., & Lestina, L. J. (1995). Strategies deaf mothers use when reading to their young deaf or hard of hearing children. *American Annals of the Deaf, 140*(4): 358–362.

Lasso, C., & Davie, B. (1987). The relationship between lexical knowledge and reading comprehension for prelingually, profoundly hearing-impaired students. *The Volta Review, 89:* pp. 211–220.

LeBerge, D., & Samuels, S. (1974). Toward a theory of automatic information processing in reading. *Cognitive Psychology, 6,* 293–323.

Lerman, A. (1976). Vocational development. In B. Bolton (Ed.), *Psychology of deaf-*

ness for rehabilitation counselors. Baltimore: University Park Press.

Lerman, A., & Guilfoyle, G. R. (1970). *The development of prevocational behavior in deaf adolescents.* Columbia: Teachers College Press.

Letourneau, N. (1972). *The effect of multiple meaning of words on the reading comprehension of intermediate grade deaf children: A comparison of two methods of teaching multiple meanings of words and their effects on reading comprehension.* New York: Unpublished doctoral dissertation. New York University.

Levin, H. M., & Rumberger, R. W. (1983, February). *The educational implications of high technology.* Institute for Research on Educational Finance and Governance, Stanford University.

Levine, E. S. (1974). Psychological tests and practices with the deaf. *Volta Review, 76,* 298–319.

Levine, E. S. (1981). *The ecology of early deafness.* New York: Columbia University Press.

Levitan, L. (1993, May). What do others call us? And what do we call ourselves? *Deaf Life,* 18–29.

Lewis, A. (1994). Inclusion. *Educational Digest, 60,* (1): pp. 71–72.

Liben, L. S. (Ed.). (1978). *Deaf children: Developmental perspectives.* New York: Academic Press.

Liberman, I., Shankweiler, D., Fischer, F., & Carel, B. (1974). Explicit syllable and phoneme segmentation in the young child. *Journal of Experimental Child Psychology, 18:* pp. 201–212.

Lichtenstein, M. J. et al. (1988). Validation of screening tools for identifying hearing-impaired elderly in primary care. *Journal of the American Medical Association, 259,* 2875–2878.

Lickona, T. (1976). Research on Piaget's theory in moral development. In T. Lickona (Ed.), *Moral development and behavior.* New York: Holt, Rinehart and Winston.

Ling, D. (1984). Early oral intervention: An introduction. In D. Ling (Ed.), *Early intervention for hearing impaired children: Oral options,* (pp. 1–14). San Diego: College-Hill Press.

Luey, H. S. (1980). Between worlds: The problems of deafened adults. *Social Work in Health Care, 5,* 253–265.

MacLeod-Gallinger, J. E. (1983, 1984, 1985, 1986). *Secondary school graduate follow-up program for the deaf.* Rochester: Rochester Institute of Technology.

Madell, J. R. (1980). Self-perceived needs of adults with hearing impairments. *Journal of the Academy of Rehabilitative Audiology, 13,* 116–121.

Magary, J. F., & Eichorn, J. R. (Eds.). (1960). *The Exceptional Child.* New York: Holt, Rinehart and Winston.

Magladery, J. W. (1959). Neurophysiology and aging. In J. E. Birren (Ed.), *Handbook of aging and the individual: Psychological and biological aspects.* Chicago: University of Chicago Press.

Maguran, M. J. (1974). Job seeking and placement. One step to a successful career. *Careers for deaf people* (pp. 36–46). Washington, DC: Department of Health, Education, and Welfare, Office of Human Development. Rehabilitation Services Administration.

Mahon, W. J. (1983). The million-unit year: 1983 hearing aid sales and statistical summary. *Hearing Journal, 36,* 9–16.

Malone, O., Jr. (1986). The adult deaf learner: A very neglected species. *Lifelong Learning: An Omnibus of Practice and Research, 10,* 8–11, 23, 30.

Maniglia, A. (1989). Implantable hearing devices. *Otolaryngologic Clinics of North America, 22* (1), 36–58.

Marieb, E. N. (1989). *Human anatomy & physiology.* Redwood, CA: Benjamin Cummings Publishing Company.

Marieb, E. N. (1989). *Human anatomy & physiology laboratory manual.* Redwood,

CA: Benjamin Cummings Publishing Company.

Marion, R. L. (1981). *Educators, parents, & exceptional children.* Rockville, MD: Aspen Systems Corp.

Martin, D. S. (Ed.). (1985). *Cognition, education, and deafness.* Washington, DC: Gallaudet College Press.

Martin, D. S. (1988). Directions for postsecondary education of hearing impaired persons. *Journal of the American Deafness and Rehabilitation Association, 22(2),* 36–40.

Martin, F. (1987). *Hearing disorders in children: Pediatric audiology.* Austin, TX: Pro-Ed.

Martin, M. D. et al. (1989, November). The diagnosis of acquired hearing loss. *ASHA, 31,* 47–50.

Mather, S. A. (1989). Visually oriented teaching strategies with deaf preschool children. In C. Lucas (Ed.), *The sociolinguistics of the deaf community* (pp. 165–187). New York: Academic Press.

Mathog, R. H., Paparella, M. M., Huff, L., Siegal, L., Lassman, F., & Bozarth, M. (1974). Common hearing disorders, methods of diagnosis and treatment. *Geriatrics, 29,* 49–88.

Matthias, V. (1981). Baltimore's job squad for the handicapped. *Rehabilitation Counseling Bulletin, 24*(4), 304–307.

Maxwell, M. M. (1979). A model for curriculum development at the middle and upper school levels in programs for the deaf. *American Annals of the Deaf, 124,* 425–432.

Maxwell, M. et al. (1977). Employment and basic skills: A program for low-achieving high school students. *American Annals of the Deaf, 122,* 563–566.

McAndrew, H. (1948). Rigidity and isolation: A study of the deaf and the blind. *Journal of Abnormal and Social Psychology, 43,* 476–494.

McClelland, D. C. (Ed.). (1982). *Education for values.* New York: Irvington Publishers.

McClure, D. P. (1972). Placement through improvement of client's job-seeking skills. *Journal of Applied Rehabilitation Counseling, 3,* 188–196.

McDaniel, E. (1980). Visual memory in the Deaf. *American Annals of the Deaf, 125,* 17–20.

McDavis, K. (1984). The effects of severity of hearing impairment and locus of control on the denial of hearing impairment in the aged. *Denial of hearing loss and the elderly.* Farmingdale, NY: Baywood Publishing Company.

McKinney, J. P. (1975). The development of values: A perceptual interpretation. *Journal of Personality and Social Psychology, 31,* 801–807.

McKinney, J. P. (1980). Moral development and the concept of values. In M. Windmiller, N. Lambert, & E. Turiel (Eds.), *Moral development and socialization.* Boston: Allyn & Bacon.

Meadow, K. (1971). Identity crisis. In P. Culton (Ed.), *Proceedings from Operation Tripod (Toward rehabilitation involvement by parents of the deaf;* pp. 26–48). Washington, DC: U.S. Department of Health, Education, and Welfare Social and Rehabilitation Service.

Meadow, K. P. (1980). *Deafness and child development.* Berkeley, CA: University of California Press.

Meadow, K. P., Greenberg, M. T., Erting, C., & Carmichael, H. S. (1981). Interactions of deaf mothers and deaf preschool children: Comparisons with three other groups of deaf and hearing dyads. *American Annals of the Deaf, 126,* 454–468.

Meier, R. (1991). Language acquisition by deaf children. *American Scientist, 79;* 60–70.

Melton, C. (1987). Trends and directions in vocational rehabilitation and their influence upon the education of deaf people. *American Annals of the Deaf, 132,* 315–316.

Meyerson, M. D. (1976). The effects of aging on communication. *Journal of Gerontology, 31*(1), 29–38.

Miles, B. (1998, December). Overview on deaf-blindness. DB-Link, The National Clearinghouse on Children Who Are Deaf Blind, pp. 1–4.

Miller, P. (1987). Learning throughout a lifetime. *American Annals of the Deaf, 132,* 312–314.

Mindel, E. D., & Vernon, M. (1971). *They grow in silence.* Silver Spring, MD: National Association for Deaf Press.

Mindel, E. D., & Vernon, M. (1987). *They grow in silence.* Boston: College-Hill Press.

Mischel, W., & Mischel, H. (1971). The nature and development of psychological sex differences. In G. Lesser (Ed.), *Psychology and educational practice.* Glenview, IL: Scott, Foresman.

Mischel, W., & Mischel, H. (1976). A cognitive social-learning approach to morality and self-regulation. In T. Lickona (Ed.), *Moral development and behavior: Theory, research and social issues.* New York: Holt, Rinehart and Winston.

Moores, D. (1996). *Educating the deaf.* Boston: Houghton Mifflin.

Moores, D. F. (1985). Reactions from the researcher's point of view. In D. Martin (Ed.), *Cognition, education, and deafness.* Washington, DC: Gallaudet College Press.

Moores, D. F. (1987). *Educating the deaf: Psychology, principals and practices.* Boston: Houghton Mifflin.

Moores, D. F., & Kluwin, T. N. (1986). Issues in school placement. In A. Schildroth & M. A. Karchmer (Eds.), *Deaf children in America.* San Diego: College-Hill Press.

Moores, D. Kluwin, T., Johnson, R., Cox, P., Blennerhassett, L. Kelly, L., Ewoldt, C.

Sweet, C., & Fields, L. (1987). *Factors predictive of literacy in deaf adolescents.* Project No. NIH-NINCDS-83-10. Final Report to National Institute on Neurological and Communicative Disorders and Stroke.

Moores, D. F., Kluwin, T. N., & Mertens, D. (1985). High school programs for the deaf in metropolitan areas. Gallaudet College Research Monograph No. 3.

Moores, D., Weiss, K., & Goodwin, M. (1978). Early education programs for hearing impaired children: Major findings. *American Annals of the Deaf, 123,* 925–936.

Morariu, J. A., & Bruning, R. H. (1984). Cognitive processing by prelingual deaf students as a function of language context. *Journal of Educational Psychology, 76,* 844–856.

Morariu, J. A., & Bruning, R. H. (1985). A contextualist perspective of language processing by prelingually deaf students. In D. Martin (Ed.), *Cognition, education, and deafness,* Washington, D.C.: Gallaudet College Press.

Morris, W. (Ed.). (1967). *The American heritage dictionary of the English language.* Boston: Houghton Mifflin.

Moses, K. L. (1985). Dynamic intervention with families. In E. Cherow (Ed.), *Hearing impaired children and youth with developmental disabilities* (pp. 82–98). Washington, DC: Gallaudet College Press.

Mow, S. (1973). How do you dance without music? In D. Watson, *Readings on deafness.* New York: New York University School of Education.

Mugny, G., dePaolis, P., & Carugati, F. (1984). Social regulations in cognitive development. In W. Doise & A. Palmonari (Eds.), *Social interaction in individual development.* Cambridge, UK: Cambridge University Press.

Murphy, J. S., & Newlon, B. J. (1987). Loneliness and the mainstreamed hearing impaired college student. *American Annals of the Deaf, 132,* 21–25.

Myerson, L. (1963). A psychology of impaired hearing. In W. M. Cruickshank, *Psychology of exceptional children and youth* (2nd ed.). Englewood Cliffs, NJ: Prentice-Hall.

Myklebust, H. R. (1950). *Your deaf child.* Springfield, IL: Charles C Thomas.

Myklebust, H. R. (1960). *The psychology of deafness.* New York: Grune & Stratton.

Nass, M. (1964). The development of conscience: A comparison of the moral judgements of deaf and hearing children. *Child Development, 35,* 1073–1080.

National Information Center on Deafness. (1990). *Deafness: A fact sheet* (085).

National Society for the Prevention of Blindness (1966). *Estimated Statistics on blindness and vision problems.* New York: Author.

Nelson, W. (1959). *Textbook of pediatrics.* Philadelphia: W. B. Saunders co.

Neugarten, B. L. (1975). The future and the young-old. *The Gerontologist 15*(11), 4–9.

Newby, H. A. (1964). *Audiology.* New York: Appleton-Century-Crofts.

Newby, H. A. (1972). The profession of audiology. In H. A. Newby (Ed.), *Audiology* (3rd ed.). New York: Appleton-Century-Crofts.

Neyhus, A. I., & Austin, G. F. (Eds.). (1978). *Deafness and adolescence. Volta Review, 80.*

NICD. (1984). NICD Publications from the National Information Center on Deafness. Washington, DC: Gallaudet University.

NICD. (1987). *Deafness: A Fact Sheet.* NICD Publications from the National Information Center on Deafness (pp. 1–6). Washington, DC: Gallaudet University.

NICD. (1990). *Deafness: A fact sheet.* (085).

Norcini, J. J., & Snyder, S. S. (1983). The effects of modeling and cognitive induction on the moral reasoning of adolescents. *Journal of Youth and Adolescence, 12,* pp. 101–115.

Norris, M., & Cunningham, D. (1981). Social impact of hearing loss in the aged. *Journal of Gerontology, 36,* 727–729.

Northcott, W. (Ed.). (1972). *Curriculum Guide: Hearing Impaired Children— Birth to Three Years and Their Parents.* Washington, D.C.: Alexander Graham Bell Association for the Deaf.

Oberman, E. (1965). *A History of Vocational Rehabilitation in America.* Minneapolis: Denison.

O'Brien, D. (1987). Reflection-impulsivity in total communication and oral deaf and hearing children: A developmental study. *American Annals of the Deaf, 132,* 213–217.

Odom, P. B., Blanton, R. L., & Laukhof, C. (1973). Facial expressions and interpretations of emotion-arousing situations in deaf and hearing children. *Journal of Abnormal Child Psychology, 1,* 139–151.

Oleron, P. (1953). Conceptual thinking of the deaf. *American Annals of the Deaf, 98,* 304–310.

Olson, G. W. (1989). *A kaleidoscope of deaf America.* Silver Spring, MD: National Association for the Deaf.

Opton, K. (1986). Dimensions of mainstreaming. *American Annals of the Deaf, 131,* 325–330.

Orlans, H. (1985). Reflections on adult hearing loss. *Adjustment to adult hearing loss.* San Diego: College-Hill Press.

Ottem, E. (1980). An analysis of cognitive studies with deaf subjects. *American Annals of the Deaf,* 564–575, Volume 125.

Otto, W. C., & McCandless, G. A. (1982). Aging and auditory site of lesion. *Ear and Hearing, 3,* 105–109.

Owens, R. (1996). *Language development: An introduction.* Boston: Allyn & Bacon.

Oyer, E. J. (1976). Exchanging information within the older family. In H. J. Oyer &

E. J. Oyer (Eds.), *Aging and communication.* Baltimore: University Park Press.

Oyer, H. J., & Oyer, E. J. (Eds.). (1976). *Aging and communication.* Baltimore: University Park Press.

Padden, C. (1990). Deaf children and literacy. Literacy lessons. Geneva: International Bureau of Education.

Pappas, D. (1985). *Diagnosis and treatment of hearing impairment in children.* San Diego: College-Hill Press.

Paul, P. (1998). *Literacy and deafness.* Boston: Allyn & Bacon

Paul, P., & Quigley, S. (1994). *Language and deafness* (2nd ed.). San Diego, CA: Singular Publishing Group.

Penrod, J. P. (1978). *Discrimination performance on a carrier phrase vs. a no carrier phrase speech discrimination task.* Paper presented at the Joint Meeting of the Tennessee/Georgia Speech and Hearing Association, Chattanooga, TN.

Peterson, C. C., & Peterson, J. L. (1989). Positive justice reasoning in deaf and hearing children before and after exposure to cognitive conflict. *American Annals of the Deaf, 134,* 277–282.

Peterson, M. (1989). Models of vocational assessment of handicapped students. *American Annals of the Deaf, 134,* 273–276.

Peterson, M., & Hill, P. (1982). *Vocational assessment of students with special needs: An implementation manual.* Commerce: Occupational Curriculum Laboratory, East Texas State University.

Peterson, R. (1973). An insight into my deaf world. *Proceedings of the National Conference on Program Development For and With Deaf People.* Washington, DC: Gallaudet College.

Pflaster, G. (1980). A factor analysis of variables related to academic performance of hearing-impaired children in regular classes. *Volta Review, 82,* 71–84.

Piaget, J. (1965). *The moral judgment of the child.* New York: The Free Press.

Pintner, R., Eisenson, J., & Stanton, M. (1941). *The psychology of the physically handicapped.* New York: Crofts & Co.

Pless, I. B., & Roghmann, K. J. (1971). Chronic illness and its consequences. *Journal of Pediatrics, 79,* 351.

Polansky, D. W. (1979). A model summer employment program for deaf youth. *American Annals of the Deaf, 124,* 450–457.

Powers, A., Elliott, R., & Funderburg, R. (1987). Learning disabled hearing-impaired students: Are they being identified? *Volta Review, 89,* 99–105.

Powers, A., Elliott, R., & Funderburg, R. (1988). Learning disabled hearing-impaired students: Teacher survey. *Volta Review, 89,* 277–286.

Quay, H. (1979). Classification. In H. Quay & J. Werry (Eds.), *Psychopathological disorders of childhood* (2nd ed.). New York: Wiley.

Quigley, S. P.(1969). *Research on some behavioral aspects of deafness.* Washington, DC: Department of Health, Education and Welfare (ERIC Document Reproduction Service No. ED 034352).

Quigley, S. P,. & Kretschmer, R. E. (1982). *The education of deaf children.* Baltimore: University Park Press.

Quigley, S., & Paul, P. (1984). *Language and deafness.* San Diego: College-Hill Press.

Quinn, L. (1981). Reading skills of hearing and congenitally deaf children. *Journal of experimental psychology, 32*(1); 139–161.

Rainer, J. D., & Altshuler, K. Z. (1966). *Comprehensive mental health services for the deaf.* New York: New York Psychiatric Institute, Columbia University.

Rainer, J. D., & Altshuler, K. Z. (1971). *Expanded mental health care for the deaf: Rehabilitation and Prevention.* Washington, DC: U.S. Government Printing Office.

Ramsdell, D. A. (1970). The psychology of the hard-of-hearing and the deafened adult. In H. Davis & R. Silverman (Eds.), *Hearing and deafness* (3rd ed.). New York: Holt, Rinehart and Winston.

Rawlings, B. W., & Jensema, C. J. (1977). *Two studies of the families of hearing impaired children.* (Ser. R., no. 5.) Washington, DC: Gallaudet College, Office of Demographic Studies.

Rawlings, B., & Karchmer, M. (Eds.). (1988). *College and career programs for deaf students.* Washington, DC: Gallaudet University Press.

Rawlings, G., & King, S. J. (1986). Post secondary educational opportunities for deaf students. In A. Schildroth & M. Karchmer (Eds.), *Deaf children in America.* San Diego: College-Hill Press.

Ray, L. (1966). The Abbe' de L'Epee'. *Deaf American, 18,* 9–11.

Reich P., & Reich, C. A. (1973). *A follow-up study of the deaf.* Unpublished manuscript, University of Toronto.

Rest, J. (1980). Development in moral judgement research. *Developmental Psychology, 16,* 251–256.

Rest, J. (1983). Morality. In J. H. Flavell & E. M. Markman, *Handbook of child psychology.* New York: Wiley.

Riekehof, L. (1978). *The joy of signing.* Springfield, MO: Gospel Publishing House.

Ries, P. (1986). Characteristics of hearing impaired youth in the general population and of students in special education programs for the hearing impaired. In A. Schildroth & M. Karchmer (Eds.), *Deaf children in America.* San Diego: College-Hill Press.

Rittenhouse, R., & Spiro, R. (1979). Conservation performance in day and residential school deaf children. *Volta Review, 81,* 501–509.

Rodda, M., & Grove, C. (1987). *Language, cognition & deafness.* Hillsdale, NJ: Lawrence Erlbaum Associates.

Rokeach, M. (1973). *The nature of human values.* New York: The Free Press.

Rosen, R. (Ed.). (1986). Life and work in the 21st century: The deaf person of tomorrow. *Proceedings of the 1986 National Association of the Deaf Forum.* Silver Spring, MD: National Association of the Deaf.

Ross, A. O. (1964). *The exceptional child in the family.* New York: Grune & Stratton.

Ross, A. O. (1980). Binaural versus monaural hearing aid amplification for hearing impaired individuals. In E. R. Libby (Ed.), *Binaural hearing and amplification,* Vol. II (pp. 1–21). Chicago: Zenetron.

Roy, H. (1962). Vocational and counseling aspects of deafness: Counseling needs and services for the deaf. *American Annals of the Deaf, 107,* 562–566.

Rusch, F. R., & Phelps, L. A. (1987). Secondary special education and transition from school to work: A national priority. *Exceptional Children, 53,* 487–492.

Russel, H. (1987). People who are disabled & employment. *American Annals of the Deaf, 132,* 317–318.

Salomone, P. R. (1971). A client-centered approach to job placement. *Vocational Guidance Quarterly, 19,* 226–270.

Saltstein, H. D., Diamon, R. M., & Belenky, M. F. (1972). Moral judgement level and conformity behavior. *Developmental Psychology, 7,* 327–336.

Sam, A., & Wright, I. (1988). The structure of moral reasoning in hearing-impaired students. *American Annals of the Deaf, 133,* 264–269.

Sanders, D. (1982). *Aural rehabilitation: A management model* (2nd ed.). Englewood Cliffs, NJ: Prentice-Hall.

Santrock, J. (1999). *Life span development.* Boston: McGraw Hill.

Santrock, J. (2000). *Psychology.* Boston: McGraw Hill.

Scarr, S. (1981). *Race, social class, and individual differences in I.Q.* Hillsdale, NJ: Erlbaum.

Schein, J. (1977). Current priorities in deafness. *Volta Review, 79,* 162–174.

Schein, J. (1989). *At home among strangers.* Washington, DC: Gallaudet University Press.

Schein, J., & Delk, M. (1974). *The deaf population of the United States.* Silver Spring, MD: National Association of the Deaf.

Schein, J., & Stewart, D. (1995). *Language in motion: Exploring the nature of sign.* Washington, DC: Gallaudet University Press.

Schick, B., & Gale, E. (1995). Preschool deaf and hard of hearing students interactions during ASL and English storytelling. *American Annals of the Deaf, 140*(4): 363–370.

Schildroth, A. N. (1976). The relationship of nonverbal intelligence test scores to selected characteristics of hearing impaired students. *Proceedings of the Third Gallaudet Symposium on Research in Deafness, 22,* (pp. 1–7.)

Schildroth, A. (1986). Hearing-impaired children under age 6: 1977 & 1984. *American Annals of the Deaf, 131,* 85–90.

Schildroth, A. (1986). Residential schools for deaf students: A decade in review. In A. Schildroth & M. Karchmer (Eds.), *Deaf children in America.* San Diego: College-Hill Press.

Schildroth, A. N. (1990). [1988–89 Annual survey]. Gallaudet University Center for Assessment and Demographic Studies. Unpublished raw data.

Schildroth, A. N., & Karchmer, M. A. (Eds.). (1986). *Deaf children in America.* San Diego: College-Hill Press.

Schelper, D. R. (1995). Reading to deaf children. Learning from deaf adults. *Perspectives in Education and Deafness, 13*(4): 4–8.

Schleper, D. R. (1995). Read it again and again . . . and again. *Perspectives in Education and Deafness, 14*(2), 16–19, 24.

Schleper, D. (1999). Principles for reading to deaf children, pp. 1–14. Retrieved November 16, 1999 from the World Wide Web: *http://www.gallaudet.edu/ponmplit/literacv/srp/15princ.html.*

Schlesinger, H. (1971). Diagnostic crises. In P. Culton (Ed.), *Proceedings from Operation Tripod (Toward rehabilitation involvement by parents of the deaf).* (pp. 20–25). Washington, DC: U.S. Department of Health, Education, and Welfare Social and Rehabilitation Service.

Schlesinger, H., & Meadow, K. (1972). *Sign and sound.* Los Angeles: University of California Press.

Schow, R. L. et al. (1978). *Communication disorders of the aged.* Baltimore, MD: University Park Press.

Schow, R. L., & Nerbonne, M. A. (1980). Hearing levels among elderly nursing home residents. *Journal of Speech and Hearing Disorders, 45(1),* 124.

Schowe, B. M. (1979). *Identity crisis in deafness: A humanistic perspective.* Tempe, AZ: The Scholars Press.

Schroedel, J. (1991). Improving the career decisions of deaf seniors in residential and day high schools. *American Annals of the Deaf, 136* (4): 330–338.

Schroedel, J. G. (1976). *Variables related to the attainment of occupational status among deaf adults.* Unpublished doctoral dissertation. New York University, New York.

Schuknecht, H. F. (1974). *Pathology of the ear.* Cambridge: Harvard University Press.

Scouten, E. L. (1984). *Turning points in the education of deaf people.* Danville, IL: Interstate Printers & Publishers.

Seagoe, M. V. (1970). *The learning process and school practice.* Scranton, PA: Chandler.

Selman, R. L. (1971). The relation of role-taking to the development of moral judgement in children. *Child Development, 42,* 79–81.

Shand, M. A. (1982). Sign-based short term coding of American Sign Language signs and printed English words by congenitally deaf signers. *Cognitive Psychology, 14,* 1–12.

Shaver, J. P., & Strong, W. (1976). *Facing value decisions: Rationale-building for teachers.* Belmont, CA: Wadsworth.

Shelfer, J. (1990, September). Interview with author. Madison, FL.

Shirinian, M. J., & Arnst, D. J. (1982). Patterns in the performance-intensity functions for phonetically balanced word lists and synthetic sentences in aged listeners. *Archives of Otolaryngology, 108,* 15–20.

Sieber, Joan E. (1980). A social learning theory approach to morality. In M. Windmiller, N. Lambert, & E. Turiel (Eds.), *Moral development and socialization.* Boston: Allyn & Bacon.

Silver, N. H. (1974). Considerations for serving the deaf client. *Rehabilitation Literature, 35(2),* 41–53.

Silverstein, R. (1986). The legal necessity for residential schools serving deaf, blind, and multi-handicapped sensory-impaired children. *American Annals of the Deaf, 131,* 78–84.

Simon, S. B., Howe, L. W., & Kirschenbaum, H. (1978). *Values clarification.* New York: Dodd, Mead.

Sisco, F., & Anderson, R. (1980). Deaf children's performance on the WISC-R relative to hearing status of parents and child rearing experiences. *American Annals of the Deaf, 125,* 923–930.

Slavin, R. E. (1988). *Educational psychology.* Englewood Cliffs, NJ: Prentice-Hall.

Sliger, S., & Culpepper, T. (1979). Vocational evaluation and deafness. *Journal of Rehabilitation of the Deaf, 13,* 1–8.

Smith, A. D. (1975). Aging and interference with memory. *Journal of Gerontology, 30,* 319–325.

Sternberg, R. J. (1985). *Beyond IQ: A triarchic theory of human intelligence.* Cambridge, England: Cambridge University Press.

Sternberg, R. J., & Detterman, D. K. (Eds.). (1986). *What is intelligence? Contemporary viewpoints on its nature and definition.* Norwood, NJ: Ablex Publishing Corporation.

Stevens, S. S., & Warshofsky, F. (1965). *Sound and hearing.* New York: Time, Inc.

Stewart, D. (1992). Initiating reform in total communication programs. *Special Education, 26(1),* 68–84.

Stewart, L. G. (Ed.). (1972). *Deafness and mental retardation.* Deafness Research & Training Center, Department of Health, Education, and Welfare.

Stewart, L. G. (1971). Problems of severely handicapped deaf: Implications for educational programs. *American Annals of the Deaf, 116,* 362–368.

Stokoe, W. (Ed.). (1980). *Sign and culture: A reader for students of American Sign language.* Silver Spring, MD: Linstock Press.

Stokoe, W. C. (Ed.). (1978). *Sign and culture, a reader for students of American Sign Language.* Silver Spring, MD: Lenstok Press.

Stokoe, W. C., & Battison, R. M. (1981). Sign language, mental health and satisfactory interaction. In L. M. Stein, E. D. Mendel, & T. Jabaley (Eds.), *Deafness and mental health* (pp. 179–194). New York: Grune & Stratton.

Stream, R. W., & Stream, K. S. (1980). Focusing on the hearing needs of the elderly. *Journal of the Academy of Rehabilitative Audiology, 13,* 104–108.

Stuckless, R. (Ed.). (1973). *Principles basic to the establishment and operation of postsecondary programs for deaf students.* Washington, D.C.: CEASD.

Sullivan, P., & Vernon, M. (1979). Psychological assessment of hearing impaired children. *School Psychology Digest, 8,* 271–279.

Supalla, T., & Newport, E. (1978). How many seats in a chair? The derivation of nouns and verbs in American Sign Language. In P. Siple (Ed.), *Understanding language through sign language research* (pp. 91–132). New York: Academic Press.

Super, D. E., & Overstreet, P. (1960). *The vocational maturity of ninth grade boys: Career pattern study.* Columbia University, New York: Teachers College Press.

Sweetow, R., & Barrager, D. (1980). Quality of comprehensive audiologic care: A survey of parents of hearing-impaired children. *ASHA, 22,* 841–847.

Taft, B. (1983). Employability of black deaf persons in Washington, DC: National implications. *American Annals of the Deaf, 128,* 453–457.

Teale, W., Hotto, S., & Sulzby, E. (Eds). (1986). *Emergent literacy.*

Tesolowski, D. G., Jarecke, W. H., & Halpin, G. (1980). Normalizing clients' attitudes and knowledge about the world of work. *Journal of Applied Rehabilitation Counseling, 11,* 196–199.

Thomas, A., & Gilhome-Herbst, K. (1980). Social & psychological implications of acquired deafness for adults of employment age. *British Journal of Audiology, 14,* 76–85.

Thrower, J. (1971). *Effects of orphanage and foster care on development of moral judgement.* Unpublished doctoral dissertation, Harvard University.

Tollefson, N. (1982). *Parental strategies for reducing learned helpless behavior among LD students.* Paper presented at the Annual Meeting of the American Psychological Association, Washington, D.C.

Tomlin, J., Spencer, L., & Flock, S. (1999). A comparison of language achievement in children with cochlear implants and children using hearing aids. *Journal of speech, language & hearing research, 42*(2): 497–512.

Tortora, G., & Anagnostakos, N. P. (1987). *Principles of anatomy and physiology.* New York: Harper & Row.

Treiman, R., & Hirsh-Pasek, K. (1983). Silent reading: Insights from second generation deaf readers. *Cognitive Psychology, 15,* 39–65.

Trelease, J. (1995). *The read aloud handbook.* New York: Penguin Books.

Trybus, R., & Karchmer, M. (1977). School achievement scores of hearing impaired children: National data on achievement status and growth patterns. *American Annals of the Deaf, 122,* 62–69.

Tsai, H., Chou, F., & Cheng, T. (1958). Changes in ear size with age, as found among Taiwanese-Formosans of Kukienese extraction. *Journal of the Formosan Medical Association, 57,* 105–111.

Tully, N. L. (1970). *A study of vocational rehabilitation counselors serving deaf clients.* Unpublished doctoral dissertation, University of Arizona.

Tweedie, D., & Shroyer, E. H. (Eds.). (1982). *The multihandicapped hearing impaired.* Washington, DC: Gallaudet College Press.

Tweney, R., Hoeman, H., & Andrews, C. (1975). Semantic organization in deaf and hearing subjects. *Journal of Psycholinguistic Research, 4,* 61–73.

Tyler, G. D. (Ed.). (1983). *Rehabilitation and human services: Critical issues for the eighties.* Silver Spring, MD: American Deafness and Rehabilitation Association.

Usdane, W. M. (1976). The placement process in the rehabilitation of the severely handicapped. *Rehabilitation Literature, 37*(6), 162–167.

Valente, M., Valenyte, M., Meister, M., McCauley, K., & Vass, W. (1994). Selecting and verifying hearing aid fittings for unilateral hearing loss. In *Strategies for selecting and verifying hearing aid fittings.* New York: Thieme Medical Publishers.

Van De Graff, K. et al. (1989). *Study notes: human anatomy & physiology.* Dubuque, IA: Wm. C. Brown Publishers.

Vandergoot, D., & Swirsky, J. (1980). Applying a systems view to placement and career services in rehabilitation: A survey. *Journal of Applied Rehabilitation Counseling, 11,* 149–155.

Veatch, D. J. (1980). A videotape series for teaching job interviewing skills. *American Annals of the Deaf, 125,* 747–750.

Vernon, M. (1967). Relationship of language to the thinking process. *Archives of General Psychiatry, 16,* 325–333.

Vernon, M. (1968). Fifty years of research on the intelligence of deaf and hard-of-hearing children: A review of literature and discussion of implications. *Journal of Rehabilitation of the Deaf, 1,* 1–12.

Vernon, M. (1969). *Multiply handicapped deaf children: Medical educational and psychological considerations.* Reston, VA: Council of Exceptional Children.

Vernon, M. (1970). Potential achievement and rehabilitation in the deaf population. *Rehabilitation Literature, 31,* 258–267.

Vernon, M. (1971). *Psychodynamics surrounding the diagnosis of deafness.* Workshop on Needs of the Hearing Impaired, St. Paul, Minnesota Crippled Children Services: Minnesota Department of Welfare.

Vernon, M. (1973). Psychological aspects of the diagnosis of deafness in a child. *The eye, ear, nose, & throat monthly, 53,* 60–66.

Vernon, M. (1982). Multihandicapped deaf children: Types and causes. In D. Tweedie & E. Shroyer (Eds.), *The multihandicapped hearing impaired: Identification and instruction* (pp. 11–27). Washington, DC: Gallaudet College Press.

Vernon, M., & Andrews, J. F. (1990). *The psychology of deafness: Understanding deaf and hard-of-hearing people.* White Plains, NY: Longman.

Vernon, M., & Hicks, D. (1980). Overview of rubella, herpes simplex, cytomegalovirus, and other viral diseases: Their relationships to deafness. *American Annals of the Deaf, 125,* 529–534.

Vernon, M., & Hyatt, C. (1981). How rehabilitation can better serve deaf clients: The problems and some solutions. *Journal of Rehabilitation, 79,* 60–62.

Vernon, M., & Koh, S. D. (1970). Early manual communication and deaf children's achievement. *American Annals of the Deaf, 115,* 527–536.

Vernon, M., & Makowsky, B. (1979). Deafness and minority group dynamics. *The Deaf American, 21,* 3–6.

Vernon, M., & Oettinger, P. (1981). Psychological evaluation of the deaf and hard-of-hearing. In L. K. Stein, E. D. Mindel, & T. Jabaley (Eds.), *Deafness and mental health* (pp. 49–64). New York: Grune and Stratton.

Vernon, M., & Rothstein, D. A. (1967). *Deafness: The interdependent variable.* Paper presented at the Congress of the World Federation of the Deaf (5th), Warsaw, Poland.

Walter, G. (1993). Some strategies for enhancing career advancement prospects: A reactant paper. *The Volta Review, 95:* 417–420.

Walter, G., MacLeod-Gallinger, J., & Stuckless, R. (1987). *Outcomes for graduates of secondary education programs for deaf students: Early findings of a cooperative national longitudinal study.* Rochester, NY: Rochester Institute of Technology.

Walter, J. B. (1982). *An introduction to the principles of disease.* Philadelphia: Saunders.

Wang, M. C., Reynolds, M. C., & Walberg, H. J. (1988). *Mildly handicapped conditions.* Oxford, England: Pergamon Press.

Wang, M. C., Reynolds, M. C., & Walberg, H. (Eds.). (1989). *Handbook of special education research and practice, Vol. 3: Low incidence conditions.* Elmsford, NY: Pergamon Press.

Wates, W. J. (1984). *A cognitive developmental approach to social problems management.* Paper presented at the International Congress of the Association of the Deaf, April, 1984.

Watson, D. et al. (Eds.). (1983). *Job placement of hearing impaired persons: Research & practice.* Little Rock, AR: Rehabilitation Research and Training Center, University of Arkansas.

Wax, T. (1987). *Managing hearing loss in later life.* Washington, DC: National Information Center on Deafness, Gallaudet University.

Wechsler, D. (1974). *Wechsler intelligence scale for children-revised.* New York: Psychological Corporation.

Wedell-Monnig, J., & Lumley, J. M. (1980). Child deafness and mother-child interaction. *Child Development, 51,* 766–774.

Weinrich, J. E. (1972). Direct economic costs of deafness in the United States. *American Annals of the Deaf, 117,* 446–454.

Welsh, W. (1993). Factors influencing career mobility of deaf adults. *The Volta Review, 95:* 329–339.

Welsh, W., & Walter, G. (1988). The effect of postsecondary education on occupational attainments of deaf adults. *Journal of the American Deafness and Rehabilitation Association, 22,* 14–22.

Welsh, W., & Walter, G. (1988). The value of a college degree to deaf adults. Rochester, NY: Rochester Institute of Technology.

Welsh, W., & Walter, G. (1989). Earnings of deaf college alumni in the United States. Rochester, NY: Rochester Institute of Technology.

White, R. (1974). Building career skills. In G. Austin (Ed.), *Careers for deaf people.* Washington, DC: Department of Health, Education, and Welfare.

Whitesell, K. M. (1991). *Reading between the lines: How one deaf teacher demonstrates the reading process.* Unpublished doctoral dissertation, University of Cincinnati.

Wilbur, R. (1979). *American Sign Language and sign systems.* Baltimore, MD: University Park Press.

Wilbur, R. (1987). *American Sign Language and sign systems.* Boston: College-Hill Press.

Windmiller, M., Lambert, N., & Turiel, E. (Eds.). (1980). *Moral development and socialization.* Boston: Allyn & Bacon.

Wolff, A. B. (1985). Analysis. In D. Martin (Ed.), *Cognition, education, and deafness.* Washington, DC: Gallaudet College Press.

Wolff, A., & Harkins, J. (1986). Multiply handicapped students. In A. Schildroth & M. Karchmer (Eds.), *Deaf children in America.* San Diego: College-Hill Press.

Wright, B. (1960). *Physical disability—A psychological approach.* New York: Harper & Row.

Wright, E. (1999). Full inclusion of children with disabilities in the regular classroom: Is it the only answer? *Social Work in Education, 21* (1), 11–22.

Wrightstone, J., Aronow, M., & Moskowitz, S. (1963). Developing reading test norms for deaf children. *American Annals of the Deaf, 108,* 311–316.

Yambert, G. B., & Van Craeynest, R. (1975). *Sign language and social networks: Grapevine communication in the deaf community.* Paper presented at the Annual Meeting of the Southwestern Anthropological Association, San Francisco, California.

Young, J. (1975). Experiential deprivation: A response. *American Annals of the Deaf, 120,* 553–554.

Youniss, J. (1981). Moral development through a theory of social construction. *Merrill-Palmer Quarterly, 27,* 385–403.

Youniss, J., & Furth, H. G. (1964). Attainment and transfer of logical connectives in children. *Journal of Educational Psychology, 55,* 357–361.

Youniss, J., & Furth, H. G. (1966). Prediction of causal events as a function of transitivity and perceptual congruency in hearing and deaf children. *Child Denial, 37,* 73–81.

Yowell, D. (1971). Cooperative improvement. In P. Culton (Ed.), *Proceedings from Operation Tripod (Toward rehabilitation involvement by parents of the deaf;* pp. 26–48). Washington, DC: U.S. Department of Health, Education, and Welfare Social and Rehabilitation Service.

Zadny, J. L., & James, L. F. (1979). The problem with placement. *Rehabilitation Counseling Bulletin, 22,* 439–442.

Zemlin, W. R. (1968, 1988). *Speech and hearing science.* Englewood Cliffs, NJ: Prentice-Hall.

Zwiebel, A., & Mertins, D. M. (1985). A comparison of intellectual structure in deaf & hearing children. *American Annals of the Deaf, 130,* 27–31.

► Index